DIAGNOSIS IN ANDROLOGY

CLINICS IN ANDROLOGY

E.S.E. HAFEZ, *series editor*

VOLUME 4

1. J.C. Emperaire, A. Audebert, E.S.E. Hafez, eds., Homologous artificial insemination, 1980. ISBN 90-247-2269-1.
2. L.I. Lipshultz, J.N. Corriere Jr., E.S.E. Hafez, eds., Surgery of the male reproductive tract, 1980. ISBN 90-247-2315-9.
3. E.S.E. Hafez, ed., Descended and cryptorchid testis, 1980. ISBN 90-247-2299-3.
5. G.R. Cunningham, W.-B. Schill, E.S.E. Hafez, eds., Regulation of male fertility, 1980. ISBN 90-247-2373-9.
6. E.S.E. Hafez, E. Spring-Mills, eds., Prostatic carcinoma: biology and diagnosis, 1980. ISBN 90-247-2379-5.
7. S.J. Kogan, E.S.E. Hafez, eds., Pediatric andrology, 1981. ISBN 90-247-2407-7.

Series ISBN: 90-247-2333-7.

DIAGNOSIS IN ANDROLOGY

edited by

J. BAIN
Toronto, Ontario, Canada

and

E.S.E. HAFEZ
Detroit, Michigan, U.S.A.

1980
MARTINUS NIJHOFF PUBLISHERS
THE HAGUE / BOSTON / LONDON

Distributors:

for the United States and Canada

Kluwer Boston, Inc.
190 Old Derby Street
Hingham, MA 02043
USA

for all other countries

Kluwer Academic Publishers Group
Distribution Center
P.O. Box 322
3300 AH Dordrecht
The Netherlands

Library of Congress Cataloging in Publication Data

Main entry under title:

Diagnosis in andrology.

  (Clinics in andrology; v. 4)
  Includes index.
  1. Men – Diseases – Diagnosis. 2. Andrology.
I. Bain, Jerald. II. Hafez, E.S.E., 1922-
III. Series.
RC875.D47   616.6'5075   80-36708

ISBN-13: 978-94-011-7513-5   e-ISBN-13: 978-94-011-7511-1
DOI: 10.1007/ 978-94-011-7511-1

TABLE OF CONTENTS

CONTRIBUTORS

BACCHUS, R.: 222 Elm Street, # 1408, Toronto, M5T 1K5, Ontario, Canada

BAIN, J.: Mount Sinai Hospital, 600 University Avenue, Toronto, M5G 1X5, Ontario, Canada

BEDARD, Y.C.: Mount Sinai Hospital, 600 University Avenue, Toronto, M5G 1X5, Ontario, Canada

BERNARDI, A.: Istituti Di Medicina Clinica dell'Universita di Padova, 35100 Padova, Via Giustiniani, 2 Padova, Italy

BUCCIANTE, G.: Istituti Di Medicina Clinica dell'Universita di Padova, 35100 Padova, Via Giustiniani, 2, Padova, Italy

BUCKSPAN, M.B.: Mount Sinai Hospital, 600 University Avenue, Toronto, M5G 1X5, Ontario, Canada

CAMPBELL, J.E.: Department of Radiology, Sunnybrook Medical Centre, 2075 Bayview Avenue, Toronto, M4N 3M5, Ontario, Canada

CHIN, J.L.: Department of Surgery, Wellesley Hospital, 160 Wellesley Street East, Toronto, M4Y 1J3, Ontario, Canada

COLE, L.J.: 99 Avenue Road, Toronto, M5R 2G5, Ontario, Canada

COLGAN, T.J.: 386 Glengarry Avenue, Toronto, M5M 1E8, Ontario, Canada

CUMMING, W.A.: Department of Radiology, Oakville Trafalgar Memorial Hospital, 327 Reynolds Street, Oakville, L6J 3L7, Canada

GARNER, P.R.: Department of Obstetrics and Gynecology, Ottawa Civic Hospital, 1053 Carling Avenue, Ottawa, K1Y 4E9, Ontario, Canada

GILBERG, K.: Organon Canada Limited, 565 Coronation Drive, West Hill, M1E 4S2, Ontario, Canada

GOLDENBERG, H.: 99 Avenue Road, Toronto, M5R 2G5, Ontario, Canada

GOLDENBERG, L.M.C.: 99 Avenue Road, Toronto, M5R 2G5, Ontario, Canada

GOTTESMAN, I.S.: 15 Coach Liteway, Willowdale, M2R 3J8, Ontario, Canada

GRAHAM, JR, S.D.: P.O. Box 2977, Duke University Medical Center, Durham, NC 27710, U.S.A.

GREYSON, N.D.: Division of Nuclear Medicine, Mount Sinai Hospital, 600 University Avenue, Toronto, M5G 1X5, Ontario, Canada

HAFEZ, E.S.E.: Department of Gynecology-Obstetrics, School of Medicine, Wayne State University, Detroit, MI, 48201, U.S.A.

JEWETT, M.A.S.: Division of Urology, Wellesley Hospital, 160 Wellesley Street East, Toronto, M4Y 1J3, Ontario, Canada

LEFEBVRE, Y.: Departments of Medicine and Medical Biochemistry, University of Calgary, Calgary, Alberta, Canada

LEIBEL, B.S.: Hospital for Sick Children, 555 University Avenue, Toronto, M5G 1X8, Ontario, Canada

LEVINE, L.S.: The New York Hospital-Cornell Medical Center, 525 East 68th Street, New York, NY 10021, U.S.A.

LUNDBERG, P.O.: Akademiska Sjukhuset, Neurologiska kliniken, 750 14 Uppsala 14, Sweden

MISKIN, M.: Division of Diagnostic Ultrasound, Mount Sinai Hospital, 600 University Avenue, Toronto, M5G 1X5, Ontario, Canada

NEW, M.I.: The New York Hospital-Cornell Medical Center, 525 East 68th Street, New York, NY 10021, U.S.A.

PANG, S.: The New York Hospital-Cornell Medical Center, 525 East 68th Street, New York, NY 10021, U.S.A.

PAULSON, D.F.: Division of Urology, Duke University Medical Center, P.O. Box 2977, Durham, NC 27710, U.S.A.

REDMAN, J.F.: Department of Urology, University of Arkansas for Medical Sciences, 4301 W. Markham, Little Rock, AK 72201, U.S.A.

SAENGER, P.: The New York Hospital-Cornell Medical Center, 525 East 68th Street, New York, NY 10021, U.S.A.

SHOKEIR, M.H.K.: Room 515, Ellis Hall, University Hospital, Saskatoon, S7N 0W0, Saskatchewan, Canada

WALFISH, P.G.: Mount Sinai Hospital, 600 University Avenue, Toronto, M5G 1X5, Ontario, Canada

FOREWORD

Despite the increasing number of andrological publications, the diagnostic aspects of andrology have received relatively little attention. In the last decade substantial progress has been made in the understanding of the fundamentals of andrology, this progress resulting from modern techniques and instrumentation in microanatomy, immunology, neurophysiology, pathology, genetics, endocrinology, biochemistry, biophysics, urology and surgery. These studies are scattered in such a wide spectrum of journals that andrologists can hardly keep abreast of the advances. There have been textbooks on the testes, male accessory organs and semen but none that have attempted to bring together the various aspects of diagnosis. Since there is an increasing literature concerning diagnostic andrology widely scattered in many different publications, we hope that a useful purpose will be served by summarizing the more pertinent material which can be made readily available to students and practitioners of andrology. This volume is an attempt to coordinate anatomical, physiological, biochemical, endocrinological, radiological, cytogenic, pharmacological and immunological techniques of diagnosis and to bring together the various medical aspects of andrology.

This volume is intended to encourage the development of basic and clinical research in andrology, to analyze modern techniques for the evaluation of male infertility, to stimulate the development of guideliness for therapeutic procedures, to recomment common norms of measurement, to promote and interchange of information and to stimulate the interest of scientists and clinicians in andrological problems.

We are grateful to the authors who have given so much of their time and talents to produce chapters of depth and breadth and who have made such a significant contribution to the andrological literature. We are also indebted to Morag M. Smith, Lori Rust and Penny Stoops for the time and patience they exhibited in typing, collation of material and in the many editorial skills necessary to put a book such as this together. Finally, we would like to thank Mr Jeffrey K. Smith of Martinus Nijhoff for his excellent cooperation in the production and publication of this volume.

J. BAIN   Toronto, Ontario, Canada
and
E.S.E. HAFEZ   Detroit, Michigan, U.S.A.

May, 1980

DIAGNOSIS IN ANDROLOGY

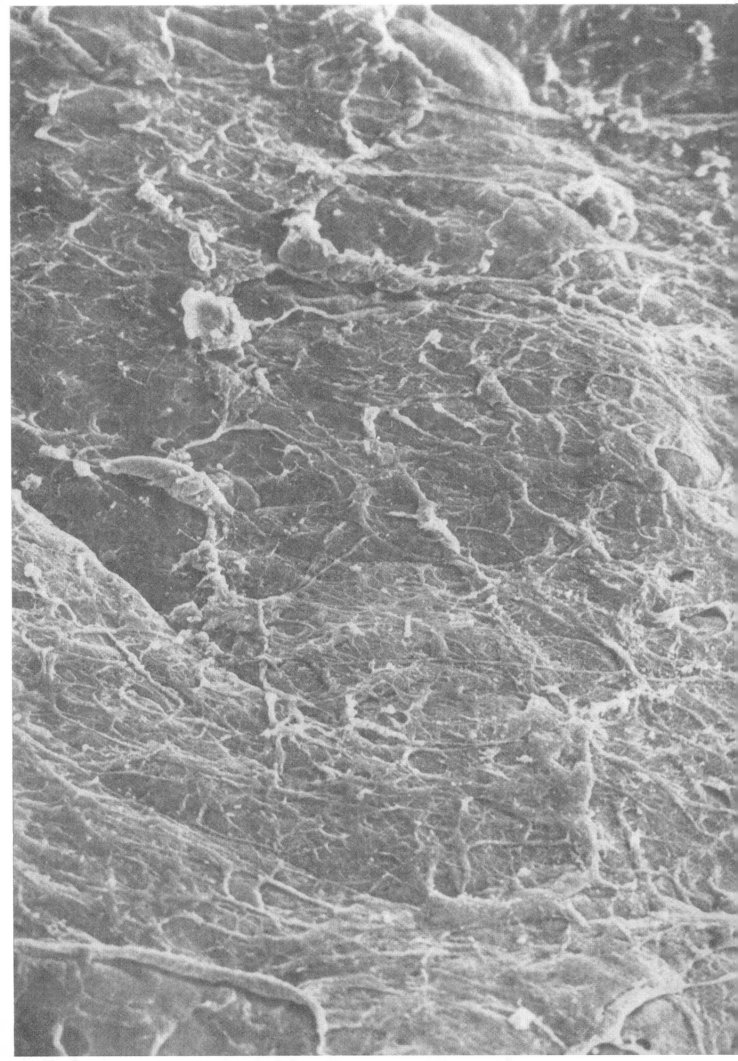

I. ENDOCRINOLOGIC AND GENETIC ASPECTS

1. DIAGNOSIS OF HYPOTHALAMIC-PITUITARY DISORDERS IN ANDROLOGY

M.H.K. SHOKEIR and Y. LEFEBVRE

The past several years, particularly the recent few, have witnessed a remarkable revolution of our understanding of the interaction of the hypothalamus and pituitary gland, the connection of the former with higher brain centers and their influence and the response of the latter to gonadal feedback and the modulation of its function thereby. In view of the recency of many of the findings, the intractable difficulty of analyzing the observed phenomena and attributing their different facets to various factors and interactive influences, and our relative ignorance of the organization of brain centers and their interdependence, our understanding of the neural and psychogenic control of hypothalamic function and expression remains far from complete.

The obvious difficulties, as well as ethical barriers which preclude or highly restrict human experimentation, particularly in the area of brain function, have forced reliance on animal data. While this appears to reflect the human situation at the lower levels in the hierarchy of organization of endocrine functions, extrapolation of the information to humans is more hazardous in the case of control of expressions of higher neural centers. it is particularly at this level that humans depart most significantly from lower animals regarding both structure and function.

Furthermore, differences between the two sexes in organization and function are suggested by the observed cyclic rhythm of the female and the more tonic activity of the male. Yet a great deal of information pertaining to pituitary-hypothalamic functional activity is derived from observations on the female. Caution has to be exercised in accepting the findings encountered in the female as representative of the male, or in extrapolating a diagnostic or therapeutic strategy found successful in the female to the male.

In this chapter, the present state of knowledge regarding the function of the pituitary, hypothalamus and higher center and their interactions will be reviewed. Because of the recency of many of the findings, as well as the fundamental nature of the research which generated these data, our review has a decidedly basic flavor.

Nevertheless, clinical application of such basic knowledge of the hypothalamic-hypophyseal-gonadal axis and its regulation is already underway, with the prospect of a vast imminent increase in the foreseeable future. Diagnosis of deficiency or excess of gonadotropic control, precise localization of such disturbance, the potential for medical management or surgical intervention, if need be, can now be based on appropriate conception of the regulatory mechanisms involved. Furthermore, the potential feasibility of fertility control in the male, via hypothalamic-hypophyseal control, looms on the horizon as a realistic possibility with far-reaching consequences. Conversely, enhancement of spermatogenesis by drug administration is already being attempted, again based on the mechanisms newly unveiled by basic research.

The multiple facets of action of brain polypeptides, including their gonadal functional control capacities, remain a highly intriguing though only partially explored area of endeavor.

The Hypothalamic-Pituitary Axis in the Normal Male Gonadal Function

The anterior pituitary and, in turn, its target organs respond to environmental changes through specialized neuro-secretory neurones located in the medial basal hypothalamus. These neurones are believed to synthesize, transport and release the hypothalamic regulatory factors that control anterior pituitary hormone secretion. They terminate on the capillaries of the hypophyseal-portal vessels and are called tuberinfundibular or tuberohypophyseal. Long hypophyseal portal vessels lie along the pituitary stalk and carry the blood-borne regulators from the hypothalamic median eminence to the pars distalis of the pituitary. Therefore, although the anterior pituitary gland does not have a direct nerve supply, the secretion of its hormones is controlled by the central nervous system.

The hypothalamus is influenced either directly or indirectly by all parts of the brain and, in turn, the hypothalamus can modify virtually all functions of the body. In this review, we shall discuss the role of the hypothalamus-pituitary axis in male gonadal function. The pituitary hormones which influence male gonadal function are luteinizing hormone (LH), follicle-stimulating hormone (FSH) and prolactin. The secretion of LH and FSH are controlled by the hypothalamic regulatory hormone LRH, which has been isolated and identified. This hormone has been variously designated luteinizing hormone-releasing factor (LRF) or gonadotropin-releasing hormone (GnRH), perhaps to stress the implication that it is responsible for the release of both LH and FSH. In this review, we shall adhere to the appelation luteinizing hormone-releasing hormone or LRH. The secretion of prolactin is controlled by prolactin release-inhibiting factor (PIF) and by prolactin-releasing factor (PRF), whose chemical structures have not yet been elucidated.

1. LUTEINIZING HORMONE-RELEASING HORMONE (LRH)

1.1. Pituitary-gonadal regulation

Androgens, which are responsible for development of male characteristics are synthesized primarily in cytosol and mitochondria of the hormone-producing cells of the testes – the Leydig cells. Some androgen synthesis takes place, in addition, in the adrenal cortex. This, however, usually proceeds at a much lower level compared with testicular production. Nevertheless, certain adrenal tumors may produce abnormally large amounts of androgens.

Testosterone, which is under the control of LH, is the major androgen secreted by the testes. In some tissues, testosterone is converted to dihydrotestosterone, which is the active androgen in those tissues. Adrenal glands secrete androgens which are less potent than testosterone, but which may engender virilizing effects if secreted in large quantities.

Maturation of the spermatozoa, which requires 70 days, depends on the sustained action of the pituitary gonadotropins, LH and FSH. LH is required for the secretion of androgens which are necessary for the maintenance of spermatogenesis. Some authors suggest that FSH is involved by feedback to the testes at specific stages in spermatid formation either during spermatogenesis or at maturation of spermatids. Others, however, noting that reduction of germinal cells leads to increased levels of FSH, suggest that maturation of spermatids results in factors regulating FSH secretion. The putative substance involved in regulating FSH secretion may be of testicular origin. A protein factor has been purified from bovine testes and has been found to cause selective decrease in levels of FSH (Keogh et al., 1976). In view of their capacity to suppress the release of FSH, these factors have been designated 'inhibin'.

FSH may regulate the concentration of androgens available to androgen target cells involved in spermatogenesis. Re-initiation of spermatogenesis in the regressed testes following hypophysectomy also requires FSH. Normally, however, FSH acts synergistically with small doses of testosterone to maintain spermatogenesis. FSH may act on the Sertoli cells to initiate biochemical events which in turn affect spermatogonial mitosis. One way this could occur would be to alter the concentration of androgens available. the testes of several mammals produce an androgen-binding protein that is secreted into the testicular fluid. this androgen-binding protein may be secreted by Sertoli cells, and its secretion is stimulated by FSH. Androgen-binding protein may serve as a regulatory mechanism for concentration of androgen from the extra-tubular testicular lymph into the seminiferous tubules.

FSH and LH are both glycoproteins and are composed of two chains, α and β, which can be dissociated under relatively mild conditions. The

β-chain determines the biological and immunological specificity for each hormone.

1.2. Hypothalamic-pituitary regulation

If androgens and the pituitary gonadotropins are considered the first and second hormonal links in gonadal function, the third is the hypothalamic luteinizing hormone-releasing hormone (LRH). LRH was isolated from porcine hypothalamic extracts (Schally et al., 1971a, b, c). Ovine LRH was isolated and found to be identical (Burgus et al., 1969). It now appears that bovine, human and rat LRH have the same structure (Mortimer et al., 1976; Schally et al., 1976). LRH is a decapeptide: pyro-Glu-His-TrpSer-Tyr-Gly-Leu-Arg-Pro-Gly-NH$_2$. This peptide stimulates the secretion of both LH and FSH in a host of animals. Although LRH does not appear to be species specific, the dogfish and goldfish LRH may be immunologically different. Furthermore, an analog of LRH, which is an effective stimulant of LH and FSH release in other species, is not effective in the bonnet monkey (Schally et al., 1976).

LRH causes increased sperm counts and production of gonadal steroids in humans and other species (Reichlin et al., 1976). Immunization of rabbits with LRH results in the production of an antiserum which, upon injection in animals, may engender infertility and gonadal atrophy (Arimura et al., 1973). Administration of anti-LRH serum to either normal or castrated rats result in lower LH and FSH levels, indicating that the decapeptide has a role in maintaining secretion of both gonadotropins (Arimura et al., 1974; Kerdelhue et al., 1975).

Schally and collaborators found that LRH is also the physiological FSH-RH (Schally et al., 1971b). Others, however, suggested that the secretion of LH and FSH may be dissociated (Cargille et al., 1969; Gay and Sheth, 1972; Stevens, 1969). Moreover, substances which would selectively influence one of the two gonadotropins have been proposed (Bowers et al., 1973). It now seems that dissociation of secretion of the two pituitary hormones may be largely explained by peripheral factors. Inhibin, for example, blocks spontaneous, and LRH-induced, secretion of FSH, but not LH (Keogh et al., 1976). In addition, there is evidence for differential feedback by sex steroids which is exerted at both pituitary and hypothalamic levels (Vale et al., 1977). It has been shown that the nature and ratio of various steroids influence LH and FSH responses to LRH differently at the levels of the pituitary (Kao and Weisz, 1975; Tang and Spies, 1975; Yen et al., 1974). FSH release due to LRH appears to be more susceptible to 17-estradiol than LH release. Dihydrotestosterone and testosterone, on the other hand, cause a greater inhibition of LH.

1.2.1. Levels of hypothalamic control of gonadal function. LRH is responsible for three aspects of male gonadal function:
1) maintenance of basal levels of secretion of the gonadotropins;
2) onset of puberty; and
3) integration of mating behavior with gonadal readiness (Martin et al., 1977a).

Males, unlike females, secrete FSH and LH in a tonic manner, with minor spiking every hour (Boyar et al., 1972b). Studies in monkeys indicate that this spiking is due to changes in secretion of LRH.

Boyar and co-workers have shown that the earliest hormonal sign of puberty is the episodic release of LH during sleep (Boyar et al., 1972a). Lesions of certain hypothalamic areas in man lead to precocious puberty (Reichlin, 1975). It has been suggested that this is because of the loss of an age-related tonic inhibitory hypothalamic influence on LRH secretion. What normally allows for this loss of inhibition of secretion of LRH is poorly understood.

In lower forms of animals, sex hormones can induce mating so that insemination can occur when the egg is ripe. In man, also, testosterone is known to be required for arousal and copulation (Davidson, 1977). The localization of LRH in areas of the brain associated with sexual behavior indicates that it may be more intimately involved in the maintenance of sexual behavior than hitherto realized (Reichlin et al., 1976).

1.2.2. Distribution of LRH. The greatest concentration of LRH is in the median eminence, as shown by microdissection, with lesser amounts in the arcuate nucleus (Palkovits et al., 1974). Although the median eminence of the rat, mouse, hamster and

guinea pig is undisputably rich in LRH, some workers report LRH in the pre-optic areas of the rat and mouse and extending in fine processes towards the median eminence (Naik, 1974; Setalo et al., 1975).

LRH has also been localized in extrahypothalamic areas. Cells rostral to the anterior commissure and the paraolfactory area have been shown to stain with anti-LRH antibody, as has the organum vasculosum of the lamina terminalis. The extent of distribution of LRH which may be also acting as a neurotransmitter affecting the sex drive remains controversial (Reichlin et al., 1976).

Normal male plasma contains less than 10pg/ml of LRH (Seyler and Reichlin, 1974). Castration and long term estrogen administration lead to increase in LRH activity, indicating feedback control on LRH secretion in man (Seyler and Reichlin, 1973). Discrepancies in plasma levels of LRH have been attributed to different chemical forms of LRH in the plasma. A metabolite of LRH has been identified in the urine (Jeffcoate and Holland, 1975). LRH has been detected in human fetuses 4-5 weeks after conception, indicating that LRH may be involved in the differentiation of the pituitary (Winter et al., 1974).

1.2.3. Cellular actions of LRH. Like other peptide hormones, the first step in the mechanism of action probably involves interaction with plasma membrane receptors and cyclic AMP turnover. Binding sites to LRH have been reported in pituitary cells and membrane fractions (Grant et al., 1973; Spona, 1973). it has been shown that LRH increases cyclic AMP in incubated anterior pituitary glands (Borgeat et al., 1972; Jutisz et al., 1972). Agonists of LRH had similar potencies in releasing LH and elevating cyclic AMP (Kaneko et al., 1973). Furthermore, LRH antagonists inhibited the secretion of LH and the rise in intracellular cyclic AMP levels which were demonstrated upon administration of LRH (Labrie et al., 1976).

1.3. Neurotransmitter-hypothalamic regulation

Noradrenergic fibers coming from the locus ceruleus of the midbrain, a region known to have connections with the limbic system, impinge on LRH neurones, and it seems reasonable that input into the limbic system should alter LRH. Although there is much evidence in experimental animals that neurones which release LRH are in turn regulated by biogenic amines (McCann, 1974), there is little evidence available to indicate a role for biogenic amines in LH or FSH control in man (Martin et al., 1977b).

2. PROLACTIN RELEASE-INHIBITING FACTOR AND PROLACTIN INHIBITING FACTOR

2.1. Pituitary-gonadal regulation

Although prolactin was discovered in 1928 as a lactogenic substance present in bovine pituitary gland. It was not until 1970 that it was clearly established that prolactin exists as a distinct hormone in man (Forsyth and Myers, 1971; Frantz and Kleinberg, 1970). It had previously been difficult to separate prolactin from growth hormone, which also has lactogenic activity. In 1971, Friesen and co-workers isolated small amounts of primate prolactin, developed a radioimmunoassay, and measured it in human plasma (Hwang et al., 1971). Recently, the entire amino acid sequence of human pituitary prolactin has been elucidated (Shome and Parlow, 1977). Interestingly, the human prolactin is identical with human growth hormone for only 16% of its sequence. However, heterogeneous forms (such as 'little' and 'big') of circulating human prolactin, resembling those of growth hormone, have been described (Rogol and Rosen, 1974; Suh and Frantz, 1974).

Circulating concentrations of prolactin increase from the twenty-fifth week of fetal life and are high at birth; thereafter, they fall to prepubertal levels by the sixth week of life (Aubert et al., 1975). In man, this low prepubertal concentration is maintained throughout life. There is a circadian rhythm of prolactin secretion; concentrations increase during night sleep, and fall by morning (Nokin et al., 1972; Sassin et al., 1972). In addition, the secretion of prolactin, like other pituitary hormones, is pulsatile, with the circulating concentrations of prolactin fluctuating every few minutes during the day (Parker et al., 1973).

Many actions have been ascribed to prolactin (Nicol, 1974). The majority of the reported effects are related to growth and reproduction. Although the administration of bovine prolactin caused water, sodium and potassium retention (Horrobin et al., 1971), recent studies indicate that prolactin is not an important osmoregulatory hormone in adult man (Baumann et al., 1977). Only its role in the control of lactation and gonadal function have been established in the human.

Although there is no longer any doubt that prolactin plays a part in male reproduction, the exact nature of this role is yet unclear. There is good evidence that while normal prolactin has a positive effect on male reproduction, high levels cause hypogonadism and sexual dysfunction.

Many of the studies, from which conclusions concerning the potential effects of normal levels of prolactin in humans have been made, have used hypophysectomized and castrated experimental animals. As there are indications that species differences exist in the actions of prolactin, caution must be exercised in extrapolating animal findings to humans.

2.2. Hypothalamic-pituitary regulation

Unlike the secretion of FSH and LH, which apparently is controlled by one hypothalamic hormone, prolactin secretion is under the dual control of a prolactin inhibitory factor (PIF) and a prolactin-releasing factor (PRF). Many types of experiments have shown the control of the pituitary prolactin secretion by the hypothalamus is mainly inhibitory; disruption of hypothalamic-pituitary connection by stalk section (Turkington et al., 1971), pituitary transplantation or placement of hypothalamic lesions produce an increase in prolactin secretion and a decrease in secretion of the other anterior pituitary hormones (Meites, 1972). These studies predicted PIF, but factors that release prolactin have also been identified in whole animals and in assay systems (Milmore and Reece, 1975; River and Vale, 1974; Tang and Spies, 1976). Although the existence of both releasing and release-inhibiting factors is not disputed, the nature of these factors remains controversial.

The chemical identity of either factor is not known with certainty. The search for each factor has been made difficult by the presence in hypothalamic fractions of substances that increase the release of prolactin, as well as those which inhibit it, resulting in neutralization or obstruction of either PIF or PRF activities (Schally et al., 1977). In addition, there is no direct method for measurement of PIF or PRF secretion. By analogy with other hypothalamic hormones, both PIF and PRF were assumed to be small polypeptides. However, the candidates for PIF now include dopamine, noradrenaline, and γ-aminobutyric acid (GABA), and acetylcholine, as well as somatostatin, and those for PRF include serotonin and histamine, as well as thyrotrophin-releasing hormone, endorphins, enkephalins, substance P and neurotensin (Lancranjan and Friesen, 1978).

2.2.1. Localization of PIF and PRF. Krulich et al. (1971) found PRF activity in the median eminence and in the basal portion of the anterior hypothalamus, whereas the lateral portions of the anterior hypothalamus exhibited a PIF activity.

2.3. Feedback control of prolactin secretion

Prolactin secretion also is regulated by two feedback mechanisms, the so-called short-loop feedback of prolactin secretion, and steroid control of prolactin release.

The self-regulation of prolactin secretion by the short-loop mechanism has been demonstrated by a decrease both in pituitary prolactin concentration and a fall in plasma prolactin levels after implants of prolactin in the hypothalamus of the rat. This effect may be mediated by a positive feedback control on dopamine turnover (Fuxe et al., 1977a, b). Oliver et al. (1977) showed that there is a retrograde blood flow from the anterior pituitary to the hypothalamus, and that prolactin can be detected in portal plasma. Similarly, LRH secretion is inhibited by prolactin feedback on the hypothalamus. This would explain why women with prolactin-secreting tumors experience amenorrhea.

Conversely, estrogens enhance prolactin secretion. The effect occurs at the pituitary and at the hypothalamus, probably through reduction of the sensitivity or number of dopamine receptors (Lancranjan and Friesen, 1978). The effect of androgens on prolactin secretion is not known.

3. DIAGNOSTIC TESTS

In addition to clinical assessment, certain investigative procedures may be carried out to establish both the nature and level of the possible lesion responsible for the observed derangement of the andrological status of the individual. For optimal utilization of such tests, the physician must decide which test he wishes done, which hormone to be assayed, or at least which function to be evaluated. The expected outcome may be deficiency or excess of a hormone, or failure or, rarely, excessive response to a stimulus, hormonal or otherwise. In general, stimulation tests are most useful when deficiency states are suspected, whereas suppression is most informative in revealing autonomous excessive production of hormones, whether partial or complete.

Hypothalamic, pituitary evaluation:

3.1. Gonadotropins

3.1.1. FSH and LH (ICSH) determination. These are quantitatively assayed when testicular failure is suspected. Their determinations help to distinguish primary testicular failure (where these pituitary gonadotropin levels are elevated) from secondary failure, whether pituitary, hypothalamic or even higher central nervous system in origin, where the pituitary gonadotropin levels are low. Fortunately, in the case of the male, there is no major episodic variation as seen in normal menstruating females during the follicular and luteal phase of the cycles. On the other hand, unlike the female situation, the correlations between spermatozoal count and FSH, and between testosterone level and LH, are comparatively poor, particularly in the former.

3.1.2. Stimulation. Clomiphene: When given to adult males in daily oral doses of 100 mg for one week, serum LH should increase by 30-300%, and FSH by 20-60%. On continued administration, a plateau is reached by the fourth week where LH reaches 200-700%, and FSH 70-350% of the baseline levels.

Conversely, when given to prepubertal males in small daily doses of 0.7 mg for one week, suppression of gonadotropins is observed. Later, in puberty, instead of suppression of gonadotropins, a rise is demonstrable on clomiphene administration.

LRH: LRH stimulates LH and FSH secretion by the pituitary, especially the former. Failure to do so following injection of LRH indicates absence of LH in the pituitary of adult males.

2.5 μg of LRH/kg body weight is injected as an intravenous bolus. Serum FSH and LH are measured at 0, 30, 60 and 90 minutes. A rise in the serum level of both gonadotropins is demonstrable which correlates with bone age, being highest between the ages of 10 and 15 years, and lowest in both infancy and adulthood. Similarly, urine samples obtained before and after LRH stimulation may be used to evaluate the pituitary response to the releasing hormone.

This test is particularly useful in distinguishing hypothalamic from pituitary disease. In both types of disorders, low serum gonadotropin levels are observed. However, there is lack of both urinary and serum response in pituitary disease, and a blunted response in hypothalamic involvement.

3.1.3. Suppression. To demonstrate the suppressibility of pituitary gonadotropin production, and thereby reveal instances of autonomous production, 100 mg of testosterone propionate is given i.m. daily to adult males in four doses. A drop of 60% and 40% should be detected in LH and FSH basal levels respectively.

3.2. Prolactin

3.2.1. Prolactin determination. Quantitative assay of fasting serum prolactin in normal adult males discloses levels ranging from 1 to 20 ng/ml, whereas females may have levels up to 25 ng/ml. Diurnal fluctuations and secretory peaks may lead transiently to values slightly above such ranges. Sleep drugs such as phenothiazines, benzodiazephines, isonazid, cannabis and reserpine, and stress, surgery and orgasm may elevate serum prolactin levels.

Some pathologic states, such as hypothyroidism, are also associated with hyperprolactinemia. The highest levels, however, are noted in pituitary tumors wherein values above 100 ng/ml are suggestive, and above 300 ng/ml are diagnostic, of such lesions.

3.2.2. Stimulation. Thyrotropic releasing hormone (TRH). (Noel et al., 1974): 100 μg of TRH is given as an intravenous bolus and serum prolactin is measured at 0, 15 and 30 minutes. Some 3- to 5-fold rise in prolactin is demonstrable between 15 and 30 minutes in males. In the case of children, appropriately smaller doses (1 μg/kg body weight) of TRH are given.

Chlorpromazine: 25 mg of chlorpromazine is given orally and serum levels of prolactin are assayed in blood samples taken at 0, 60 and 90 minutes. An approximately three-fold increase in serum prolactin is observed at 60-90 minutes. No such rise is demonstrable in hypothalamic disease. In children, the dose should be reduced, to 0.4 mg/kg body weight.

3.2.3. Suppression. L-dopa: 500 mg of L-dopa is given orally to fasting adult males, with blood samples drawn at 0, 1, 2 and 3 hours. A 50% decline in serum prolactin should be at 1, 2 or 3 hours from baseline levels. This test is not uniformly successful, however, in distinguishing functional hyperprolactinemia from autonomous prolactin-secreting tumors.

TRH stimulation may lead to transient hypertension, whereas the chlorpromazine test is beset with the risk of hypotension. L-dopa administration is attended with the risk of vertigo and nausea, which may be relieved by recumbency. Moreover, caution should be exercised in giving it to patients with cardiac disease.

3.3. Triple-bolus test

This test attempts to evaluate the pituitary response to three stimuli, namely, TRH, LRH and insulin. The response to the first stimulus (TRH) manifests in the production of TSH (thyroid-stimulating hormone) and prolactin; to the second (LRH) in the release of FSH and LH; and to the third (insulin) in the release of growth hormone (GH) and adreno-corticotrophic hormone (ACTH).

The first and second components of the test have already been described. Insulin hypoglycemia is achieved after an overnight fast by giving crystalline-zinc insulin as an intravenous bolus in a dose of 0.1 units/kg body weight. The amount of insulin may be reduced in children or in patients suspected of certain disorders, such as the inability to mobilize

catecholamines, glucagon and cortisol. It may be increased in patients suspected of certain conditions of increased peripheral resistance to insulin, such as acromegaly, obesity, diabetes or Cushing's syndrome. Blood samples for hormone and glucose determination are drawn at 0, 15 and 60 minutes. The blood glucose should fall by at least 50% of the fasting level for the results to be meaningful (in exceptional circumstances, the advent of pronounced adrenergic signs may suffice to consider the stimulus adequate despite less than 50% blood glucose fall). Growth hormone should increase by two- to three-fold over basal levels, with a rise of more than 8 ng/ml.

A 10 μg/100ml increment in plasma cortisol is observed, and more than 20 μg/100 ml 30 minutes after the maximum fall of blood glucose is recorded in individuals with normal ACTH pituitary production and a normal glucocorticoid response by the adrenal cortex.

Throughout the test, the patient's mental status should be continuously assessed by a physician. However, the test should not be terminated by oral or intravenous glucose until the patient is evidently obtunded, or at least 30 minutes have elapsed from the maximum drop of blood glucose.

The triple-bolus test attempts to appraise the thyrotropic, adrenotropic and gonadotropic responsiveness of the pituitary, as well as its ability to produce growth hormone and prolactin when provoked by appropriate stimuli.

4. CLINICAL COMMENTS

The assay of pituitary hormones has enabled the diagnosis or confirmation of diagnosis of many andrological disorders. In primary gonadal failure, whether due to genetic, including chromosomal, causes or environmentally-induced damage of the testes, both gonadotropins, FSH and LH, are substantially elevated. For instance, in XXY Klinefelter's syndrome, a sex chromosomal anomaly, and XY-gonadal dysgenesis, a genetically determined autosomal recessive disorder, primary testicular failure leads to uninhibited anterior pituitary gonadotropin production with demonstrably high quantitative levels of both FSH and LH, especially the former.

Similarly, high gonadotropin levels may be found in testicular atrophy following mumps orchitis, vascular infarction, traumatic or surgical ablation, and post-irradiation atrophy. FSH usually rises with LH, sometimes following suit as a later development. The term castrate levels is often coined to denote such abnormally high pituitary gonadotropin production when testicular function is impaired or abolished.

A similar, albeit less striking, rise in gonadotropin levels is encountered in disorders of qualitative or quantitative deficiency of the androgen-binding receptors in the cellular cytosol, the extreme case being the sex chromosomal-XY, phenotypic female testicular-feminization-syndrome patients. Perhaps more relevant, however, are the more numerous examples of partial deficiency of the androgen-binding receptors among phenotypic males, such as Reifenstein's syndrome and other forms of male pseudohermaphroditism. The proposed basis for the observed elevated gonadotropin levels in these conditions is the quantitative deficiency or qualitative defect of the receptors in the pituitary cytosol itself, with diminished response to feedback inhibition by testicular hormones. The gonadotropin levels may also be elevated when a secreting pituitary adenoma autonomously produces gonadotropic hormones.

Conversely, in chromophobe adenoma and other more destructive lesions, as well as surgical and radiological ablation of the hypophysis, pituitary tropic hormone output is dramatically curtailed, with broad endocrine consequences including both hypogonadism and infertility. The latter two features, of course, result from gonadotopin deficiency. Such deficiency is also observed in familial hypogonadotropic hypogonadism, an autosomal recessive disorder, in which a monotropic pituitary defect limited to gonadotropins occurs. In this respect, the disorder is akin to that of monotropic defect of growth hormone demonstrated in ateliotic dwarfs. It manifests in the male by absence or gross deficiency of secondary sex characteristics and disproportionately long extremities. Clomiphene administration fails to bring about any change in this condition – another evidence in favor of a basic pituitary defect.

In Kallmann's syndrome, an X-linked disorder in which anosmia and occasional midline facial cleft-ing are associated with hypogonadism and infertility, a similar deficiency of gonadotropin production is noted. The location of the lesion is, however, less certain, with a hypothalamic defect and reduction of LRH secretion being a likely prospect (Males et al., 1973). Testicular biopsy specimens from such patients reveal decreased numbers of germ cells, and a spermatogenic state at the primary spermatocyte stage. Leydig cells are not readily histologically identifiable.

Prolactin secretion was found to be abnormally elevated in several clinical disorders, for example, in males with the XXY syndrome (Price et al., 1978). The manifestations included marked gynecomastia and galactorrhea in addition to the physical, intellectual and psychological features of XYY syndrome itself. Significant hyperprolactinemia might also be the outcome of an autonomously functioning adenoma, with all the metabolic and morphological effects, including gynecomastia and galactorrhea, in the male.

The role of LRH in sexual arousal in the human male has recently generated considerable interest. The available data strongly suggest that LH, and to a lesser extent FSH, production is increased on sexual arousal (LaFerla et al., 1978). The underlying mechanism is believed to be cortical stimulation evoking excitatory impulses through the amygdala and other areas of the limbic system to the hypothalamus. The latter, in turn, responds by augmenting the release of LRH. Quantitative assay of gonadotropins and LRH may thus be of value in the diagnostic evaluation of cases of male impotence.

4.1. Therapeutic implications

Although this chapter is devoted to the diagnostic evaluation of hypothalamic-pituitary disorders in the male, a brief mention of some therapeutic trials helps place such discussion in perspective and provides some of the relevance of such diagnostic effort.

Apart from the diagnostic applications noted for hypophyseal and hypothalamic hormones, therapy for several conditions has been attempted utilizing hypophyseal, hypothalamic hormones or their analogs. For example, LRH was given for the treatment of undescended testes in prepubertal boys with unilateral cryptorchidism, with encouraging results (full descent in one-third, and partial descent in another third) (Pirazzoli et al., 1978). LRH and its analogs have also been used to enhance libido in men. D-Leucine-6-LRHEA (longer acting LRH analog) administration to normogonadotropic oligoasthenospermic patients did not, however, enhance the number, viability, motility or forward progression of spermatozoa (Schwarzstein et al., 1978). This contrasts with earlier reports in which synthetic LRH appeared to promote spermatogenesis in normogonadotropic oligoasthenospermic males (Schwarzstein et al., 1975).

LRH analog D-Trp[6] LRH has been effectively used to treat anovulatory women and induce ovulation, followed by successful conception, even among those who had been previously unresponsive to clomiphene therapy (Jaramillo et al., 1978). It is tempting, therefore, to suggest the application of this analog to males with impotence, hypogonadism or oligospermia in whom primary testicular or pituitary lesions have been ruled out.

Clomiphene citrate, which is now believed to exert most of its action on the hypothalamic-hypophyseal level by binding competitively to the steroid receptors, thereby counteracting the negative feedback of the circulating testosterone, has been employed in the management of patients with oligospermia. In all subjects, both normal and those with idiopathic oligospermia thus treated, a marked rise of LRH, gonadotropins and testosterone levels were ascertained (Masala et al., 1978). Moreover, increased number, viability and motility of spermatozoa were recorded.

Combining more than one modality of therapy such as clomiphene and LRH, or one of its analogs, is another avenue which has been pursued recently in the treatment of some andrological conditions such as oligoasthenospermia, especially when associated with diminished libido. The latter appears to be enhanced with LRH or one of its longer acting analogs.

The above knowledge has enabled a more rational approach in the endocrine management of males following surgical, radiological and medical treatment of pituitary lesions, particularly tumors. Replacement therapy may not only include testosterone administration, but also LH and FSH supplementation (usually in the form of human chorionic gonadotropin and extracts from urine of postmenopausal women). The suggested therapy ensures a more physiological redress of the sexual endocrine deficit. Not only will potency be retained or restored, but also oligoazoospermia (a sequel of hypophysectomy) may either be mitigated or partially reversed.

5. CONCLUDING REMARKS

In this chapter, we attempt to cover the current understanding of the regulatory mechanisms of the hypothalamic-hypophyseal-gonadal axis in the normal male, and the possible causes and impact of departure from normal in various disease states. We feel that such understanding is imperative if one is to use effectively the available technological tools for the diagnosis of the pertinent andrological disorders.

Figure 1 depicts the hierarchy which encompasses the higher centers of the central nervous system, the hypothalamus, the anterior pituitary and the gonads, and which is implicated in the regulation of the manufacture and release of human gonadotropins in the male.

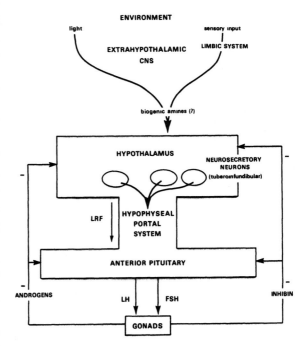

Figure 1. Regulation of release of LH and FSH.

Table 1. Hypothalamic-pituitary-gonadal profile in some andrological disorders.

Disorder	Hypothalamic hormone (LRH)	Pituitary gonadotropins (LH and FSH)	Testosterone	Lesion	Etiology	Mechanism	Pathogenesis
Klinefelter's XXY syndrome	Elevated?*	Elevated	Generally diminished	Primary gonadal	Genetic	Chromosomal – one or more extra X chromosome with or without mosaicism	Morphologic and functional abnormalities of the seminiferous tubules and Leydig cells
Gonadal dysgenesis (XY)	Elevated?	Elevated	Diminished	Primary gonadal	Genetic	Autosomal recessive inheritance	Failure of normal testicular development
Testicular feminization complete and partial	Elevated?	Elevated	Normal, even occasionally increased	End-organ unresponsiveness, complete or partial	Genetic	X-linked recessive inheritance	Deficiency or defect of cytosol androgen receptors complete or partial
Reifenstein's syndrome	Elevated?	Elevated	Normal, even occasionally increased	Partial end-organ unresponsiveness	Genetic	X-linked recessive inheritance	Partial deficiency or defect in cytosol androgen receptors
Male pseudo-hermaphroditism	Elevated?	Elevated	Normal or even occasionally increased	Partial end-organ unresponsiveness	Genetic	X-linked recessive inheritance	Partial deficiency or defect in cytosol androgen receptors
Testicular atrophy	Elevated?	Elevated	Diminished	Primary gonadal	Environmental agents	a-infections e.g. mumps orchitis; b-vascular infarction, e.g. torsion; c-traumatic; d-surgical ablation; e-tumors; f-post irradiation	Damage to both spermatogenic and endocrine elements of the testes
Chromophobe adenoma of the pituitary	Elevated?	Diminished	Diminished	Secondary hypogonadism	Neoplastic	Destruction of gonadotropin secreting cells	Secondary functional and structural deficiency in the testes, both spermatogenic and endocrine elements

Hypophysectomy	Elevated?	Diminished	Diminished	Secondary hypogonadism	Surgical or radiological ablation	Destruction of gonadotropin secreting cells	Secondary functional and structural deficiency in the ates, both spermatogenic and endocrine elements
Hypogonadotropic hypogonadism (pituitary)	Elevated?	Diminished	Diminished	Secondary hypogonadism due to monotropic defect in gonadotropin production	Genetic	Autosomal recessive inheritance	Secondary functional and structural deficiency of the testes both spermatogenic and endocrine elements
Kallmann's syndrome	Diminished	Diminished	Diminished	Hypothalamic lesion agenesis of the olfactory lobes, bulbs, and tracts, mid-line facial defects in some patients, unilateral renal agenesis in a few	Genetic	X-linked inheritance mostly recessive though occasionally expressed in females (partial dominance)	Defect in LRH production with secondary hypogonadism involving both spermatogenic and endocrine elements of the testes
Hypogonadotropic hypogonadism (hypothalamic)	Diminished	Diminished	Diminished	Secondary hypogonadism due to deficiency of hypothalamic production or LRH	Genetic	Autosomal recessive	Defect in LRH production with secondary hypogonadism involving both spermatogenic and endocrine elements of the testes

* The reason for the query (?) is that recent studies cast some doubt on the technical aspects of LRH determination in serum and its by-products in the urine of man. However by extrapolation of animal studies where experimentally induced comparable conditions were found to be associated with elevated LRH in the hypothalamus and in the hypothalamic-pituitary portal circulations enhanced LRH production is anticipated in man in these disorders.

Figure 2 portrays the corresponding present state of knowledge regarding the control of prolactin synthesis and release. Both diagrams emphasize: a) the multiplicity of levels subject to regulation, b) the intricate relationship between various hormones and neural messengers (neurotransmitters), and c) the intimate association between the hypothalamus and external environmental stimuli as mediated partly by the extra hypothalamic nervous system and, partly, by the chemical composition of the

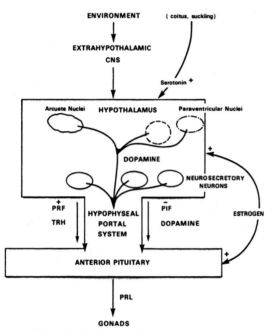

Figure 2. Regulation of prolactin secretion.

internal body milieu. The system, thus characterized, is an example of exquisite homeostatic control.

The site of synthesis, triggers for synthesis and release, mode of action, pattern of regulation, stimulatory and inhibiting agents, and degradation of pituitary and hypothalamic hormones were also reviewed.

Therapeutic applications of the hypothalamic hormone LRH and its synthetic analogs in the management of various andrological disorders, such as undescended testes, impotence and oligo-asthenospermia, have also been briefly outlined. The proposed use of inhibin in the control of male fertility (de Krester, 1974) is a tantalizing and probably realistic possibility with potentially significant implications in population control, as well as in specific clinical or social situations.

Table 1 attempts to summarize the relevant hypothalamic, pituitary and gonadal findings in a number of representative andrological disorders.

It is eminently likely that with the rapid advances, and the application of more sophisticated methodology and critical analysis to the field much of what is included in this chapter will be modified or altered outright. Nevertheless, it is hoped that it lays the scientific foundation for thorough evaluation for individuals with suspected andrological disorders regarding their hypothalamic-pituitary-gonadal axis.

REFERENCES

Arimura A, Sato H, Kumasaka T, Worobec RB, Debeljuk L, Dunn J, Schally, AV (1973) Production of antiserum to LH-releasing hormone (LH-RH) associated with gonadal atrophy in rabbits: development of radioimmunoassays for LH-RH. Endocrinology 93: 1092.

Arimura A, Debeljuk L, Schally AV (1974) Blockade of the preovulatory surge of LH and FSH and of ovulation by anti-LH-RH serum in rats. Endocrinology 95: 323.

Aubert ML, Grumbach MM, Kaplan SL (1975) The ontogenesis of human fetal hormones. III. Prolactin. J Clin Invest 56: 155.

Baumann G, Marynick SP, Winters SJ, Loriaux DL (1977) The effect of osmotic stimuli on prolactin secretion and renal water excretion in normal man and in chronic hyperprolactinemia. J Clin Endocrinol Metab 44: 199.

Borgeat P, Chavancy G, Dupont A, Labrie F, Arimura A, Schally AV (1972) Stimulation of adenosine 3′:5′-cyclic monophosphate accumulation in anterior pituitary glands in vitro by synthetic luteinizing hormone-releasing hormone. Proc Nat Acad Sci USA 69: 2677.

Bowers CY, Currie BL, Johansson KNG, Folkers K (1973) Biological evidence that separate hypothalamic hormones release the follicle stimulating and luteinizing hormones. Biochem Biophys Res Commun 50: 20.

Boyar R, Finkelstein J, Roffwarg H, Kapen S, Weitzman E, Hellman L (1972a) Synchronization of augmented luteinizing hormone secretion with sleep during puberty. N Eng J Med 287: 582.

Boyar R, Perlow M, Hellman L, Kapen S, Weitzman E (1972b) Twenty-four hour pattern of luteinizing hormone secretion in normal men with sleep stage recording. J Clin Endocrinol Metab 35: 73.

Burgus R, Dunn TF, Desiderio D, Guillemin R (1969) Structure moléculaire du facteur hypothalamique hypophysiotrope TRF d'origine ovine: mise en évidence par spectrométrie de masse de la séquence PCA-His-Pro-NH₂. C R Acad Sci Paris (Sér D) 269: 1970.

Cargille CM, Ross, GT, Yoshini T (1969) Daily variations in plasma follicle stimulating hormone, luteinizing hormone and progesterone in the normal menstrual cycle. J Clin Endocrinol Metab 29: 12.

Davidson JM (1977) Neurohormonal bases of male sexual

CPSIA information can be obtained
at www.ICGtesting.com
Printed in the USA
LVOW09s1622190217
524744LV00002B/3/P

2. GENETIC AND CHROMOSOMAL EVALUATION
IN ANDROLOGY

M.H.K. Shokeir

Genetic assessment plays a crucial diagnostic role in andrology. The information gleaned therefrom may be relevant in elucidating the etiology, defining the prognosis and guiding the therapy of suspected andrological disorders. These may include, among others: hypogonadism, infertility, precocious or delayed sexual development, sexual and psychosocial difficulties and antisocial sexual behaviour. Four modalities of diagnostic investigations contribute to an appropriate genetic assessment in andrology: clinical, cytogenetic, biochemical and radiological.

1. CLINICAL EVALUATION

1.1. History

As in other areas of medicine, substantial information can be obtained by history-taking, including family history. For example, a patient with the complaint of hypogonadism who volunteers that he cannot smell (anosmia) strongly suggests Kallmann's syndrome. A history of delayed puberty, hypogonadism and infertility in brothers, sisters or other family members favours an inherited form of hypogonadism whereas a history of mumps, particularly if complicated by orchitis, is obviously critical to the diagnosis of testicular dystrophy.

The age of sexual maturity in other family members such as siblings, parents, uncles, aunts, etc. is often helpful in distinguishing physiological delay of sexual maturity from pathological disorders. The information is even more useful when it pertains to male relatives. For the individual himself, age at puberty, nature and frequency of sexual activity, rate of growth in stature and increase or fluctuation in body weight, major changes in appe-

tite, rapid visual impairment are all germane findings towards the assessment of males with possible andrological disorders.

Recent deterioration of vision is particularly significant and should suggest the possibility of a pituitary lesion whereas major changes in appetite, sleep or urine output (without increased thirst) may indicate potential hypothalamic damage. Increased appetite and polyphagia, intense thirst with polydipsia, polyuria, weight loss, and pruritis may signal the advent of diabetes mellitus – a disorder occasionally associated with impotence and other features of hypogonadism.

In expressing the family history it is often helpful to (a) depict the findings in a diagrammatic form by drawing a pedigree of the family and kindred, (b) to elicit in depth and detail similar complaints, features, or related manifestations in other family members, rather than the usual general, often perfunctory, enquiry about common or chronic disorders.

1.2. Examination

The height/span difference may suggest whether the observed hypogonadism is prepubertal and of long standing or of more recent onset. In Klinefelter's (XXY) syndrome or the autosomal recessive hypogonadotropic hypogonadism not only tall stature but increased span over height are often noted (difference of 5 cm or more) whereas in testicular atrophy due to adult mumps orchitis, radiation, or vascular damage neither tall stature nor increased span is observed. In the XYY syndrome the increased height, which is almost invariably seen, is not associated with limb/trunk linear-length disproportion.

Short stature along with hypogonadism with or

(1976) Hypothalamic hormones. Annu Rev Physiol 38: 389.

Rivier C, Vale W (1974) In vivo stimulation of prolactin secretion in the rat by thyrotropin-releasing factor and related peptides and hypothalamic extracts. Endocrinology 95: 978.

Rogol AD, Rosen SW (1974) Prolactin of apparent large molecular size: the major immunoreactive prolactin component in plasma of a patient with a pituitary tumor. J Clin Endocrinol Metab 38: 714.

Sassin JF, Frantz AG, Weitzman ED, Kaplen S (1972). Human prolactin: 24 hour pattern with increased release during sleep. Science 177: 1205.

Schally AV, Arimura A, Baba Y, Nair RMG, Matsuo H, Redding TW, Debeljuk L, White WF (1971b) Isolation and properties of the FSH and LH-releasing hormone. Biochem Biophys Res Commun 43: 393.

Schally AV, Arimura A, Kastin AJ, Matsuo H, Baba Y, Redding TW, Nair RMG, Debeljuk L, White WF (1971a) Gonadotropin-releasing hormone: one polypeptide regulates secretion of luteinizing and follicle-stimulating hormones. Science 173: 1836.

Schally AV, Kastin AJ, Coy DH (1976) LH-releasing hormone and its analogs: recent basic and clinical investigations. Int J Fertil 27: 1.

Schally AV, Nair RMG, Redding TW, Arimura A (1971c) Isolation of the luteinizing hormone and follicle-stimulating hormone-releasing hormone from porcine hypothalami. J Biol Chem 246: 7230.

Schally AV, Redding TW, Arimura A, Dupont A, Linthicum GL (1977) Isolation of gamma-amino butyric acid from pig hypothalami and demonstration of its prolactin release-inhibiting (PIF) activity in vitro. Endocrinology 100: 681.

Schwarzstein L, Aparichio NJ, Turner D, Calamera JC, Mancini R, Schally A (1975) Use of synthetic luteinizing hormone-releasing hormone in treatment of oligospermic men: a preliminary report. Fertil Steril 26: 331.

Schwarzstein L, Aparichio NJ, Turner D, DeTurner EA, Premoli F, Schally AV (1978) D-leucine-6-luteinizing hormone ethylamide in the treatment of normogonadotropic oligasthenospermia. Fertil Steril 29: 332.

Setalo G, Vigh S, Schally AV, Arimura A, Flerko B (1975) LH-RH-containing neural elements in the rat hypothalamus. Endocrinology 96: 135.

Seyler LE Jr, Reichlin S (1973) Luteinizing hormone-releasing factor (LRF) in the blood of men induced by castration or estrogen treatment. Clin Res 21: 502.

Seyler LE Jr, Reichlin S (1974) Episodic secretion of luteinizing hormone-releasing factor (LRF) in the human. J. Clin Endocrinol Metab 39: 471.

Shome B, Parlow AF (1977) Human pituitary prolactin (hPRL): the entire linear amino acid sequence. J Clin Endocrinol 45: 1112.

Spona J (1973) LH-RH stimulated gonadotropin release mediated by two distinct pituitary receptors. FEBS Lett 35: 59.

Stevens VC (1969) Comparison of FSH and LH patterns in plasma, urine and urinary extracts during the menstrual cycle. Clin Endocrinol Metab 29: 904.

Suh HK, Frantz AG (1974) Size heterogeneity of human prolactin in plasma and pituitary extracts. J Clin Endocrinol Metab 39: 928.

Tang LKL, Spies HG (1975) Effects of gonadal steroids on the basal and LRF induced gonadotropin secretion by cultures of rat pituitary. Endocrinology 96: 349.

Tang LKL, Spies HG (1976) Effects of hypothalamic-releasing hormones on LH, FSH, and prolactin in pituitary monolayer cultures. Proc Soc Exp Biol Med 151: 189.

Turkington RW, Underwood LE, Van Wyk JJ (1971) Elevated serum prolactin levels after pituitary stalk section in man. N Engl J Med 285: 707.

Vale W, Rivier C, Brown M (1977) Regulatory peptides of the hypothalamus. Annu Rev Physiol 39: 473.

Winter AJ, Eskay RL, Porter JC (1974) Concentration and distribution of TRH and LRH in the human fetal brain. J Clin Endocrinol Metab 39: 960.

Yen SSC, Vandenberg G, Siler TM (1974) Modulation of pituitary responsiveness to LRF by estrogen. J Clin Endocrinol Metab 39: 170.

behavior. In: Greep RO, ed. Reproductive physiology. Baltimore University Park Press.

Forsyth IA, Myers RP (1971) Human prolactin. Evidence obtained by the bioassay of human plasma. J. Endocrinol 51: 157.

Frantz AG, Kleinberg DL (1970) Prolactin: evidence that it is separate from growth hormone in human blood. Science 170: 745.

Fuxe K, Hokfelt T, Eneroth P, Gustafsson JA, Skett P (1977) Prolactin-like immunoreactivity: localization in nerve terminals of rat hypothalamus. Science 196: 899.

Fuxe K, Lofstrom A, Agnati L, Hokfelt T, Johansson O, Eneroth P, Gustafsson JA, Skett P, Jeffcoate S, Fraser H (1977b) Functional morphology of the median eminence. In: Hubinont PO, l'Hermite M, Robyn C eds. Clinical reproductive endocrinology, p 41. Basel: Karger.

Gay VL, Sheth NA (1972) Evidence for a periodic release of LH in castrated male and female rats. Endocrinology 90: 158.

Grant G, Vale W, Rivier J (1973) Pituitary binding sites for (^{3}H)-labelled luteinizing hormone releasing factor (LRF). Biochem Biophys Res Commun 50: 771.

Horrobin DF, Lloyd IJ, Lipton A, Burnstyn PG, Durkin N, Muiruri KL (1971) Actions of prolactin on human renal function. Lancet ii: 352.

Hwang P, Guyda H, Friesen H (1971) A radioimmunoassay for human prolactin. Proc Natl Acad Sci USA 68: 1902.

Jaramillo CJ, Charro-Salgado A, Perez-Infante V, Del Campo GL, Coy DH, Schally AV (1978) Clinical studies with D-Trp[6]-luteinizing hormone-releasing hormone in anovulatory women. Fertil Steril 29: 418.

Jeffcoate SL, Holland DT (1975) Further studies on the nature of the immunoreactive luteinizing hormone-releasing factor. (LH-RH)-like peptide in human urine. Acta Endocrinol 78L: 232.

Jutisz M, Kerdelhue B, Berault A, Paloma de la Llosa M (1972) On the mechanism of action of hypothalamic gonadotropin releasing factors. In Saxena BB, Beling CG, Gandy HM eds. Gonadotropins, p 64. New York: Wiley Interscience.

Kaneko T, Saito S, Oka H, Oda T, Yanaiharo N (1973) Effect of synthetic LH-RH and its analogs on rat anterior pituitary cyclic AMP and LH and RSH release. Metabolism 22: 77.

Kao LWL, Weisz J (1975) Direct effect of testosterone and its 5 alpha-reduced metabolites on pituitary LH and FSH release in vitro: change in pituitary responsiveness to hypothalamic extract. Endocrinology 96: 253.

Keogh EJ, Lee VWK, Rennie GC, Burger HG, Hudson B, Krester DM de (1976) Selective suppression of FSH by testicular extracts. Endocrinology 98: 997.

Kerdelhue B, Catlin S, Jutisz M (1975) Short and long term effects of anti-LH-RH serum administration on gonadotropic regulation of the female rat. In Motta M, Crosignani PG, Martini L eds. Hypothalamic hormones: chemistry, physiology, pharmacology and clinical uses, p 43. New York: Academic Press.

Krester DM de (1974) The regulation of male fertility: the state of the art and the future possibilities. Contraception 9: 562.

Krulich L, Illner P, Fawcett CP, Quijada M, McCann SM (1971) Dual hypothalamic regulation of growth hormone secretion. In Pecile A, Muller EE, eds. Growth and growth hormone, p 306. Amsterdam: Excerpta Medica.

Labrie F, Pelletier G, Borgeat P, Drouin J, Ferland L, Belanger A (1976) In Martini L, Ganong WF eds. Frontiers in neuroendocrinology, Vol 4, p 63. New York: Raven Press.

LaFerla JJ, Anderson DL, Schalch DS (1978) Psychendocrine response to sexual arousal in human males. Psychosom Med 40 (2): 166.

Lancranjan I, Friesen HG (1978) The neural regulation of prolactin secretion. In Lederis K, Veale W, eds. Current studies of hypothalamic function (1978), p 131. Basel: Karger.

Males JL, Townsend JL, Schneider RA (1973) Hypogonadotropic hypogonadism with anosmia – Kallman's syndrome: a disorder of olfactory and hypothalamic function. Arch Intern Med 131: 501.

Masala A, Delitala G, Algna S, Devilla L, Lotti G (1978) Effect of clomiphene citrate on plasma levels of immunoreactive luteinizing hormone-releasing hormone, gonadotropin and testosterone in normal subjects and in patients with oligospermia. Fertil Steril 29: 424.

Martin JB, Reichlin S, Brown GM (1977a) Extrahypothalamic regulation of hypophysiotrophic function. In Martin JB, Reichlin S, Brown GM, eds. Clinicaneuroendocrinology, p 38. Philadelphia: F.A. David.

Martin JB, Reichlin S, Brown GM (1977b) Biogenic amines and gonadotropin regulation. In Martin JB, Reichlin S, Brown GM, eds. Clinical neuroendocrinology, p 102. Philadelphia: F.A. David.

McCann SM (1974) In Greep RO, Astwood EB, eds. Handbook of physiology, Sect 7: Endocrinology, Vol 4, p 489. Baltimore: Williams & Wilkins.

Meites J (1972) Recent studies on functions and control of prolactin secretion in rats. Rec Progr Horm Res 28: 471.

Milmore JE, Reece RP (1975) Effects of porcine hypothalamic extract on prolactin release in the rat. Endocrinology 96: 732.

Mortimer CH, McNeilly AS, Rees LH, Lowry PJ, Gilmore D, Dobie HG (1976) Radioimmunoassay and chromatographic similarity of circulating endogenous gonadotropin releasing hormone and hypothalamic extracts in man. J Clin Endocrinol Metab 43: 882.

Naik DV (1974) Immunohistochemical and immunofluorescent localization of LH-RF neurons in the hypothalamus of rat. Anat Rec 178: 424.

Nicol CS (1974) Physiological actions of prolactin. In Knobil E, Sawyers WH, eds. Handbook of physiology, Vol 4, p 283. Baltimore: Williams & Wilkins.

Noel LG, Dimond RC, Wartofsky L, Earle VJ, Frantz AG (1974) Studies of prolactin and TSH secretion by continuous infusion of small amounts of TRH. J Clin Endocrinol Metab 39: 6.

Nokin J, Vekemans M, l'Hermite M, Robin C (1972) Circadian periodicity of serum prolactin concentration in man. Br Med J 3: 561.

Oliver C, Mical RS, Porter JC (1977) Hypothalamic-pituitary vasculatore: evidence for retrograde blood flow in the pituitary stalk. Endocrinology 101: 598.

Palkovits M, Arimira A, Brownstein M, Schally AV, Saavedra JM (1974) Luteinizing hormone-releasing hormone (LH-RH) content of the hypothalamic nuclei in rat. Endocrinology 95: 554.

Parker DC, Rossman LG, VanderLaan EF (1973) Sleep-related myctohemeral and briefly episodic variation in plasma prolactin concentrations. J Clin Endocrinol Metab 36: 1119.

Pirazzoli P, Zapulla F, Bernardi F, Villa MP, Aleksandrowicz A, Scandola A, Standari P, Cicognani A, Cacciari E (1978) Luteinizing hormone-releasing hormone nasal spray as therapy for undescended testicle. Arch Dis Child 53: 235.

Price WH, Renton WB, Campbell WA (1978) Prolactin secretion in XXY males. Lancet ii: 50.

Reichlin S (1975) Regulation of the hypophysiotropic secretions of the brain. Arch Intern Med 135: 1350.

Reichlin S, Saperstein R, Jackson IMD, Body AE III, Patel Y

Table 4. Men with epididymitis and prostatitis, divided according to sperm count categories.

Count (million/ml)	Number in each group	Percentage within each group
0	8/101	7.9
> 0- 5	8/109	7.3
> 5-20	10/144	8.0
>20-40	9/135	6.7
>40	9/333	2.7

Table 6. Sperm counts in men with cryptorchidism.

Count (million/ml)	Unilateral: number in each group	%	Bilateral: number in each group	%
0	5/101	4.9	7/101	6.9
> 0- 5	7/109	6.4	3/109	2.8
> 5-20	8/144	5.6	2/144	1.4
>20-40	1/135	0.7	4/135	4.4
>40	6/333	1.8	0/333	0

ceeded 40 million/ml which was associated with a decreased incidence of varicocele (Table 5). Varicoceles were present in 192 out of the 822 men or 23.3% of the total number of men.

Hydroceles and spermatoceles were felt to be unrelated to fertility. The only significant chromosomal abnormalities found were nine cases of Klinefelter's syndrome, all of which were azoospermic.

Table 5. Sperm count and motility in men with varicoceles.

		Number in each group	Percentage within each group
Sperm count (million/ml)	0	25/101	24.8
	> 0- 5	29/109	26.6
	> 5-20	54/144	37.5
	>20-40	35/135	25.9
	>40	48/333	14.4
Motility (%)	0	33/134	24.6
	> 0- 5	14/57	24.6
	> 5-10	20/45	44.4
	>10-20	33/97	34.0
	>20-30	37/123	30.1
	>30-40	23/110	20.9
	>40	30/246	12.2

Van Zyl et al. (1975) and Dubin and Amelar (1971) found that cryptorchidism was not associated with a sperm count of greater than 20 million/ml. In our study, we found six males with a past history of unilateral cryptorchidism having sperm counts greater than 40 million/ml. Also, there were four males in the study with a history of bilateral cryptorchidism who had sperm counts of 20-40 million/ml. However, with unilateral cryptorchidism, 20/27 males (74%) were oligospermic, and with bilateral cryptorchidism, 12/16 (75%) were. Cryptorchidism is therefore a significant factor in infertility (Table 6).

One final aspect of our study involved testicular

biopsies in 44 males with azoospermia. In a male with azoospermia, obstruction of the vas deferens must be ruled out, for this is a potentially reversible cause of infertility. Of 34 biopsies that were available, 19 revealed Sertoli cells only, 7 showed maturation arrest, 6 had atrophic tubules, and only 2 cases of vasal obstruction were found.

5. HORMONAL ANALYSES

It has been shown that gonadotropin releasing hormone, produced in the hypothalamus, is responsible for the release of FSH and LH by the pituitary gland. These hormones then act on the testes, LH having its action on the Leydig cells to produce testosterone and FSH acting on Sertoli cells to enhance spermatogenesis. The testis in turn modulates pituitary and hypothalamic release of hormone by a negative feedback pathway. Testosterone has been shown to inhibit the LH pathway and it is believed that the seminiferous tubules produce a substance, inhibin, which modulates the secretion of FSH.

Studies have shown elevated FSH levels in oligospermic males with an inverse correlation between sperm count and FSH (Rosen and Weintraub, 1972; Hunter et al., 1974; Christiansen, 1975). Testis histology has also been used to show an inverse relationship between germinal cells and FSH (de Kretser et al., 1974; Franchimont et al., 1972). Nankin and Troen (1976) reported elevated FSH titers in oligospermia with the highest titers in those males with sperm counts <5 million/ml.

LH levels in oligospermic males have been variously reported as being normal (Rosen and Weintraub, 1972), or elevated (Christiansen, 1975; Hunter et al., 1974; Nankin and Troen, 1976; Rosen and Weintraub, 1972). From these studies as well as

from our own lab (Bain, 1978), it has been suggested that seminiferous tubular insufficiency, as evidenced by oligospermia or azoospermia, may also be associated with a partial insufficiency of Leydig cell function, both of these two dysfunctional states being manifested by mean elevations of serum FSH and LH.

Testosterone is the physiological feedback inhibitor of LH in males. The serum testosterone levels in oligospermic males in three reports were not found to be significantly different from control levels (Lawrence and Swyer, 1974; Rosen and Weintraub, 1972; Wieland et al., 1974). However, Troen et al. (1970) and Purvis et al. (1975) found plasma testosterone levels to be lower in some oligospermic males. Nankin and Troen (1976) again confirmed these latter two reports and demonstrated a significantly lower mean testosterone value in males with less than 5 million/ml. Urry et al. (1976) found significantly lower plasma T levels both in the group with azoospermia and with counts of less than 10 million/ml.

In our laboratory we have measured serum T and dihydrotestosterone (DHT) (Bain, 1978) and have found that although the azoospermic males (450 ng/dl) and those with sperm counts less than 5 million/ml (507 ng/dl) do have lower T levels, these are not significantly different from the males with sperm counts of more than 20 million/ml (525 ng/dl). There were, as well, no differences in serum DHT (range 58-62 ng/dl for all groups).

Serum androgen levels may not accurately reflect androgenic activity within the seminiferous tubules; seminal plasma levels of T and DHT although possibly having several sources may nonetheless be more indicative of intratesticular conditions. Pazzagli et al. (1974) found the testicular vein concentration of T to be 200 times greater than circulating levels and felt this reflected the high local concentration of testosterone in the testis. Mean seminal plasma testosterone levels revealed no difference among males with different sperm counts (Bain et al., 1979). However, mean seminal plasma DHT levels rose with increasing sperm counts. As the sperm counts decreased from greater than 40 million/ml to 0 the DHT level fell progressively so that the azoospermic males had seminal levels 30% of the value of those men with counts greater than 40 million/ml.

LHRH administered intravenously has the ability to cause a release of LH and FSH from the pituitary gland. Wollesen et al. (1976) studied responses of FSH and LH to LHRH administered to normal males. They found that the peak gonadotropin response occurred 30 minutes after the LHRH injection and that 100 μg increased LH by 4-8 times and FSH by 1-2 times baseline values.

Franchimont et al. (1973), Isurugi et al. (1973), Mecklenburg and Sherins (1974) and Nankin and Troen (1976), have all studied the LH, FSH response to LHRH in men with varying sperm counts. In general it was found that men with severe oligospermia or azoospermia have increased LH and FSH baseline levels and have a larger incremental gonadotropin response to LHRH than men with normospermia.

We administered 100 μg LHRH to azoospermic, oligospermic (sperm count less than 20 million/ml) and normospermic men (sperm count greater than 20 million/ml) and measured their LH and FSH responses (Bain et al., 1978). It was noted that the LH response was not different among the groups but the azoospermic and severely oligospermic groups (sperm count less than 5 million/ml) did have significantly increased FSH responses. These results suggest bicompartmental testicular insufficiency in oligo-azoospermia.

6. FURTHER INVESTIGATION WITH SPECIAL TESTS

The history and physical examination will determine the nature and extent of the investigation of the infertile male. Systemic disease as well as specific endocrine disease must be ruled out. It may be necessary to measure parameters of renal, hepatic and thyroid function as well as hemoglobin, white blood count and other biochemical indices. A urinalysis should always be done. The request for radiological studies and more extensive pituitary function tests will depend on the clinical and biochemical findings. Other chapters of this book discuss a wide variety of investigative procedures that may be helpful in the diagnosis of the etiology of male subfertility.

7. THERAPEUTICS

If during the history, physical examination or biochemical workpup some abnormality is found, obviously the treatment will be directed to correct this. This would include such problems as genitourinary infections, varicocele, pituitary tumor, psychological problem, thyroid disease or another systemic illness. If a chromosmal abnormality is detected, there s usually no treatment to increase fertility but testosterone may be given for Leydig cell dysfunction.

To find an identifiable and correctable problem in a male with infertility is uncommon. Consequently treatment can only be empiric at best. Male infertility still awaits a therapeutic mode with a high success rate. Exogenous thyroxine or triiodothyronine and vitamin E have been tried to increase fertility but claims of success are unsubstantiated and their role in male infertility is questionable. Prolonged treatment with human menopausal urinary gonadotropins and HCG is occasionally effective when a deficiency of LH and FSH is the cause of infertility. Clomiphene citrate, acting at the level of the hypothalamus to cause an increased release of LHRH and hence LH and FSH from the pituitary gland has been used in the treatment of oligospermia with unregarding results (Palti, 1970; Schellen and Beek, 1974).

Weekly testosterone injections given over a period of time will induce azoospermia by virtue of its suppression of LH and FSH. After the testosterone is discontinued, sperm counts return to former values and in some cases a rebound phenomenon occurs in which counts rise to levels higher than baseline (Heller et al., 1950; Rowley and Heller, 1972). A few investigators have attempted to use LHRH in idiopathic oligospermia and azoospermia with somewhat encouraging results (Schwartzstein, 1975). Because LHRH has a short half-life, it has to be injected frequently or infused intravenously, although long-acting analogues are now being studied.

8. CONCLUDING REMARKS

The male factor in infertility is significant, but unfortunately in the majority of instances a specific cause cannot be clearly delineated. However, rational diagnostic procedures are warranted to define those entities for which there is specific treatment and to uncover those entities which are subtle or subclinical. Occasionally the investigator may be regaded in bringing to light such entities as hyper- or hypothyroidism, hyperprolactinemia or some systemic disorder that was not previously suspected. Perhaps one of the most important aspects of undertaking a rational diagnostic protocol is the alleviation of the anxieties and frustrations of the patient. Even if no specific diagnosis is made, even if no effective treatment can be recommended, at the very least the patient is made aware that every reasonable diagnostic and therapeutic avenue has been explored. Male subfertility and infertility continues to challenge us as we have yet so much to learn. It remains a persistent dilemma.

ACKNOWLEDGEMENTS

The authors are grateful to Tammy Rosenthal for collation of some of the data presented in this chapter, Ingrid Foldes and her staff in the Division of Cytology at the Mount Sinai Hospital for the semen analyses, Morag Smith for typing the manuscript, and to Carmela Schonberg for technical assistance.

REFERENCES

Amelar RD (1966) Interfertility in men. Philadelphia: F.A. Davis.

Bain J (1978) Neuroendocrine parameters of male fertility and infertility. In: Bain J, Hafez ESE, Barwin BN eds. Progress in reproductive biology – andrology, Vol 3. Basel: Karger.

Bain J, Duthie M, Keene J (1979) Relationship of seminal plasma testosterone and dihydrotestosterone to sperm count and motility in man. Arch Androl 2: 35.

Bain J, Moskowitz JP, Clapp JJ (1978) LH and FSH response to gonadotropin releasing hormone (GnRH) in normospermic, oligospermic and azoospermic men. Arch Androl 1: 147.

Christiansen P (1975) Studies on the relationship between spermatogenesis and urinary levels of FSH and LH in oligospermic males. Acta Endocrinol 78: 192.

de Kretser DM, Burger HG, Hudson B (1974) Relationship between germinal cells and serum FSH levels in males with infertility. J Clin Endocrinol Metab 38: 787.

Dubin L, Amelar RD (1971) Etiologic factors in 1294 consecutive cases of male infertility. Fertil Steril 22: 469.

Eliasson R (1971) Standards for investigations of human semen. Andrologie 3: 49.

Eliasson R (1975) Analysis of semen. In: Behrman SJ, Kistner RW, eds. Progress in infertility, 2nd edn. Boston: Little, Brown.

Freund M (1962) Interrelationships among the characteristics of human semen and factors affecting semen specimen quality. J Reprod Fertil 4: 143.

Freund M (1963) Effects of frequency of emission on semen output and an estimate of daily sperm production in man. J Reprod Fertil 6: 269.

Freund M (1968) Performance and interpretation of the semen analysis. In: Roland M, ed. Management of the infertile couple. Springfield: Charles C. Thomas.

Freund M, Peterson RN (1976) Semen evaluation and fertility. In: Hafez ESE ed. Human semen and fertility regulation in men, p 349. St. Louis: Mos BV.

Freund M, Wiederman J (1966) Factors affecting the dilution, freezing and storage of human semen. J Reprod Fertil 11: 1.

Guess WL, Jacob J, Autian J (1967) A study of polyvinyl chloride blood bag assemblies. I. Alteration of contamination of ACD solutions. Drug Intelligence 1: 120.

Heller CG, Nelson WO, Hill IB, Henderson E, Maddock WD, Jungck EC, Paulsen CA, Mortimer GE (1950) Improvement in spermatogenesis following depression of human testis with testosterone. Fertil Steril 1: 415.

Hunter WM, Edmon P, Watson GC, McLean N (1974) Plasma LH and FSH levels in subfertile males. J Clin Endocrinol Metab 39: 740.

Inchiosa MA Jr (1965) Water soluble extractives of disposable syringes: nature and significance. J Pharm Sci 54: 1379.

Isurugi K, Wakahayashi K, Fukutani K, Takayasu H, Tomaoki BD, Okada M (1973) Responses of serum LH and FSH levels to synthetic LHRH in various forms of testicular disorders. J Clin Endocrinol Metab 37: 533.

Jaeger RJ, Rubin RJ (1970) Plasticizers from plastic devices – extraction, metabolism and accumulation by biological systems. Science 170: 460.

Janich J, MacLeod J (1970) The measurement of human spermatozoan motility. Fertil Steril 21: 140.

Kjessler B (1973) Chromosomal constitution and gamete production in 1000 males attending an infertility clinic. In: Hasegawa T, Ebling FJ, Henderson IW, eds. Fertility and sterility. Amsterdam: Excerpta Medica.

Lawrence DM, Swyer GIM (1974) Plasma testosterone and testosterone binding affinities in males with impotence, oligospermia, azoospermia and hypogonadism. Br Med J 1: 349.

MacLeod J (1965a) Seminal cytology in presence of varicocele. Fertil Steril 16: 735.

MacLeod J (1965b) The semen examination. Clin Obstet Gynecol 8: 115.

MacLeod J (1973) The parameters of male infertility. In: Hospital practice. New York: H.P. Publishing.

MacLeod J, Gold RZ (1951) Male factor in fertility and infertility. II. Spermatozoan counts in 1000 men of known fertility and in 1000 cases of infertile marriage. J Urol 66: 436.

MacLeod J, Hotchkiss RS (1946) Semen analysis in 1500 cases of sterile marriage. Am J Obstet Gynecol 52: 34.

MacNaughton MC (1973) Treatment of female infertility. Clin Endocrinol Metab 2: 545.

Macomber D, Sanders MR (1929) Spermatozoa count. New Engl J Med 200: 981.

Mecklenburg RS, Sherins RJ (1974) Gonadotropin response to LHRH in men with germinal aplasia. J Clin Endocrinol Metab 38: 1005.

Miskin M, Bain J (1978) Use of diagnostic ultrasound in evaluation of testicular disorders. In: Bain J, Hafez ESE, Barwin BN eds. Progress in reproductive biology – andrology, Vol 3, p 117. Basel: Karger.

Nankin HR, Troen P (1976) Endocrine profiles in idiopathic oligospermic males. In: Hafez ESE, ed. Human semen and fertility regulation in men, p 370. St. Louis: Mosby.

Palti Z (1970) Clomiphene therapy in defective spermatogenesis. Fertil Steril 21: 838.

Paulsen CA (1974) The testes. In: Williams RH, ed. Textbook of endocrinology, p 323. Philadelphia: W.B. Saunders.

Pazzagli M, Borreli D, Forti G, Serio M (1974) Dihydrotestosterone in human spermatic venous plasma. Acta Endocrinol 76: 388.

Purvis K, Brenner PF, Landgren, BM, Cekan Z, Diczfalusy E (1975) Indices of gonadal function in the human male. Plasma levels of unconjugated steroids and gonadotropins under normal and pathological conditions. Clin. Endocrinol Metab 4: 237.

Rosen SW, Weintraub BD (1972) Monotropic increase of serum FSH correlated with low sperm count in young males with idiopathic oligospermia and aspermia. J Clin Endocrinol Metab 32: 410.

Rowley MJ, Heller CG (1972) The testosterone rebound phenomenon in the treatment of male infertility. Fertil Steril 23: 98.

Schellen TMCM, Beek JJHMJ (1974) The use of clomiphene treatment for male sterility. Fertil Steril 25: 407.

Schwartzstein LLK, Aparico NJ, Turner, D, Calamera JC, Mancini R, Schally AV (1975) Use of synthetic LHRH in the treatment of oligospermic men: a preliminary report. Fertil Steril 26: 331.

Söltz-Szöts J (1973) Urethritis nongonorrhoica des mannes, diagnose et thérapie. Berlin: Springer Verlag.

Troen P, Yanaihara T, Nankin H, Tominaga T, Leuer H (1970) Assessment of gonadotropin therapy in infertile males. In: Rosemberg E, Paulsen CA eds. The human testis, p 591. New York: Plenum.

Tyler ET (1951) Semen studies and fertility. JAMA 146: 307.

Tyler ET, Singher HO (1956) Male infertility – status of treatment, prevention, and current research. JAMA 160: 91.

Urry RL, Cockett ATD, Dougherty KA (1976) Correlation between FSH, LH, testosterone and 5-hydroxyindole acetic acid with sperm cell concentration. J Urol 116: 332.

Van Zyl JA, Menkveld R, Kotze TJ van W, Retief AE, Van Niekerk WA (1975) Oligozoospermia: a seven-year survey of the incidence, chromosomal aberrations, treatment and pregnancy rate. Int J Fertil 20: 129.

Van Zyl JA, Menkveld R, Retief AE, Van Niekerk WA (1976) Oligospermia. In: Hafez ESE, ed. Human semen and fertility regulation in men, p 363, St. Louis: Mosby.

Wieland RG, Zorn EM, Miles K, Hallberg MC (1974) Endocrinologic evaluation of oligospermic males: determination of dihydrotestosterone and estradiol. Clin Res 22: 634A.

Williams WW (1964) Sterility: the diagnostic survey of the infertile couple, p 9. Springfield: Charles C. Thomas.

Wqllesen F, Swerdloff RS, Odell WD (1976) LH and FSH responses to LHRH in normal adult males. Metabolism 25: 845.

7. TESTICULAR BIOPSY: STRUCTURAL ASPECTS

M.B. BUCKSPAN, Y.C. BEDARD and T.J. COLGAN

In North America approximately 15% of marriages are barren (MacLeod, 1971, Simmons, 1956) and male factor infertility accounts for half of these cases (Paulsen, 1974; Reame and Hafez, 1975). The investigative protocol of infertile males includes semen analysis, testicular biopsy and endocrinologic evaluation. From these determinations a broad clinical pathologic classification has evolved, made up of three groups: the pre-testicular, testicular and post-testicular causes (Wong et al., 1973a).

The pre-testicular causes of infertility are related to decreased testicular stimulation due to hypogonadotropism which is a natural state in the pre-pubertal testis but is pathologic in the post-pubertal state. In these cases the testicle fails secondarily. The testicular causes are related to primary testicular endorgan failure and this group makes up the largest numbers of patients subjected to testicular biopsy. The remaining causes are post-testicular and consist mainly of obstruction of the conduit system from the testis. The list of conditions included in these three groups of causes of infertility is presented in Table 1.

1. TECHNIQUE

In order to preserve the delicate histologic architecture of the testis, an open biopsy should be performed. These is no role for needle biopsy of testis in these cases. Generally unilateral testicular biopsy is performed. However, if there is a gross discrepancy in size or consistency bilateral biopsy is indicated (Posinovec, 1976).

The biopsy is performed on an outpatient basis, in the operating room under general anesthesia. Complete regard for normal operating room technique is mandatory. The anterior aspect of the testicle is fixed in position and the skin, dartos and testicular tunics are incised. Using gentle digital pressure the testicular tubules are extruded through a small incision in the tunica albuginea and the specimen is immediately immersed in Bouin's solution, which offers a more rapid penetration and fixation of tissues than formalin, thus preventing any significant distortion of the tubular architecture. The incised tissues are approximated with 3-O chromic atraumatic sutures and the patient discharged within 2 hours to resume normal activities within 24 hours.

Vasography should not precede or be performed at the time of testicular biopsy. It is indicated to localize the site of the ductal obstruction in those azoospermic patients with a normal or mildly

Table 1. Etiologic classification of male infertility.

PRE-TESTICULAR
1. Hypogonadotrophic hypogonadism
    a) Prepubertal
    b) Post-pubertal
2. Estrogen excess – endogenous
                  – exogenous
3. Androgen excess – endogenous
                  – exogenous
4. Glucocorticoid excess – endogenous
                        – exogenous

TESTICULAR
1. Maturation arrest
2. Hypospermatogenesis
3. Sertoli cell only
4. Klinefelter's syndrome
5. Mumps orchitis
6. Chemical or physical agents

POST-TESTICULAR
1. Obstructive
    a) Congenital – absence of vasa
                 – absence of epididymis
    b) Acquired – post-inflammatory
    c) Idiopathic

J. Bain and E.S.E. Hafez (eds.), Diagnosis in andrology, 87-92. All rights reserved.
Copyright © 1980 by Martinus Nijhoff Publishers bv, The Hague/Boston/London.

hypospermatogenic biopsy. Vasography is contra-indicated in oligospermic patients in that the technique itself can lead to obstruction of the vasa resulting in secondary azoospermia.

When vasography is indicated a biopsy or aspiration of the epididymal head is recommended to exclude obstruction at the level of the efferent ductules. Obstruction at this level precludes surgical correction or vasography.

2. MORPHOLOGY – INTERPRETATION

2.1. Qualitative assessment

As with any other biopsy the microscopic assessment of a testicular biopsy should cover all components, including the seminiferous tubules and the intertubular tissues. In addition to a normal picture a testicular biopsy can reveal changes which are classified as: hypospermatogenesis, maturation arrest, Sertoli-cell-only syndrome and Klinefelter's syndrome.

2.2. Normal

The seminiferous tubules are composed of germinal epithelium. Sertoli cells and the basement membrane. In the germinal epithelium spermatogenesis progresses in six steps from spermatogonia to mature spermatozoa and proceeds from the basement membrane of the tubules to the lumen (Clermont, 1963) (Fig. 1a). Because spermatogenesis occurs in waves of activity along the seminiferous tubule, a cross-section of a single tubule may only show groups of cells at the same stage of maturation. Therefore the final assessment of spermatogenesis should be based on the examination of many seminiferous tubules.

The Sertoli cells are large with pale nuclei located within the seminiferous tubules. They abut onto the basement membrane and mature spermatozoa are noted to adhere to these cells. Their role is probably to nourish the mature spermatozoa. However, they may be partially responsible for the coordination and the progressive step-wise maturation process of spermatogenesis.

The intertubular component of the testis is made up of a fine connective tissue stroma with sup-porting vascular and lymphatic vessels, and the occasional lymphocyte and plasma cell. Interstitial cells are distributed randomly throughout the intertubular tissue and are morphologically variable, with large polyhedral cells predominating. It is these large interstitial cells originally described by Leydig which are thought to be the cells capable of biosynthesis of androgens.

2.3. Hypospermatogenesis

In these biopsies we note a proportional quantitative decrease in numbers of germinal cells. Spermatogenesis occurs through all stages and a decrease may be mild, moderate or severe (Fig. 1b). Peritubular fibrosis may be a prominent feature in the severe cases but the interstitial cells are unremarkable. An overall thinning of the germinal epithelium is a notable feature although some spermatozoa may be seen within the tubular lumen.

2.4. Maturation arrest

This condition represents a halt in the normal progression of spermatogenesis. The arrest is usually abrupt and specific occurring at an early stage of maturation, such as at the stage of the formation of primary spermatocytes or later at the level of spermatids (Fig. 1c). No alteration is noted in the basement membrane, the Sertoli cells or the interstitial cell components.

The stage at which the maturation arrest occurs is constant in individual patients but does vary from patient to patient. The final histologic result is similar in all cases, i.e. the absence of mature spermatozoa with premature sloughing and destruction of the immature forms within the tubular lumen.

2.5. Sertoli-cell-only syndrome (absence of germ cells)

The biopsy reveals a complete absence of germ cells in this disorder, in association with a decrease in diameter of the seminiferous tubules (Fig. 1d). The tubules are lined only by Sertoli cells which appear histologically normal, the Leydig cell population is normal, and peritubular fibrosis may be present but is not a prominent feature.

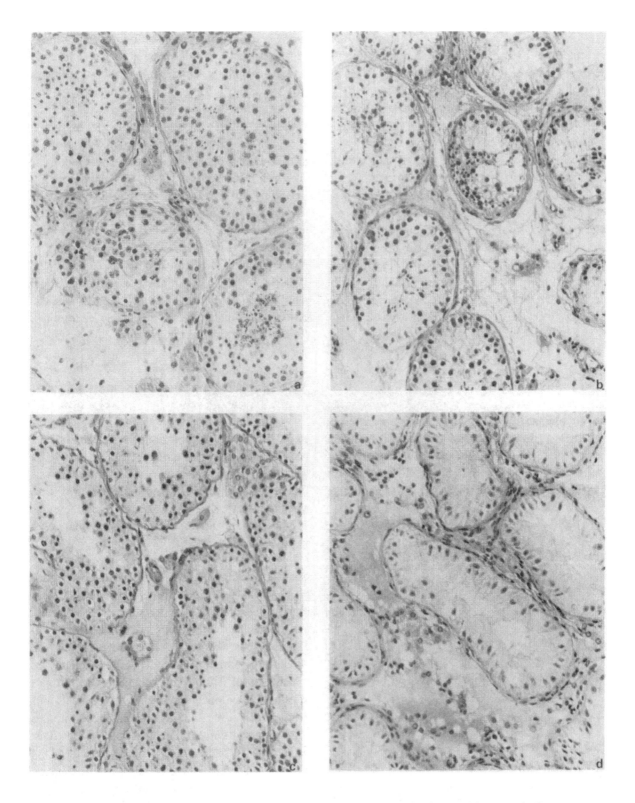

Figure 1. (a) Normal testicular biopsy. The seminiferous tubules show active spermatogenesis progressing step-wise from spermato-gonium to spermatozoa. Note the normal width of the tubular basement membrane and the small collections of interstitial cells. × 300. (b) Severe hypospermatogenesis. All stages from spermatogonia to mature sperms are present but the total number of cells at each stage is reduced. × 300. (c) Maturation arrest. All tubules show a halt in the progression of the spermatogenesis at the level of spermatids resulting in an absence of spermatozoa. × 300. (d) Sertoli cells only. The germ cells are completely absent. × 300.

2.6. Klinefelter's syndrome

In this condition there is a gradual failure of spermatogenesis, with a progressive fibrous obliteration of tubules and a marked hyperplasia of Leydig cells. This histologic picture, which is also known as sclerosing tubular degeneration, is seen in the presence of 47 XXY chromosomal karyotype and occasionally in infertile men with a normal chromosomal karyotype. There is a varying picture in the histology of the seminiferous tubules with early hypospermatogenesis to maturation arrest and Sertoli cell only. In the end stage, the germinal cells and Sertoli cells disappear progressively, leaving seminiferous tubules with diffusely hyalinized basement membranes (Fig. 2). Early in the development of this syndrome the changes do not affect all tubules equally and the histologic picture is patchy (Becker, 1972).

2.7. Quantitative assessment

Since the defect noted in some testicular biopsies is predominantly a reduction in the number of different germ cells, several quantitative analyses have been developed. Roosen-Runge (1956) estimated the volume rather than the number of germ cells but realized that this method is not applicable

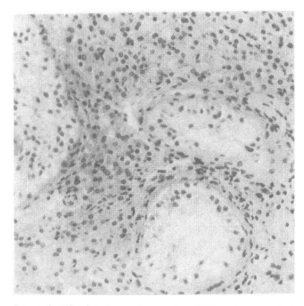

Figure 2. Klinefelter's syndrome. In addition to a marked hyperplasia of Leydig cells, note three tubules lined by Sertoli cells only.

to the analysis of spermatids. Methods of calculating germ cells per cross-sectional area of seminiferous tubules have been reported by Steinberger and Tjioe (1968), Leonard et al. (1972) and de Kretser et al. (1974). However, the necessity of counting many tubules and the artifactual tubular shrinkage due to fixation, limit the usefulness of these techniques. Recently, Skakkeback et al. (1973a) have proposed an interesting method, using the ratio of each germ cell type to the number of Sertoli cells. This method is based on the observations that, both in animals and humans, the Sertoli cells do not divide after sexual maturity (Steinberger and Steinberger, 1971) and are resistant to hormonal influences and irradiation (Rowley and Heller, 1971). This technique however is predominantly for research and has not gained wide acceptance in clinical practice, probably because it is too laborious and time consuming.

3. CLINICAL AND ENDOCRINE CORRELATIONS WITH MORPHOLOGY

In patients with testicular biopsies showing normal histology or hypospermatogenesis, the testes are usually of normal size and studies of endocrine function are normal. Maturation arrest is also associated with testes of normal size and the gonadotropins are usually normal or minimally elevated (de Kretser et al., 1974).

In the Sertoli-cell-only syndrome the patients are usually well masculinized with normal secondary sex characteristics. The testicles are small and softer than normal and endocrine evaluation reveals normal testosterone, indicating adequate Leydig cell function, but elevated FSH in response to the absence of spermatogenesis (de Kretser et al., 1974).

The clinical features of Klinefelter's syndrome are noted after puberty. The testes are small and firm. Leydig cell function decreases to varying degrees and a eunuchoid appearance is noted in these patients. There are variations in the development of secondary sex characterisitcs and circulating testosterone is usually low. The plasma gonadotropins are classically elevated even in patients with normal testosterone levels.

The endocrine findings observed in the various conditions are summarized in Table 2.

Tabel 2. Correlation between morphology and gonadotropins.

Morphology	Gonadotropins
Normal	Normal
Hypospermatogenesis	Normal or elevated
Maturation arrest	Normal or elevated
Sertoli cell only	Markedly elevated (FSH only)
Klinefelter's syndrome	Markedly elevated

4. RELATIVE FREQUENCIES OF THE VARIOUS MORPHOLOGICAL GROUPS

During the period 1971-1979, 142 testicular biopsies were performed for male infertility at Mount Sinai Hospital in Toronto, Canada. The distribution of the morphological pictures observed is presented in Table 3. Slightly more than half of the biopsies show hypospermatogenesis. The remainder revealed in descending order of frequency normal histology, Sertoli-cell-only and maturation arrest. Klinefelter's syndrome was seen in only four cases.

Table 3. Testicular biopsies 1971-1979, Mount Sinai Hospital.

Hypospermatogenesis	69
Normal	29
Sertoli cell only	17
Maturation arrest	15
Klinefelter's syndrome	4
*Unsatisfactory	8
Total	142

* Unsatisfactory refers to inadequate amount or severe crushing artifacts.

Other series of testicular biopsies have been reported (Nelson, 1953; Sniffen et al., 1950; Wong et al., 1973a, b). Sniffen et al. reported a majority of normal biopsies since their series included predominantly patients with ductal obstruction. In our series obstruction was also associated with normal histology or mild hypospermatogenesis. Using much broader indications for biopsy, Nelson presented the largest series with 622 cases. Although his histologic classification is different, when his descriptions are compared to our categories, the distribution of his cases appears fairly similar to ours. In Wong's series, maturation arrest was more commonly observed than in ours.

5. ETIOLOGY

The etiologic factors responsible for each condition are largely unknown. However, a definite etiology can be established in some cases. Normal or mild hypospermatogenesis is seen in post-testicular obstruction. Irradiation and drugs are responsible for some cases of maturation arrest and hypospermatogenesis, and exhibit dose-dependent effects (Clarke and Resnick, 1978; Sherins and Devita, 1973). At levels greater than 600 rads, radiation probably causes irreparable damage to spermatogenesis. Cyclophosphamide and chlorambucil are the most common drugs associated with infertility (Clarke and Resnick, 1978). Mumps orchitis results in the destruction of the germinal tubular epithelium and residual varying degrees of tubular atrophy (Craig, 1975; Wong et al., 1973a). Tuberculosis may damage spermatogenesis after spread from an epididymal infection, but the presence of typical tubercles facilitates the diagnosis (Craig, 1975). More recently, decreased spermatogenic activity with loss of spermatocytes and spermatogonia has been noted in pesticide workers exposed to 1-2-dibromo-3-chloropropane (DBCP) (Marshall et al., 1978). Various inherited defects may present a heterogenous morphology such as Sertoli-cell-only in Del Castillo's syndrome, maturation arrest in Rosewater's syndrome and tubular atrophy and sclerosis in Reifenstein's syndrome (Craig, 1975). Chromosomal abnormalities have been implicated in some cases of Sertoli-cell-only syndrome with the presence of XYY karyotype (Skakkebaek et al., 1973b) but too few cases have been studied to implicate these abnormalities in a cause and effect relationship. In Klinefelter's syndrome an XXY chromosomal pattern is the most common abnormality, but variations exist where chromosomal mosaicism such as XY and XXY cell lines are noted in the same patient (Paulsen et al., 1968) and the clinical picture depends on the presence of an abnormal number of X chromosomes in the testicular tissue. Environmental factors such as temperature have been implicated (MacLeod and Hotchkiss, 1941; Van Demark and Free, 1970). Alcohol, nicotine, caffeine, and sexual excesses have been postulated as possible causes of infertility (Simmons, 1956).

6. INDICATIONS FOR TESTICULAR BIOPSIES

The role of testicular biopsy in the investigation of male infertility has been redefined in recent years. The primary indication for testicular biopsy is the azoospermic patient with normal sized testes. In these cases, the biopsy can distinguish between obstructive azoospermia and those patients with primary testicular failure. This distinction can then direct subsequent investigation to vasography or extensive endocrine or genetic evaluation and treatment (Charny, 1940; Hotchkiss, 1942; Sniffen et al., 1950). In cases of hypogonadotropic hypogonadism treated with testosterone, the testicular biopsy is useful prior to embarking on prolonged and expensive hormonal treatment to stimulate spermatogenesis. Testicular biopsy has also been used to establish prognosis only in the post-radiotherapy or chemotherapy patient who remains azoospermic between 4 months and 5 years post-treatment (Clarke and Resnick, 1978).

The role of testicular biopsy is more controversial in oligospermic patients. In the past, biopsy had been advocated in oligospermia to establish prognosis, exclude partial obstruction of the ejaculatory ducts, and assess a treatment regimen (Charny, 1940, 1963; Cunningham, 1978). In our experience, testicular biopsy in oligospermia is not very informative. The availability of hormonal assays to identify the pre-testicular infertile patient has made biopsy essentially non-contributory. Partial obstruction resulting in oligospermia has not been convincingly demonstrated. Finally, the assessment of the therapeutic efficacy of any hormonal program can be achived by seminal fluid analyses only.

REFERENCES

Amelar RD, Dubin L (1977) The management of idiopathic male fertility. J Reprod Med 18: 191.

Becker KL (1972) Clinical and therapeutic experiences with Klinefelter's syndrome. Fertil Steril 23: 568.

Charny CW (1940) Testicular biopsy. JAMA 115: 1429.

Charny CW (1963) Reflections on testicular biopsy. Fertil Steril 14: 610.

Clarke, SJ, Resnick MI (1978) Infertility following radiation and chemotherapy. Urol Clin N Am 5: 537.

Clermont Y (1963) The cycle of the seminiferous epithelium. Am J Anat 112: 35.

Craig JM (1975) The pathology of infertility. In: Sommers SD ed. Genital and mammary pathology decennial 1966-1975, p 149. New York: Appleton-Century-Crofts.

Cunningham GR (1978) Medical treatment of the subfertile male. Urol Clin N Am 5: 537.

de Kretser DM, Burger HG, Hudson B (1974) The relationship between germinal cells and serum FSH levels in males with infertility. J Clin Endocrinol Metab 38: 787.

Hotchkiss RS (1942) Testicular biopsy in the diagnosis and treatment of sterility in the male. Bull NY Acad Med 18: 600.

Leonard JM, Leach RB, Couture M, Paulsen CA (1972) Plasma and urinary follicle-stimulating hormone levels in oligospermia. J Clin Endocrinol Metab 34: 209.

MacLeod J (1971) Human male infertility. Obstet Gynecol Surv 26: 335.

MacLeod J, Hotchkiss RS (1941) The effect of hyperpyrexia upon spermatozoa counts in man. Endocrinology 28: 780.

Marshall S, Whorton D, Krauss R, Palmer W (1978) Effect of pesticides on testicular function. Urology 11: 257.

Nelson WO (1953) Interpretation of testicular biopsy. JAMA 151: 449.

Paulsen CA (1974) The testis. In: Williams RH, ed. Textbook of endocrinology, p 323. Philadelphia: W.B. Saunders.

Posinovec J (1976) The necessity for bilateral biopsy in oligo- and azoospermia. Int J Fertil 21: 189.

Van Demark NL, Free MJ (1970) Temperature effects. In: Johnson AD, Gomes WR, Vandencek NL, eds. The testis, Vol 3, p 233. New York: Academic Press.

Wong TW, Straus FH, Warner NE (1973a) Testicular biopsy in the study of male infertility. I. Testicular causes of infertility. Arch Pathol 95: 151.

Wong TW, Straus FH, Warner NE (1973b) Testicular biopsy in the study of male infertility. II. Post-testicular causes of infertility. Arch Pathol 45: 160.

Wong TW, Straus FH, Warner NE (1974) Testicular biopsy in the study of male infertility. III. Pretesticular causes of infertility. Arch Pathol 98: 1.

Reame NE, Hafez ESE (1975) Hereditary defects affecting fertility. N Engl J Med 292: 675.

Roosen-Runge EC (1956) Quantitative investigations on human testicular biopsies. I. Normal testis. Fertil Steril 7: 251.

Rowley MJ, Heller CG (1971) Quantitation of the cells of the seminiferous epithelium of the human testis employing the Sertoli cell as a constant. Z Zellforsch 115: 461.

Shane JM, Schiff I, Wilson EA (1977) The infertile couple. Clin Symp (CIBA) 29.

Sherins RJ, DeVita VT (1973) Effects of drug treatment for lymphoma on male reproductive capacity. Studies of men in remission after therapy. Ann Intern Med 79: 216.

Simmons FA (1958) Medical progress. Human infertility. N Engl J Med 255: 1140.

Skakkeback NE, Hammen R, Phillip J, Rebbe H (1973a) Quantification of human seminiferous epithelium. III. Histological studies on 44 infertile men with normal chromosome complements. Acta Pathol Microbiol Scand A 81: 97.

Skakkeback NE, Hutton M, Jacobsen P et al. (1973b) Quantification of human seminiferous epithelium. II. Histological studies in eight 47XYY men. J Reprod Fert 32: 391.

Sniffen RC, Howard RP, Simmons FA (1950) The testis. Arch Pathol 50: 285.

Steinberger A, Steinberger E (1971) Replication pattern of Sertoli cells in maturing rat testes in vivo and in organ culture. Biol Reprod 4: 84.

Steinberger E, Tjioe DY (1968) A method for quantitative analysis of human seminiferous epithelium. Fertil Steril 19: 960.

8. TESTICULAR BIOPSY: FINE STRUCTURE

E.S.E. HAFEZ

The importance of evaluation of testicular biopsies with light microscopy in the diagnosis of the male infertility, particularly when azoospermia is present, is well established. However, available information about the ultrastructural findings in such cases is limited. Testicular biopsies examined by light microscopy show a wide range of histological characteristics ranging from severe hypospermatogenesis to relatively normal-appearing germinal epithelium.

Extensive studies have been conducted on the structural and ultrastructural characteristics of the testicular biopsy and spermatogenesis in man (Camatini et al., 1978; Carr et al., 1968; Dym, 1977; Fawcett et al., 1970, 1971, 1976; Fawcett and Phillips, 1979; Holstein et al., 1973; Pedersen and Rebbe, 1974; Ross et al., 1971; Rowley and Heller, 1971; Schulze, 1974; Skakkeback and Heller, 1973a, b; and Sohval et al., 1973).

1. METHODOLOGY AND EVALUATION

Testicular biopsies are fixed in Karnovsky's fixative buffered with cacodylate for 2-4 hr and transferred to 2% osmium tetroxide in collidine buffer for 90 min. For lanthanum tracer technique (Neaves, 1973), testicular biopsies are immersed in a fixative containing 1% lanthanum and 2% glutaraldehyde in 0.1 M cacodylate buffer and left standing at room temperature for 5 hr. The specimens are postfixed in 1% osmium tetroxide in 0.1 M collidine buffer containing 1% lanthanum for 3-5 hr. Specimens are dehydrated in a graded concentration of ethanol and embedded in Epon. Thin sections, cut on an ultramicrotome, are observed by transmission electron microscopy. Evaluation of testicular biopsy by light microscopy should pre-

cede any evaluation of the biopsy using transmission electron microscopy.

1.1. Quantitative evaluation of the biopsy

There are two methods of quantitation of functional morphology of the cells in the seminiferous tubule employing the Sertoli cell as a constant; a) the whole tubular cross-sections and side areas of longitudinally cut tubules are used; b) segments of tubules are counted with recognizable cell associations (Rowley and Heller, 1971). There are remarkable constancies of cell count between biopsies of different individuals.

1.2. Stereology

Stereology is a method of obtaining quantitative information of structural changes at the light and electron microscopic level. The basic principles of stereology are outlined below. Stereologic techniques can be used to obtain structural data from histologic and electron micrographs of intact tissue and cells. A stereologic model, which provides information on the structure of the epididymis has been developed for the rat epididymal head (Bartsch et al., 1978). The model consists of morphologically defined space and membrane compartments of the rat epididymal head and the principal cells. The alterations, induced in the principal cell of the epididymal head after long-term hypophysectomy, were studied by electron microscopy. The results presented are relative to a cubic centimeter of epididymal tissue, a cubic centimeter of principal cells and principal cell cytoplasm.

To establish structure-function relationships, these morphological methods should be completed by quantitative techniques which would yield ob-

jective and reproducible values for any morphological structure, allowing statistically defined comparisons. This can be achieved by stereological methods.

Stereology is based on geometric probability and allows for quantitation of three-dimensional cross-sections (Elias et al., 1971; Weibel, 1969, 1974; Weibel et al., 1966). Morphometry is the application of stereologic axioms so that the volume (V), surface (S), and number (N) of cells or cell organelles can be quantitated (Fig. 1).

Several components of the cell can be evaluated quantitatively, e.g. the nucleus, the rough and smooth endoplasmic reticulum, the Golgi apparatus, the mitochondria, lysosomes and the secretory droplets. The volume, surface area or number of a component are expressed as the density per unit volume in a given reference space (Bartsch et al., 1978):

Volume density (V_{Vi}) = Volume of the component i within the unit volume of a given reference space.

Surface density (S_{Vi}) = Surface of the component i within the unit volume of a given reference space.

Numerical density (N_{Vi}) = Number of the component i within the unit volume of a given reference space.

By application of appropriate calculations (Rohr et al., 1976) these densities can be related to different reference spaces: unit volume of tissue, unit volume of epithelial (= principal) cells, unit volume of epithelial cell cytoplasm or the absolute volume of an average epithelial cell. The selection of the appropriate reference spaces is of primary importance in correlating morphological and biochemical parameters.

The following cell components of testicular biopsies can be evaluated using stereological techniques:

I. Interstitial cells, density and location of Leydig cells.
II. Peritubular connective tissue.
III. Seminiferous tubules: lumen, germinal cells, Sertoli cells.
   A. Nucleus.

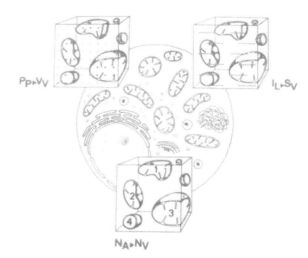

Figure 1. Measurements of the three main parameters. Top left: volume density (V_v) – the fraction of test points (P_p) which lie over profiles of a given particle equals volume density (V_v). Tp right: surface density (S_V) – from the intersection (I_L) of membrane traces with test lines, the surface density (S_V) is calculated. Bottom: numerical density (n_V) – number of profiles (1-4) in the test areas (n_A) is converted to n_V by a formula which includes correction factors for shape and inhomogenous distribution (Bartsch et al., 1978).

B. Cytoplasm.
   1. ground substance.
   2. vacuoles.
   3. rough endoplasmic reticulum.
   4. mitochondria.
   5. lysosomes.
   6. secretory droplets.
   7. Golgi complex-vacuoles, vesicles, saccules.

2. SEMINIFEROUS TUBULES

2.1. Germ cells

Remarkable developmental changes take place in the seminiferous tubules from birth to puberty (Tables 1 and 2; Figs. 2 and 3).

Spermatogenesis involves remarkable structural and ultrastructural differentiation, including spermatogonial stem cell renewal, the two meiotic reduction divisions and the process of spermiogenesis, where the young round spermatids differentiate into mature spermatids. The fine structural characteristics of germ cells are summarized in Table 3.

The ratio between germinal cells and Sertoli cells

is 9 or 10:1 (Rowley and Heller, 1971; Skakkebaek and Heller, 1973a). The ratio of different types of spermatogonia is as follows: 2AL:6AD:1AP, with occasional B cells (Siew et al., 1977). Spermatocytes outnumber spermatogonia 10:7 to 9:5 (Clermont, 1963; de Kretser, 1969).

A major portion of the cytoplasm of the sperm is eliminated prior to its release into the tubular lumen. The excess cytoplasm (residual cytoplasm) is separated from the neck and proximal flagellar regions at the time of sperm release. Once freed, this residual cytoplasm is transported to the base of the seminiferous tubule where it is degraded by the Sertoli cell. The excess of cytoplasm is also eliminated at the head of the spermatid.

2.1.1. Cellular relationship. Long tubular projections of the spermatid with bulbous endings, the tubulobulbar complexes, form by invaginating into the Sertoli cell. The bulbous and tubular portions are devoid of organelles and are in direct continuity with the cytoplasm surrounding the head of the spermatid. Tubulobulbar complexes formed during spermiation undergo phagocytosis by the Sertoli cell. Upon the regression of tubulobulbar processes the perinuclear space around the head shrinks to allow a close relationship of the spermatid plasma membrane and acrosome around the nucleus.

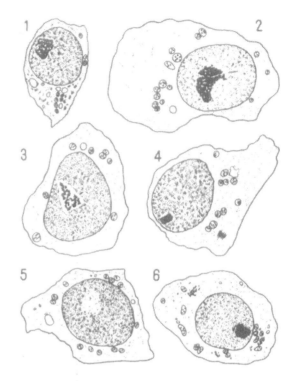

Figure 2. Various types of germ cells. 1: Gonocyte; 2: fetal spermatogonia; 3: transitional spermatogonia; 4: A_p spermatogonia; 5: a_d spermatogonia; 6: B spermatogonia (Hadziselimovic, 1977).

Table 1. Ultrastructural differentiation of the human testis (Bartsch et al., 1978).

Stage	Seminiferous tubules	Peritubular connective tissue	Interstitial tissue
Neonate (1 yr)	Made of two types of gonocytes (primitive germ cells); located in center of tubule with tendency to migrate toward basement membrane; oval shaped; spermatogonia and Sertoli cells; contacting basement membrane most common.	Composed of the basement membrane, of one layer, a collagen fiber zone, and fibroblasts; fibroblast form concentric rings around tubule.	Fetal Leydig cells are well developed.
4 yr	Gonocytes are absent; spermatogonia A and B, spermatocytes and primary Sertoli cells complete the transformation to S_a and S_b types. S_a type is most common.	Certain widening without quantitative changes: basement membrane still consists of one layer without knob formation; collagen fiber layer is wider and cellular layers is composed of fibroblasts; fibroblasts differentiate into myofibroblasts.	Precursors of Leydig cells grouped around vessels at 4-8 yr of age.
Puberty	Tubules acquire a lumen; development of all stages until spermatozoa with a few degenerating cells; Sertoli cells increase 4-5 times in size and increase in number; sperm appear with full development of Sertoli cells; tubules acquire certain contractility.	Under the influence of FSH and LH ultrastructural changes occur; basement membrane becomes multilayered with knob formation; collagen fibers run in an orderly fashion.	Leydig cells well differentiated with remarkable increase in smooth endoplasmic reticulum; Reinecke's crystalloids are absent.

Table 2. Comparative morphological characteristics of seminiferous tubules and Sertoli cells in prepubertal and pubertal testis (Furuya et al., 1978).

	Prepubertal	*Pubertal*
Seminiferous tubule		
Diameter	60-105	100-200
Spermatogonia count*	8-18	105-244
Spermatocyte-sperm	Absent	Absent Present
Lumen	Absent	Absent Present
Sertoli cell		
Shape	Cuboidal or Columnar	Radially elongated
Nucleus	Oval	Irregularly infolded
Endoplasmic reticulum	Moderate	Abundant
Lipid droplet	Seldom	Regularly present
Cytoplasmic filament and microtubule	Moderate	Abundant

* Total number of spermatogonia per 20 transverse tubular sections.

2.2. Sertoli cells

The nucleus is irregularly shaped and its membrane presents numerous pores. The inner aspect of the nuclear membrane is electron dense due to the presence of a fibrous lamina. The outer aspect presents a concentric arrangement of 50 Å cytoplasmic filaments (Fig. 4). The chromatin is dispersed with some perichromatin granules (Bustos-Obregon and Esponda, 1977). Micro-tubules are abundant in Sertoli cells at certain stages of the spermatogenic cycle. With the elongation of the spermatids, their long axis becomes perpendicular to the basement membrane; their nucleus is located in a deep recess in the Sertoli cell, and most of the cytoplasm is displaced caudally around the base of the flagellum, extending toward the lumen of the seminiferous tubule. Owing to the syncytial nature of the developing germ cells, the residual lobules of spermatid cytoplasm are connected to one another by intercellular bridges which result from incomplete cytokinesis in the germ cell divisions of spermatogenesis (Fawcett, 1975).

The nucleolus consists of a tripartite complex; the central portion is Feulgen-negative, the lateral structures (heteropyknotic bodies or satellite karyosomes) are Feulgen-positive.

The mitochondria are numerous, generally very long and have lamellar cristae generally oriented

transversely. In the basal cytoplasm they are randomly oriented, 'cup-shaped' and contain vesicular crystals (Fig. 5). The Golgi complex consists of a few short parallel cisternae and small vesicles. There are numerous lysosomes, autophagic and heterophagic vacuoles and lipid droplets. These lipid droplets vary according to a true 'lipid cycle' which corresponds to the cycle of seminiferous epithelium. Sertoli cells contain two types of crystals: 1) Charcot-Bottcher crystalloids, 10-25 μm long and 2-3 μm thick, and 2) smaller 'spangaro' crystals 1-5 μm long and about 1 μm thick.

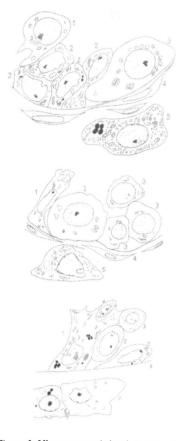

Figure 3. Ultrastructural development of the human testis after 2 months, 4 years, and 13 years. *Top:* 2-month-old normal testicle – 1: gonocyte; 2: fetal Sertoli cells (S_f); 3: fetal spermatogonia; 4: fibroblasts; 5: Leydig cells. *Middle:* 4-year-old normal testicle – 1: S_b Sertoli cells; 2: fetal spermatogonia; 3: S_a Sertoli cells; 4: fibroblasts; 5: Leydig cells. *Bottom:* 13-year-old normal testicle – 1: S_c Sertoli cells; 2: primary spermatocytes; 3: secondary spermatocytes; 4: spermatids; 5: A_p spermatogonia; 6: peritubular connective tissue; 7: Leydig cells (Hadziselimovic, 1977).

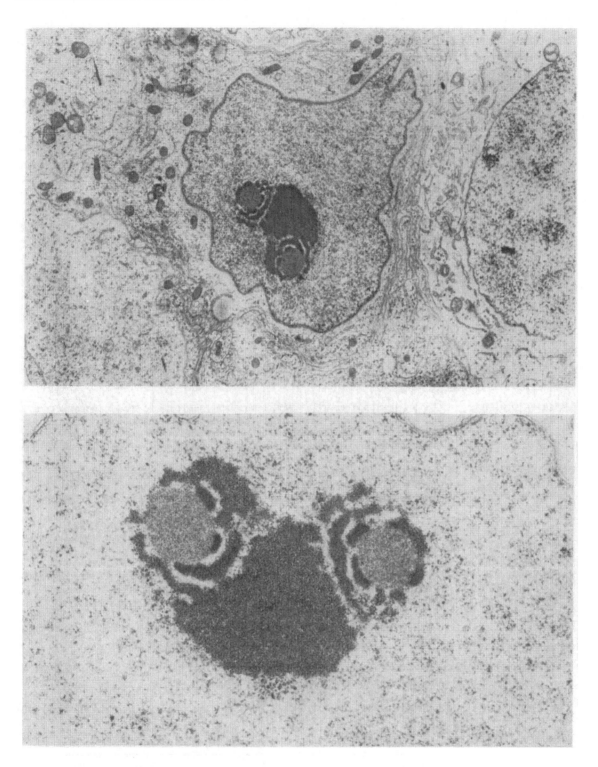

Figure 4. Sertoli cell nucleolus, exhibiting the three zones. (a) is formed by the intermixing of 60-80 Å fibers and 200 Å granules ('pars granular'); (b) are dense cords composed of fine fibrils ('pars fibrilar'); (c) is a less dense, spherical zone, formed by 70 Å fibers ('light zones' or 'fibrillar centers'). *Top:* ×9,900; *Bottom:* ×22,500. (Courtesy Professor Edwardo Bustos.)

In the depths of the apical invaginations of Sertoli cells there are parallel bundles of filaments which appear to course circumferentially in the thin layer of cytoplasm between the inner surface of the cell membrane and a fenestrated cisterna of endoplasmic reticulum. In this zone the filaments develop during condensation of spermatid nucleus and thus seem to represent a peculiar device for maintaining attachment of the Sertoli cell; each cell has subsurface cisternae and bundles of filaments connected with its opposed membranes. These arrangements represent extensive and unique junctional complexes involving two adjacent Sertoli cells. The outer leaflets of the membranes are 150-200 Å apart, but in some areas they approach to within 20 Å of one another, recalling the gap junctions of other cellular types.

Junctional specializations between the Sertoli

Table 3. Fine structural characteristics of germ cells in testicular biopsies (Bustos-Obregon and Holstein, 1973; Clermont, 1963; de Kretser, 1969; de Kretser et al., 1975; Dym and Cavicchia, 1978; Fabbrini and Hafez, 1979; Rowley and Heller, 1971; Siew et al., 1978).

Cell type	Structural characteristics
SPERMATOGONIUM AL (long)	A long, very flat cell with extensive attachment to basal lamina. Its nucleus is also long and irregular; nucleolus peripheral, on the nuclear membrane with diffuse nucleonema; mitochondria in groups connected by bars and associated with nucleus away from basal lamina; tubular cristae; glycogen, crystalloids of Lubarsch and lamellar bodies.
SPERMATOGONIUM AD (dark)	Long and flat with less contact to basement membrane; nucleus long and oval; nucleolar mitochondria are similar to the AL type; plate-like and tubular cristae; glycogen and Lubarsch crystals; small amount of smooth and rough endoplasmic reticulum.
SPERMATOGONIUM AP (pale)	Round cell with less contact to basement membrane; round or ovoid nucleus; peripheral nucleolus differentiated into a pars amorpha and nucleonema; mitochondria connected only in pairs and never attached to nucleus; cristae are plate-like; endoplasmic reticulum smooth and granular; single strands; myelin-like arrays in cytoplasm.
SPERMATOGONIUM B	Pear-shaped with least contact (2 μm) to basement membrane; spherical nucleus with chromatin granules within nuclear membrane; nucleolus central with a nucleonema and a pars amorpha; single mitochondria; plate-like cristae; Golgi apparatus more elaborate with myelin-like arrays.
SPERMATIDS Sb_1	Golgi and centrioles begin a caudal migration; acrosomal vesicle closely applied to nucleus extending over about one third of its surface; acrosomal granule centrally situated within the vesicle.
SPERMATID Sb_2	Caudal migration of centrioles and axial filament completed – they are lodged in juxtaposition to abacrosomal pole of nucleus; nucleus moves rostrally from central position of previous stages and its acrosomal pole is closely applied to cell membrane; nuclear shape more elongated.
SPERMATID Sc	Maturation of nucleoplasm begins; central condensations of more coarse and dense chromatin granules.
SPERMATID Sd_1	Formation of larger and more electron dense chromatin granules; reduction in nuclear volume gives rise to a pear-shaped head.
SPERMATID Sd_2	Chromatin forms a homogeneous electron dense mass; sperm head resembles arrowhead or is spatulate.
Differentiated spermatid	Acrosomic granules are redistributed to form acrosomal contents; well developed smooth endoplasmic reticulum in close association with Golgi apparatus; acrosomal cap associated with full formation of reorientation of anterior pole of nucleus towards base of seminiferous tubules; elongation and condensation of nucleus; axonemal complex of sperm tail is initiated by centriolar complex during 'Golgi' phase of spermiogenesis.
Mature spermatid	Remarkable alterations in smooth endoplasmic reticulum.
BASEMENT MEMBRANE	A homogeneous moderately electron dense layer, 0.3-0.4 μm thick, in direct contact with the base of the spermatogonia and Sertoli cells; membrane may protrude into tubule indenting these cells.

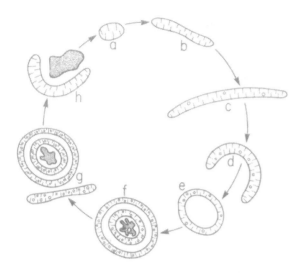

Figure 5. Ultrastructural changes of mitochondria of Sertoli cells during the cycle of seminiferous epithelium in the rat. The mitochondria change their shape from ovoidal to circular. a-c correspond to stages 5-14, according to Clermont. f-h correspond to stages 1-4 (DeMartino, 1968).

cells have both gap and tight junctions, as judged by uranyl acetate staining, electron-opaque tracer and freeze-fracture techniques (Dym, 1973; Dym and Fawcett, 1970; Nagano and Suzuki, 1976a, b). These gap junctions gradually disappear in the course of the postnatal development of the testis, while the tight junctions appear to increase in size and number. In the mature testis, special tight junctions are characterized by three components: (a) multiple punctata pentalaminar membrane fusions; (b) subsurface cisternae of endoplasmic reticulum oriented in parallel with the Sertoli cell plasma membrane; and (c) bundles of microfilaments between the Sertoli cell plasma membrane and the associated subsurface cisternae (Fawcett, 1975; Fawcett et al., 1976).

Sertoli cells actively participate in the spermatogenic process; they undergo cyclical changes of the endoplasmic reticulum, mitochondria, the 'cycle of glycogen' and the 'cycle of lipids'. There is a close relationship between quantity and location of the glycogen and the stage of the spermatogenic cycle (Fabbrini et al., 1969). Glycogen accumulates during the first stage, whereas there is a sharp decrease in the amount of Sertolian glycogen in the second, third and sixth stages. For example, glycogen accumulates in the dark spermatogonia only before the transformation of spermatogonium A into spermatogonium B (Fabbrini et al., 1969).

There is an increase of lipid content immediately after spermiation due to phagocytosis of residual bodies.

Sertoli cells act as 'bridge cells' between the interstitial blood vessels and the germ cells (Vilar et al., 1962). Exchange between Sertoli cells and germ cells is strongly suggested by the conspicuous mobilization of spermatid mitochondria at the cell surface in some stages and by the aggregation of Sertoli cell smooth reticulum immediately adjacent to the heads of maturing spermatids (Fawcett, 1975).

2.3. Blood-testis barrier

Complicated interdigitation-like junctions between the immature Sertoli cells are apparent in the prepubertal testis. In pubertal testis, junctional specializations between Sertoli cells are composed of membrane fusions, bundles of microfilaments and associated cisternae. These tight junctions block the deep penetration of lanthanum into the seminiferous tubules. The lanthanum-filled Sertoli junctions show characteristic features of membrane fusions. The blood-testis barrier is established shortly before or after the spermatogonia proliferate to give rise to primary spermatocytes (Furuya et al., 1978).

The initiation of the blood-testis barrier in the human testis seems to depend on gonadotropins, but the maintenance of this barrier is not. An effective blood-testis barrier is maintained in azoospermic cases and the infertility is not attributable to altered Sertoli-Sertoli junctions.

Near the peritubular membrane around the seminiferous tubules, tight junctions between Sertoli cells divide the seminiferous epithelium into two compartments: (a) a 'basal compartment' between the junctions and basal lamina, and (b) an 'adluminal compartment' between the junctions and lumen of tubule (Dym, 1973; Dym and Cavicchia, 1978).

A physiological barrier characterized by Sertoli-Sertoli occluding junctions acts as the blood-testis barrier.

The Sertoli cell acts as a 'bridge cell' between the interstitium and germinal cells except for spermatogonia and preleptotene spermatocytes (Vilar et al., 1962). The junctional complexes divide the Sertoli cell into two compartments: a basal or external

compartment, connected with the spermatogonia and preleptotene spermatocytes; and an apical or adluminal compartment containing the other more mature germinal cells. All substances from the blood that reach the base of the epithelium have direct access to the external compartment; but they have to be transported through the Sertoli cell cytoplasm to reach the apical compartment, because of the presence of the junctional complexes which bar the extracellular route (Fabbrini and Hafez, 1980). It would appear that the areas of fusion of the opposing Sertoli cell membranes represent low-resistance pathways for cell-to-cell communication.

The barrier function of the peritubular smooth muscle cells is a part of the blood-testis barrier, similar to the blood-brain barrier. A barrier certainly exists at the level of the Sertoli cells, which

have unique ultrastructural characteristics.

There is a barrier at the level of the peritubular smooth muscle cells, the function of which is hormone-dependent (Fawcett et al., 1969).

2.4. Tubular wall

The tubular wall is a complex structure made of five layers: a typical basement membrane next to the basal surface of the Sertoli cell; an internal acellular layer, containing collagen fibers, glycoproteins and hyaluronic acid; an internal cellular layer made of spindle-shaped cells (myoid cells or 'peritubular smooth muscle cells' – p.s.m. cells); and an external cellular layer consisting of fibroblast (Fig. 6). The acellular layers probably act as a cushion against microtrauma and variations in hydrostatic and/or osmotic pressure whereas the basement membrane

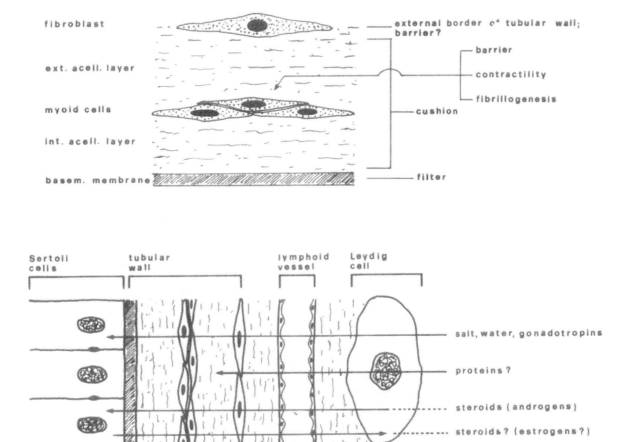

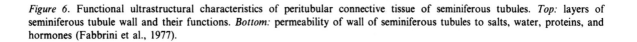

Figure 6. Functional ultrastructural characteristics of peritubular connective tissue of seminiferous tubules. *Top:* layers of seminiferous tubule wall and their functions. *Bottom:* permeability of wall of seminiferous tubules to salts, water, proteins, and hormones (Fabbrini et al., 1977).

probably constitutes a sort of selective filter for some proteins (Fabbrini and Hafez, 1979). The fibroblasts probably participate in the barrier mechanism. The peritubular connective tissue is made up of regularly alternating 2-6 (variable) layers of collagen fibers and myoid cells (contractile) beneath the basement membrane. The external surface is covered by a basement membrane and it may be in close association with some microfibrillar material.

3. INTERSTITIAL TISSUE

The space between the seminiferous tubules, which is filled with an irregular meshwork of loose connective tissue containing Leydig cells (Fig. 7), fibroblasts, macrophages, mast cells and nonmyelinated nerve cells, occupies one third of the testicular volume. The fine structural characteristics of Leydig cells as compared to Sertoli cells are shown in Table 4.

4. FINE STRUCTURAL ANOMALIES

Characteristic anomalies in the firm structure of germ cells, Sertoli cells, peritubular connective tissue, Leydig cells and other testicular compartments are summarized in Table 5. Some of the common anomalies include parenchymatous degeneration, a diminution of mature germ cells, abnormalities in the formation of spermatids, and phagocytosis of spermatids by the prominent Sertoli cells (Siew et al., 1978).

Spermatidic arrest is one of the causes of oligoazoospermia, often secondary to toxic or traumatic factors or to decreased gonadotropin stimulation. Developmental anomalies of the acrosome are extremely frequent. Some ultrastructural characteristics of pathological aspects of the testes in infertile men are summarized in Table 6.

Abnormalities were found in the lamina propria and basement membrane of the tubule in blood

Table 4. Fine structural characteristics of Sertoli cells and Leydig cells (Bustos-Obregon and Esponda, 1977; Bustos-Obregon and Holstein, 1973; Christensen, 1975; de Kretser, 1967, 1968; Fawcett, 1975).

	Sertoli cell	*Leydig cell*
General characteristics	Tall and columnar, extending from base of epithelium to tubule lumen; laterally directed cytoplasmic processes causing intimate wrapping around spermatogonia with elaborate infolding of cytoplasmic membranes and ingested sperm cell elements, especially spermatids. Three types of prominent vacuoles: a) small clear vacuoles, b) small, faintly eosinophilic vacuoles, c) large lucent vacuoles with a dark rim (Schulze cell type III).	Found in clusters in close proximity to blood vessels but separated from them by perivascular fibrosis; polygonal in form, 15-20 μm in diameter, surrounded by a typical plasmalemma thrown into folds or microvilli. Most prominent organelle is abundant smooth endoplasmic reticulum consisting of interconnected membrane tubules, 800-1200 Å in diameter.
Cytoplasmic organelles	Mitochondria are numerous, long and slender; mitochondria in basal cytoplasm are randomly oriented, whereas those in the supranuclear columnar portion of cell are parallel to cell axis; multiple separate Golgi elements scattered through the basal cytoplasm in supranuclear region.	Scattered patches of rough endoplasmic reticulum interconnect with smooth endoplasmic reticulum. Mitochondria are elongated or rounded and contain cristae of lamellar or, less frequently, tubular formation; intramitochondrial granulation uncommon; Golgi complex well developed, connected with two centrioles and situated at one pole of nucleus; Golgi elements consist of 4-6 flattened sacs closely pressed together, with small vesicles at their periphery; cytoplasm contains lipid droplets, Reinke crystals, microtubules and microfilaments, lysosomes, digestive vacuoles (secondary lysosomes), and residual bodies (late secondary lysosomes) containing pigment.
Nucleus	Infolded in shape; karyosomes and peripheral clumps of heterochromatin that characterize nuclei or most somatic cell types are lacking; nuceloplasm homogeneous with large proportion of euchromation with fine fibrogranular texture.	Large, oval or round with a thin peripheral rim of heterochromatin, broken only at the sites of pores through the nuclear envelope; one or two prominent nucleoli.

vessels and in spermatids. The diminished blood supply in, and increased denseness of, the peritubular connective tissue and the interstitial tissue cause impared functions of both the interstitial cells and the germinal epithelium.

Ultrastructural differences between the descended and cryptorchid testis are shown in Table 7. Fine structural characteristics are shown for germ cells (Fig 8), Sertoli cells (Fig. 9) and Leydig cells (Fig. 10).

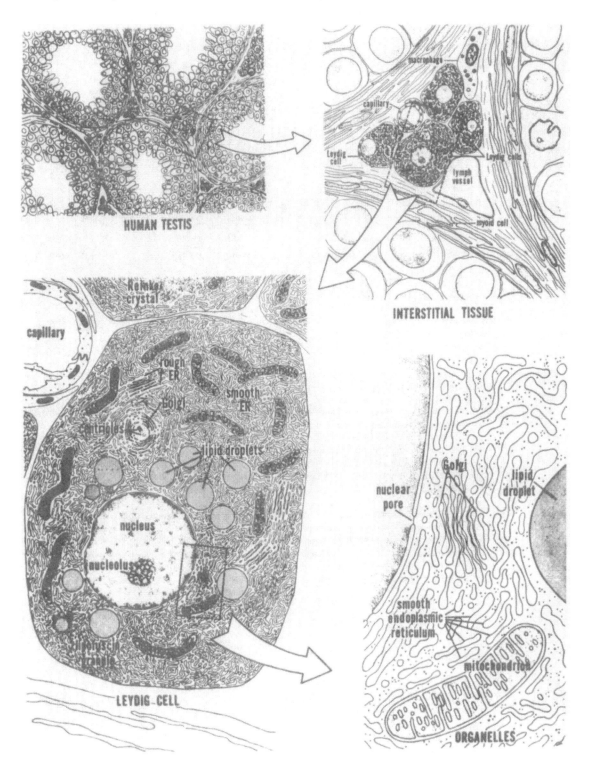

Table 5. Fine structural anomalies in testicular biopsies associated with male infertility (Nistal and Paniagua, 1978; Siew et al., 1977, 1978).

Structure or type of anomaly	Structural characteristics
Acrosomal	Complete absence of acrosome in ejaculates with a high percentage of round-headed spermatozoa; acrosomal cap not attached to the nucleus; acrosomal vesicle overlays the nucleus with little or no granular material; ballooning of acrosomal vesicle.
Division of nucleus (multi-nucleated forms)	Anomalies of nuclear division characterized by multinucleated cells; early spermatids connected by intercytoplasmic bridges.
Nuclear fine structure	Anomalies in nuclear morphology – rounded or pear-shaped – associated with delayed maturity; abnormal extension of acrosomal pole with tapering of nucleus; tapering of abacrosomal pole; asynchronous development of acrosome and of nucleus.
Spermatid formation	Late spermatids with spherical nucleus with chromatin of medium density; rough endoplasmic reticulum Golgi complex are hypoplastic in spermatids; depression of nuclear surface at the contact area with the acrosomic vesicle and absence of true acrosomic cap; asynchrony between stage of development of acrosomal cap and degree of maturation of nucleus; nuclear immaturity with a delay in progression of the spherical vesicular morphology of earliest spermatids (Sa stage of spermiogenesis) to homogeneous electron-dense-type mature cell (Sd2); deficiences in the nuclear envelope leading to communication chromatin and cytoplasm; abnormal increased glycogen content in cases of spermatidic arrest due to inadequate Sertoli utilization of energy sources.
Sperm formation	Tail, detached from nucleus, is lying within cytoplasm of Sertoli cell; presence of irregular mitochondria only around rostral portion of middle piece; caudal section of middle piece is bare; absence of annulus at its junction with principal piece.
Basement membrane	Increased reduplication and infolding of the tubular basement membrane.
Peritubular connective tissue	(a) A thickening due to increase in width of collagen layers; or an increase in the number of collagen fibers; (b) Increase in fine microfibrils and basement membrane-like material; (c) Or regular distribution of collagen and myoid cells; (d) Irregular arrangement of collagen bundles; collagen fibers are seen in longitudinal, tangential, and cross-section, indicating loss of polarity.
Blood vessels	Thickening of the arteriolar walls and endarteritis obliterans; varying degrees of perivascular fibrosis.

Figure 7. Location and fine structure of human Leydig cells. Leydig cells, source of testosterone, occur in clusters in the interstitial tissue between the seminiferous tubules (*upper left*). In addition to Leydig cells, interstitial tissue (*upper right*) also contains macrophages, fibroblasts, and other components of connective tissue, as well as capillaries and lymph vessels, which carry androgen to other parts of the body. Seminiferous tubules are surrounded by a boundary layer of flattened myoid cells. Within the cytoplasm of an individual Leydig cell (*lower left*), the most abundant organelle is the smooth endoplasmic reticulum (smooth ER), although small patches of rough endoplasmic reticulum (rough ER) also occur. Mitochondria are common. The Golgi complex consists of Golgi elements that are clustered at one pole of the nucleus but also extend elsewhere in the cytoplasm. Two centrioles lie within the Golgi area. Lipofuscin pigment granules and other lysosomal stages are present, as are peroxisomes (not illustrated). The number of lipid droplets and Reinke crystals varies from cell to cell. The nucleus contains a thin peripheral rim of heterochromatin and a prominent nucleolus. The cell is enclosed in a plasma membrane. In a selected area of cytoplasm (*lower right*), some of the organelles are seen in greater detail. The smooth endoplasmic reticulum is shown as it appears in thin sections viewed with the electron microscope; in three dimensions, however, it is actually a network of interconnecting tubules. Ribosomes occur between tubules but are not attached to membranes. Some cristae in the mitochondrion are tubular, others are lamellar. A Golgi element consists of several closely packed, flattened sacs and accompanying vesicles. The nucleus is surrounded by a nuclear envelope composed of two membranes. The envelope is penetrated here and there by nuclear pores (Christensen, 1975).

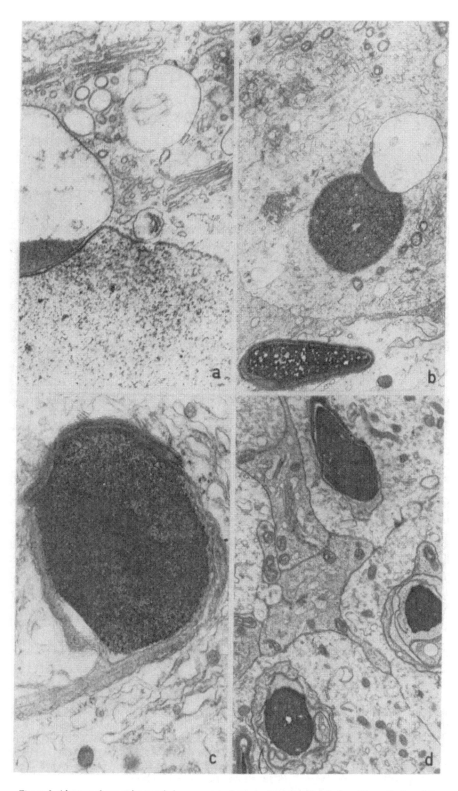

Figure 8. Abnormal spermiogenesis in azoospermic men. a) At the Golgi-phase the majority of the early spermatids have developing acrosomes which show morphological changes. b) Acrosomal material may become irregularly distributed and the abnormalities may have several patterns, the most frequent being greatly swollen vesicles. c, d) During the nuclear elongation phase distortions of the acrosomal cap and underlying nuclear region are evident and spermatids equipped with distorted acrosomal caps give rise to sperm with abnormal head morphology (Camatini, 1979).

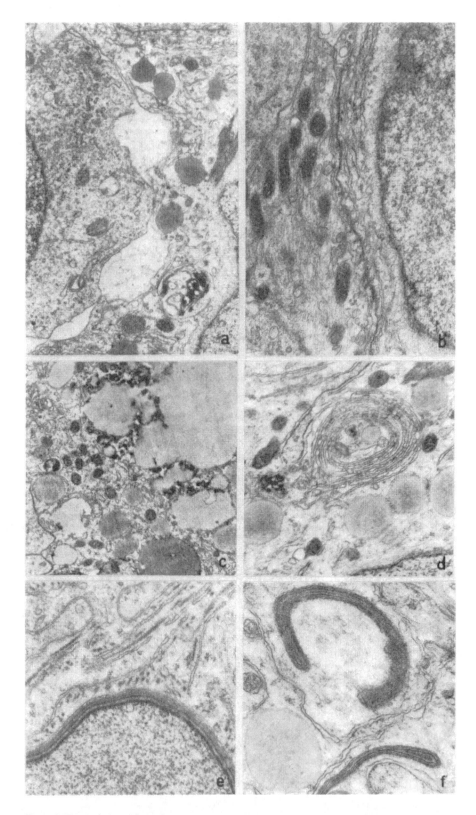

Figure 9. Transmission electron micrographs of Sertoli cells in azoospermia. a) Charcot-Buttcher's crystalloids. b) Note prominent junctional complexes linking adjacent Sertoli cells. c) Note large number of various lipid inclusions and lipofuscin bodies growing. d) Note presence of lamellar bodies. e) Sertoli cell relationship reveals that junctional specializations adapt to the distortions of the acrosomal cap, undergoing the same deformation. f) Phagocytotic activity was demonstrated by the presence of degenerating germ cells in the cytoplasm, or of portions of them. Note the presence of an acrosome vesicle (Faleri and Franchi, 1979).

Table 6. Some ultrastructural characteristics of pathological aspects of the human testes of infertile men (Barham et al., 1976; Castellani-Ceresa and Berruti, 1979; Camatini, 1979; Castellani-Ceresa et al., 1978; Faleri and Franchi, 1979; Furuya et al., 1979; Re et al., 1979).

Syndrome	Some ultrastructural characteristics of testicular biopsy
Obstructed deferent ducts	Mature sperm surrounded by Sertoli cells and occupying deep niches in the sides of supporting cells, thus denoting altered spatial organization within the tubules; alteration in spermatid-Sertoli cell relationship reveals that junctional specializations adapt to the distortions of the acrosomal cap, undergoing the same deformation; Sertoli-Sertoli junctions are normal; polymorphic content of cytoplasm includes lysosomes and lipid droplets of various sizes and electron densities; phagocytotic activity, demonstrated by presence of degenerating germ cells in the cytoplasm.
Obstructive azoospermia or absence of deferent ducts	Developmental anomalies of the acrosome during the Golgi-phase of spermiogenesis, e.g. atypical Golgi complexes, loss or deformed head caps; course of spermatogenesis does not differ significantly from normal until after the completion of meiosis; early spermatids show abnormal acrosome at Golgi-phase; acrosomal material may become irregularly distributed; swollen vesicles in acrosome; Sertoli cells are characterized by glycogen accumulation, vacuolization of cytoplasm and large number of various lipid inclusions and lipofuscin bodies, giving the cytoplasm the vacuolated appearance.
Idiopathic spermatidic arrest	Modification in the smooth endoplasmic reticulum of Sertoli cell cytoplasm characterized by the presence of dilated cisternae, which causes ultrastructural biochemical modification of the germinal epithelium.
Hypogonodotropic enuchoidism	The seminiferous tubules are filled mainly with immature Sertoli cells, with a few spermatogonia; no lumen formation.
Cryptorchidism	Thickening of the basement membrane, which appears as a homogeneous or a multilaminar structure, due to thickening of the internal and external acellular layers and of the intertubular vessels which is itself due to accumulation of collagen fibers and microfibrillar material.

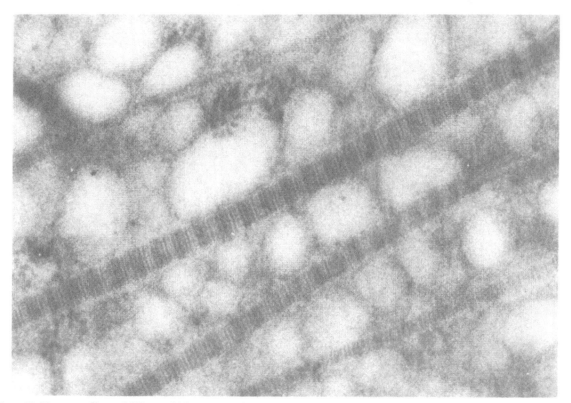

Figure 10. Numerous fibers of different thicknesses are visible in the cytoplasm of a pathological human Leydig cell. All fibers show the typical periodism of collagen. (Courtesy Dr. C. DeMartino.)

Table 7. Ultrastructural differences between descended and cryptorchid testis (Bartsch et al., 1978).

Morphometrical parameters	Normal testis	Cryptorchid testis
Number of Sertoli cell nuclei, cu/cm	1461×10^6	1617×10^6
Single cell volume, cu	491	429
Volume density of spermatogonia, cu/cm	0.0056	0.0021
Volume density of degenerating cells	0.0012	0.0018

REFERENCES

Barham SS, Berlin JD, Brackeen RB (1976) The fine structural localization of testicular phosphatases in man: the central testis. Cell Tiss Res 166(4): 497.

Bartsch G, Overholzer M, Holliger O, Wever J, Weber A, Rohr HP (1978) Sterology: a new quantitative morphological method to study epididymal function. Andrologia 10: 31.

Bustos-Obregon E, Esponda P (1977) Ultrastructure of the nucleus of human Sertoli cells in normal and pathological testes. Andrologia 1: 19.

Bustos-Obregon E, Holstein AF (1973) On structural patterns of the lamina propria of human seminiferous tubules. Z Zellforsch 141: 413.

Camatini M (1979) Abnormal spermiogenesis in azoospermic men. Arch Androl II, Suppl I.

Camatini M, Franchi E, Faleri M (1978) Ultrastructure of acrosomal malformations in men with obstructive azoospermia. Arch Androl 1: 203.

Carr I, Clegg EJ, Meedk GA (1968) Sertoli cells as phagocytes. J Anat 102: 501.

Castellani-Ceresa L, Berruti G (1979) Cytochemistry of the testis of infertile men. Arch Androl II, Suppl I.

Castellani-Ceresa L, Chiara F, Cotelli F (1978) Fine structure and cytochemistry of the morphogenesis of round-headed human sperm. Arch Androl I, 291.

Christensen AK (1975) Leydig cells. In: Hamilton DW, Greep RO, eds. Handbook of physiology, sect 7: Endocrinology, Vol V. Washington: American Physiological Society.

Clermont Y (1963) The cycle of the seminiferous epithelium in man. Am J Anat 112: 35.

De Kretser DM (1967) The fine structure of the testicular interstitial cells in men of normal androgenic status. Z Zellforsch 80: 594.

De Kretser DM (1968) Crystals of Reinke in the nuclei of human testicular interstitial cells. Experientia 24: 587.

De Kretser DM (1969) Ultrastructural features of human spermiogenesis. Z Zellforsch 98: 477.

De Kretser DM, Kerr JB, Paulsen CA (1975) The peritubular connective tissue in the normal and pathological human testis. An ultrastructural study. Biol Reprod 12: 317.

DeMartino C (1968) In Conti E, Fabbrini A, Gl: Spogonadismi maschili, Pozzi L, ed. Rome.

Dym M (1973) The fine structure of the monkey (*Macaca*) Sertoli cell and its role in maintaining the blood-testis barrier. Anat Rec 175: 639.

Dym M (1977) The role of the Sertoli cell in spermatogenesis. In: Yates R, Gordon M, eds. Male reproductive system pp 155-169. New York: Raven Press.

Dym M, Cavicchia JC (1978) Functional morphology of the testis. Biol Reprod 18: 1.

Dym M, Fawcett DW (1970). The blood-testis barrier in the rat and the physiological compartmentation of the seminiferous epithelium. Biol Reprod 3: 308.

Elias HA, Henning A, Schwartz DE (1971) Stereology: application to biomedical research. Physiol Rev 51: 158.

Fabbrini A, Hafez ESE (1980) Testis-Epididymis. In: Hafez ESE, ed. Human reproduction: conception and contraception. Hagerstown: Harper & Row.

Fabbrini A, Re M, Conti C (1969) Glycogen in normal human testis: a histological and histochemical study. J Endocrinol 43: 499.

Fabbrini A, Santiemma V, Bellocci M, Francavilla S, Francavilla F, Micali F (1977) Cyproterone acetate and seminiferous tubule wall. In: Martini L, Motta M, eds. Androgens and antiandrogens. New York: Raven.

Faleri M, Franchi E (1979) Ultrastructure of Sertoli cells in testicular pathology. Arch androl II, Suppl I.

Fawcett DW (1975) Ultrastructure and function of the Sertoli cell. In: Hamilton DW, Greep RO, eds. Handbook of physiology, endocrinology, sect 7, Vol V, Washington: American Physiological Society.

Fawcett DW, Anderson WA, Phillips DM (1971) Morphogenetic factors influencing the shape of the sperm head. Dev Biol 26: 220.

Fawcett DW, Gilula NB, Aoki A (1976) Recent observations on the organization of the seminiferous epithelium. In: Kurosumi K, ed. Gunma Symp. Institute of Endocrinology, Gunma University, Maebashi, Japan. Endocrinology 13: 49.

Fawcett DW, Heidger PM, Leack LV (1969) Lymph-vascular system on the interstitial tissue of the testis as revealed by electron microscopy. J Reprod Fertil 19: 109.

Fawcett DW, Leak LV, Heidger PM (1970) Electron microscopic observations on the structural components of the blood-testis barrier. J Reprod Fertil Suppl 10: 105.

Fawcett DW, Phillips DM (1969) Observations on the release of spermatozoa and on changes in the head during passage through the epididymis. J Reprod Fertil Suppl 6: 405.

Furuya S, Kumamoto Y, Ikegaki S (1979) Blood-testis barrier in men with hypogonadotropic eunuchoidism and postpuberal pituitary failure. Arch Androl II, Suppl I.

Furuya S, Kumamoto Y, Sugiyam S (1978) Fine structure and development of Sertoli junctions in human testis. Arch Androl 1: 211.

Hadziselimovic F (1977) Cryptorchidism-ultrastructure of normal and cryptorchid testis development. Berlin: Springer-Verlag.

Holstein AF, Schirren C, Schirren CG (1973) Human spermatids and spermatozoa lacking acrosomes. J Reprod Fertil 35: 489.

Nagano T, Suzuki F (1976a) Freeze-fracture observations on the intercellular junctions of Sertoli cells and of Leydig cells in the human testis. Cell Tiss Res 166: 37.

Nagano T, Suzuki F (1976b) The postnatal development of the junctional complexes of the mouse Sertoli cells and revealed by freeze-fracture. Anat Rec 185: 403.

Neaves WB (1973) Permeability of Sertoli cell tight junctions to lanthanum after ligation of ductus deferens and ductuli efferentes. J Cell Biol 59: 559.

Nistal M, Paniagua R (1978) Morphogenesis of round-headed human spermatozoa lacking acrosomes in a case of severe teratozoospermia. Andrologia 10: 49.

Pedersen H, Rebbe H (1974) Fine structure of round headed human spermatozoa. J Reprod Fertil 37: 51.

Re M, Carpino F, Familiari G, Iannitelli M, Vicari A, Fabbrini A (1979) Electron microscopical characteristics of idiopathic arrest. Arch Androl II, Suppl I.

Rohr HP, Oberholzer M, Bartsch G, Keller M (1976) Morphometry in experimental pathology: methods, baseline, data and applications. Int Rev Exp Pathol 15: 233.

Ross A, Christie S, Kerr MG (1971) An electron microscope study of a tail abnormality in spermatozoa from a subfertile man. J Reprod Fertil 24: 99.

Rowley MJ, Berlin JD, Heller CG (1971) The ultrastructure of four types of human spermatogonia. Z Zellforsch 112: 139.

Rowley MJ, Heller CG (1971) Quantitation of the cells of the seminiferous epithelium of the human testis employing the Sertoli cell as a constant. Z Zellforsch 115: 461.

Schulze C (1974) On the morphology of the human Sertoli cell. Cell Tiss Res 153: 339.

Siew S, Troen P, Nankin HR (1977) Ultrastructure of testicular biopsies from infertile men. In: Troen P, Nankin HR, eds. The testis of normal and infertile men. New York: Raven Press.

Siew S, Troen P, Nankin HR (1978) Ultrastructural study of human testicular biopsies in infertility. In: Yates RD, Gordon M, eds. Male reproductive system: fine structure analysis by scanning and transmission electron microscopy. New York: Masson.

Skakkebaek NE, Heller CG (1973a) Quantification of human seminiferous epithelium. I. Histological studies in 44 infertile men with normal chromosome components. Acta Pathol Microbiol Scand (A)81: 97.

Skakkebaek NE, Heller CG (1973b) Quantification of human seminiferous epithelium. II. Histological studies of twenty-one fertile men with normal chromosome complements. J Reprod Fertil 32: 379.

Sohval AR, Gabrilove JL, Churg J (1973) Ultrastructure of Leydig cell paracrystalline inclusions, possibly related to Reinke crystals in normal human testis. Z Zellforsch 142: 13.

Vilar O, Perez del Cerro MI, Manami RE (1962) The Sertoli cell as a 'bridge-cell' between the basal membrane and the germ cells. Exp Cell Res 27: 158.

Weibel ER (1969) Stereological principles for morphometry in electron microscopic cytology. Int Rev Cytol 26: 235.

Weibel ER (1974) Selection of the best methods in stereology. J Microsc 100: 261.

Weibel Er, Kistler GS, Scherle WF (1966) Practical sterological methods for morphometric cytology. J Cell Biol 30: 23.

9. INGUINAL HERNIA AND HYPOSPADIAS

J.F. REDMAN

1. INGUINAL HERNIA

1.1. Definition

In men an inguinal hernia is a protrusion of a viscus, either in whole or in part, through an actual opening or a weakness in the inguinal abdominal wall.

Various terms have been used to describe hernias of the inguinal region which are important to understand prior to a discussion of their diagnosis. The most frequently occurring terms applied to hernias are indirect inguinal, direct inguinal, pantaloon, sliding, strangulated, Richter's, and femoral hernia.

1.1.1. Indirect inguinal hernia.
An indirect inguinal hernia always occurs with the protrusion of a viscus into the patent processus vaginalis, the vestigial remnant of the peritoneal envelope which accompanies the testicle through the internal ring in its progress to the scrotum (Fig. 1). The internal ring is for practical purposes a hole in the transversalis fascia. The processus accompanies the spermatic cord and is found, when present, from the internal ring to the level of the testicle in an anterio-medial relationship with the spermatic cord structures (Fig. 2). The serosal sac is held to the cord structures by the fascial-like investments of tissue layers derived from the abdominal wall (Fig. 3). From outside in they include the external spermatic fascia derived from the external oblique fascia, the cremasteric muscle and fascia derived from the internal oblique muscle and fascia, the internal spermatic fascia derived from the transversalis fascia, and the tela subserosa or subserous fascia which is contiguous from the abdominal wall and contains the preperitoneal fat. A lipoma or large protrusion of preperitoneal fat through the internal ring may clinically behave as an indirect inguinal hernia.

1.1.2. Direct inguinal hernia.
A direct inguinal hernia is a protrusion of a viscus through either an acquired, traumatic or iatrogenic weakness in the abdominal inguinal wall medial to the internal ring and lateral to the pubic tubercle. Traditionally, the area of occurrence of the direct inguinal hernia is termed Hesselbach's triangle which is bounded laterally by the inferior epigastric vessels, medially by the outer border of the rectus sheath, and caudally by the inguinal ligament (Fig. 4). Generally, the direct inguinal hernia will not have a small neck but rather will represent a diffuse bulge. The layers of the abdominal wall will be represented in the wall of the direct hernia. In direct hernias the preperitoneal layer is important in that a considerable collection of fat may be present in the layers giving substance to the hernia mass.

1.1.3. Pantaloon hernia.
The concomitant ipsilateral occurrence of both an indirect and a direct inguinal hernia gives the gross appearance of a pair of pants with the confluence of the legs straddling the interior epigastric vessels, hence, the term pantaloon hernia. A similar term occasionally applied is saddlebag hernia.

1.1.4. Sliding hernia.
A sliding hernia is one in which a partially retroperitoneal viscus such as the colon or bladder slides and becomes itself a portion of the hernia sac, the remainder of the sac being composed of the peritoneum. This variety of sliding hernia is termed a parasacular sliding hernia and comprises 95% of sliding hernias. A herniation of the large bowel per se is not synonymous with a sliding hernia.

J. Bain and E.S.E. Hafez (eds.), Diagnosis in andrology, 109-119. All rights reserved.
Copyright © 1980 by Martinus Nijhoff Publishers bv, The Hague/Boston/London.

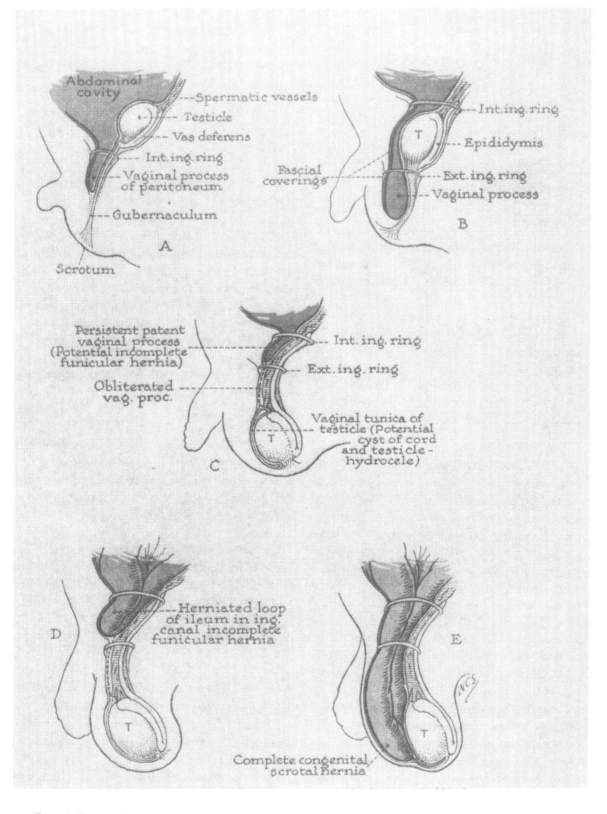

Figure 1. Descent of the testis as related to various types of indirect inguinal hernias. (Reproduced from Jones TS, Shepard WC (1945) A manual of surgical anatomy, 63. Philadelphia: W.B. Saunders.

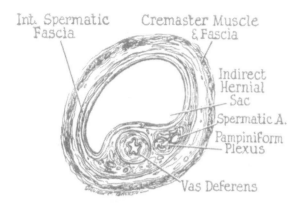

Figure 2. Diagrammatic cross-section of spermatic cord showing unvarying portion of indirect sac. (Reproduced from Zimmerman LM, Anson BJ (1967) Anatomy of the abdominal wall. In: Anatomy and surgery of hernia, 127. Baltimore: Williams & Wilkins.

1.1.5. Strangulated hernia and incarcerated hernia. These terms are included to clarify their meaning. A strangulated hernia refers to the protrusion of a viscus which has undergone a constriction of its vascular circulation. Incarceration merely refers to the fact that the contents of the hernia sac cannot be reduced back into the peritoneal sac of the abdomen.

1.1.6. Richter's hernia. A Richter's hernia refers to a peculiar type of protrusion in which less than a full circumference of a loop of bowel herniates. Generally, this condition is acquired. It may occur at any age but most usually over the age of 50.

1.1.7. Femoral hernia. Because of the close proximity of femoral and inguinal hernias a discussion of femoral herniation usually accompanies those of the groin. By definition the femoral hernia is a protrusion of a viscus through the femoral ring and a small space located just medial to the femoral vein. The mechanism of occurrence of femoral hernias is not as clear as that of the inguinal region. The femoral hernia does not carry with it the coverings of the abdominal wall with the exception of the transversalis fascia.

1.2. Signs and symptoms

1.2.1. General. In general, the signs and symptoms of inguinal hernias are related to a swelling or a bulge in the inguinal region either at rest or accom-

panied by an action which increases intra-abdominal pressure. Pain may occasionally be an associated symptom of an inguinal hernia. Signs and symptoms of intestinal obstruction may herald the presence of an inguinal hernia.

1.2.2. Indirect inguinal hernia. In both children and adults the presence of an inguinal swelling or bulge is known to the patient or parents prior to presentation to a physician. In adults particularly medical attention is delayed because of a lack of symptoms, a lack of time, or because of fear. The patient may note that there is discomfort where there was none before or note an inability to reduce the mass or a change in consistency of the mass which should suggest the development of complications.

Any condition which may produce sudden or chronic intra-abdominal pressure may produce indirect herniation or may exaggerate a pre-existing herniation. Historically, these sudden increases in pressure may be related to lifting, straining at stool or micturition, a sudden fall or slip, vomiting, crying or coughing. Gradual increases in pressure may be associated with chronic coughing or straining at stool or with voiding. With these signs and symptoms further investigation may disclose previously undiagnosed obstructive lesions of the large bowel, chronic obstructive lung disease or bronchiogenic carcinoma, obstructive lower urinary tract disorders, or ascites related to hepatic failure or carcinomatosis.

Sharp acute pain radiating down to the testicle particularly with coughing may suggest a small indirect inguinal hernia. A chronic nagging sensation of pressure may suggest a large longstanding indirect hernia or a direct hernia. Pain occurring in a right-sided hernia which had been previously asymptomatic should raise the possibility of acute appendicitis. All patients presenting a sign and symptom of a small bowel obstruction should undergo a careful examination for an inguinal hernia (Hardy, 1977).

In patients with an indirect inguinal hernia pain will occur in approximately 50% of cases whereas a visible swelling will be present in about 75%.

Men over age 50 with a large inguinal hernia extending into the scrotum should be suspected of having a concomitant herniation of the bladder.

1.2.3. Direct inguinal hernia. Most of the signs and symptoms of direct inguinal herniations are similar to those of indirect herniations and indeed the two conditions can coexist in 10-25% of adult cases (Koontz, 1963). A previous history of inguinal surgery in persons with groin symptoms may suggest a direct herniation. An inguinal mass or bulge which lessens or disappears following voiding may suggest a direct herniation with the bladder being the protruding viscus.

1.2.4. Femoral or Richter's hernia. Patients with signs and symptoms of small bowel obstruction should be examined carefully for a femoral hernia or Richter's hernia which may appear anywhere in the groin region. Femoral hernias are most commonly noted by the patient as a bulge below the inguinal ligament, but they also may be noted above the ligament with an appearance much like that of a direct or indirect inguinal hernia (Zimmerman, 1967).

1.3. Physical examination

1.3.1. General. Usually an inguinal or femoral hernia may be diagnosed without difficulty on physical examination merely by inspection with the identification of a visible swelling. The diagnosis of

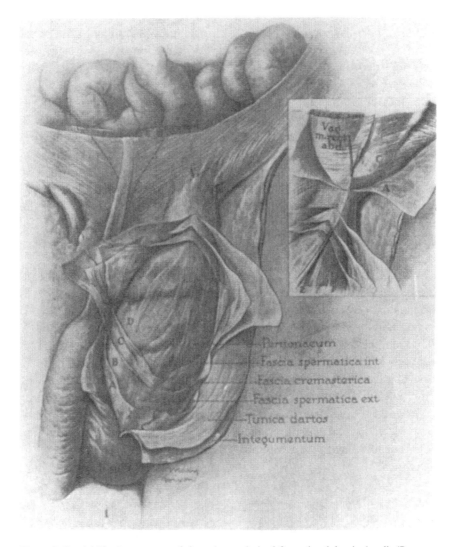

Figure 3. Fascial-like investments of tissue layers derived from the abdominal wall. (Reproduced from Ashley FL, Anson FJ (1941) The anatomy of the region of inguinal hernia. *Bull W School* 15: 117.

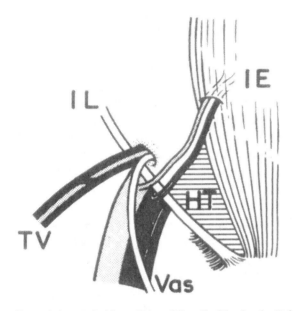

Figure 4. Anatomical boundaries of Hesselbach's triangle. (Reproduced from Clain (1973, p 266 – see refs.).)

an inguinal hernia by physical examination may however be more subtle, and various techniques of examination are required to disclose the protrusions. The differentiation of the various herniations of the groin likewise requires particular attention to fine points of diagnostic technique.

The proper physical examination requires time and thoroughness. The areas for examination should be fully exposed and the place of examination should be comfortable. Gentleness and warm hands are appreciated by the patient.

1.3.2. Techniques of examination. The initial portion of the physical examination involves inspection of the inguinal region. This examination is carried out with the patient in both the upright and recumbent positions.

With the patient standing visible swellings may be noted in one or both groins (Fig. 5). This may or may not extend to the scrotum. If the swelling is small or if none are noted, the patient is asked to stand erect and then either cough, strain, or blow his nose. Sustained straining usually is more efficacious in eliciting a bulge than a maneuver which produces is sudden intra-abdominal pressure. Each inguinal region is again inspected carefully with each increase in intra-abdominal pressure for an impulse indicating a protrusion. Similarly if a

swelling is noted on standing, the patient is asked to lie supine and by either coughing, straining, or blowing of the nose, intra-abdominal pressure is increased and the area of the first appearance of the bulge is noted.

Following inspection of the groin, the next step in examination for a hernia is palpation. Various techniques have been described to facilitate the examination. The patient is examined first in the standing position. The examiner may be seated in front of the patient or may be standing behind the patient and somewhat beside him on the right for a right-sided examination or on the left for the left-sided examination. A common technique employed is that of invaginating the scrotal skin on the ipsilateral side with the examining finger (Fig. 6). Often the examiner's little finger is used to negotiate the confines of the external inguinal ring. If the external inguinal ring is large, it is at times possible to palpate the internal ring also. With the finger so placed the patient is asked to cough, strain, or blow his nose and the impulse of the bulging sac is appreciated. A technique described by Zieman em-

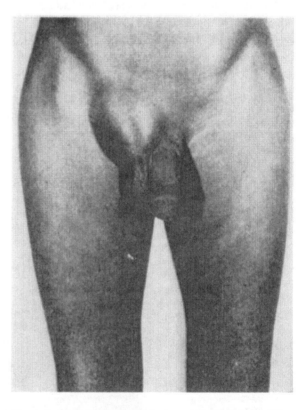

Figure 5. Right inguinal hernia in young adult male. (Reproduced from Zimmerman and Anson (1967, p 152 – see refs.).)

ploys the fingers of one hand (Zieman, 1940) (Fig. 7). The index finger is placed over the inguinal canal including the external ring, the middle finger is placed over Hesselbach's triangle and the ring finger is placed over the femoral canal. With a sudden increase in intra-abdominal pressure or straining, an impulse may be felt in the respective areas indicating either an indirect, direct, or femoral herniation. In addition to palpating for impulses indicative of protrusions, fascial defects should also be noted. It has been suggested that for this portion of the examination the finger should be rotated so that the fingernail rests against the cord and the fingertip itself will be in a position to palpate a subtle fascial defect. If the finger is introduced so that the pulp of the finger is against the cord, it has been suggested that the nail will abut against the ring and the defect will be missed.

Obvious lumps or masses or swellings should be noted along the course of the cord both in the scrotum and in the inguinal canal. The examiner should attempt to get above the swelling; if able to do so, it is obvious that the protrusion or mass does not emanate from the inguinal canal.

The remainder of the physical examination is done with the patient in a supine position. If the swelling is not acute, an attempt is made to reduce the swelling by lightly manipulating the swelling to

and fro until the contents return to the abdominal cavity. The contents of the protrusion may be ascertained during this maneuver. Omentum will give a doughy impression to the fingers. Bowel will usually be a bit difficult at first to reduce but then will slide rather easily into the peritoneal cavity usually accompanied by characteristic gurgling sounds. If a hernia has been irreducible by the patient for several weeks or months, no attempt should be made to try and reduce it. A hydrocele of the cord or an incarcerated hernia will not reduce. Following the reduction of the mass, the defect from which the protrusion came may be palpated and its location noted. With sustained straining, coughing, or sitting the protrusion can be palpated again to assure its origin.

For scrotal protrusions, transillumination is often employed. Usually fluid sacs, such as hydroceles, transilluminate the best. Certainly transillumination is invaluable in differentiating solid lesions in the scrotum.

1.3.3. Special considerations and examinations. In some instances, particularly in children, the patient may have intermittent signs and symptoms suggestive of a protrusion but the diagnosis is not forthcoming with the usual examination techniques. It has been suggested in adults that lifting

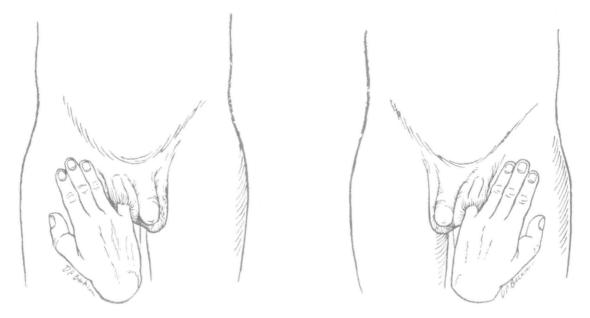

Figure 6. Examination for inguinal hernia. Finger invaginated into canal, right hand on right side and left hand on left. (Reproduced from Zimmerman and Anson (1967, p 153 – see refs.).)

or rapid walking for several blocks may be helpful in producing a protrusion. In children, running or jumping may accomplish the same end. Rolling of the cord gently between the index finger and thumb may at times be helpful in eliciting the diagnosis of an occult hernia. When the hernia is reduced, the cord on the side with the hernia will be thickened. In children particularly the sensation of silk rubbing on silk, the so-called 'silk sign', may suggest a hernial sac.

The presence of an undescended testicle should alert the physician to suspect a hernial sac since such sacs have been reported to be concomitant with undescended testes in 85-95% of cases.

In cases of femoral hernias examination may reveal instead a saphenous vein varix in the fossa ovalis. The differential may be difficult; however, a bluish discoloration and the presence of a saphenous varicosity more distally may be helpful findings.

Approximately one-third of all small bowel ob-

structions are due to hernias or various types, the great majority of which are incarcerated groin hernias.

A radiographic examination, the herniogram, has been employed to diagnose occult hernias (Nyhus and Condon, 1978). This examination has been particularly useful to children who have a demonstrable lesion on one side and in whom the question of contralateral surgical exploration is considered. The examination is accomplished by the intraperitoneal injection of a radio-opaque contrast medium suitable for intravenous administration. The patient ia rolled from side to side and placed in an erect position allowing the contrast medium to flow into the hernial protrusion. A radiograph will demonstrate a characteristic diverticulum of the serosal sac into the groin.

1.4. Differential diagnosis

There are several differential diagnoses to be

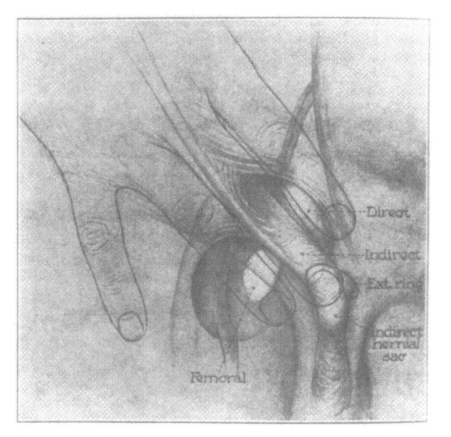

Figure 7. Relationship of the various hernias to the examining fingers. (Reproduced from Zieman (1940, p 1874 – see refs.).).

reckoned with in dealing with herniations of the groin.

An initial consideration is the differentiation of a direct from an indirect inguinal hernia. Initially inspection alone will give the diagnosis by virtue of the protrusion either through the internal ring or through Hesselbach's triangle. Lindsey has enumerated several differentiating features of direct and indirect inguinal hernias (Lindsey, 1961) (Table 1). It should be mentioned that a large external ring does not always indicate the presence of a hernia nor does it herald the potential for a hernia.

Often it is necessary to differentiate a scrotal swelling from a significant herniation. If the examiner can get above the scrotal swelling then it is not usually true that the swelling is a herniation. It should be stated, however, that particularly in children a small caliber patent processus vaginalis may accompany a discrete non-reducible scrotal swelling. Lipomas of the cord may well masquerade as an inguinal herniation and the distinction may not be made until the time of surgery.

All hernial protrusions from the region of the inguinal canal do not actually issue from the inguinal canal. Femoral hernias may pursue a cephalad course and be rather difficult to differentiate from an inguinal herniation, particularly if the protrusion is not reducible and an impulse cannot be perceived to emanate from a particular area.

Femoral hernias may also be mimicked by a saphenous vein varix at the level of the fossa ovalis or by one or more lymph nodes in the femoral canal (Clain, 1973).

2. HYPOSPADIAS

2.1. Definition

Hypospadias by definition is a developmental anomaly in which the urethral meatus is located proximal to the tip of the penis. Embryologically this is simplistically explained as a failure of closure of the urethral folds over the urethral groove. Hypospadias may be classified according to the location of the urethral meatus. Terms commonly applied to designate their location are glanular or balanitic, coronal, penile, penoscrotal, scrotal, and perineal. A rather consistent anomaly that coexists with the proximal location of the urethral meatus is a ventral curvature of the penis which is also termed chordee (Fig. 8). A variant of hypospadias is the so-called chordee without hypospadias. The incidence of hypospadias is one in every 300-400 male births.

2.2. Physical findings

The diagnosis of hypospadias is generally made in the newborn nursery with the initial examination of the child. The most constant finding is that of the curious hooded prepuce (Fig. 9). The prepuce generally fails to reunite ventrally and the hood is therefore more exaggerated by the relative abundance of skin on the dorsum of the penis. In some cases the prepuce is joined ventrally in the presence of a hypospadiac meatus. In others the prepuce is complete ventrally but a dorsal cutaneous hump exists in the presence or absence of a hypospadiac

Table 1. Differentiating features of direct and indirect inguinal hernia. (Reproduced from Lindsey, 1961.).

Features	Indirect	Direct
Age	Younger	Older
Abdominal wall	Normal	Weak
External ring	Not necessarily enlarged until late stage of large hernia	Always enlarged
Position	Oblique in groin; frequently scrotal	Localized near external ring; seldom scrotal
Shape	Ovoid, pear-shaped, or fusiform	Dome-shaped, or globular
Bilateral?	About one-quarter of cases	Over one-half of cases
Inguinal canal	Posterior wall firm	Posterior wall weak
Relation to cord	In front or on outer side	Above and to inner side
History	? Congenital	Strain; chronic or recurrent increase in intra-abdominal pressure

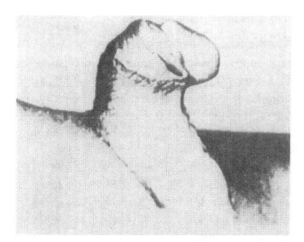

Figure 8. Ventral curvature or chordee associated with hypospadias.

meatus which is quite reminiscent of the dorsal hooded prepuce. When a dorsal cutaneous hump exists with or without a hypospadiac meatus, close attention should be given to trying to ascertain the coexistence of a ventral penile curvature.

A further characteristic finding in a patient with hypospadias is the widened, flattened appearance of the glans penis. When noted, the examiner should search further for the hypospadiac meatus and the presence of a ventral curvature on erection.

As mentioned the meatus may be located in one of many sites. The meatus is examined by any technique which will allow the meatus to gape open. If the meatus is located near the glans, the glans may be grasped on each side and drawn out laterally. Frequently, what appears to be a meatus will be found to be only the cleft fossa navicularis and the meatus is indeed located more proximally. On the shaft the skin just proximal to the meatus is grasped between thumb and finger and drawn outward which allows the meatus to gape open. With these techniques a seemingly stenotic urethral meatus is often found to be quite adequate.

The urethra is variously encased in the corpora spongiosa. Frequently, in its distal portion the corpora spongiosa flares laterally and the urethra proceeds as an epithelial tube covered only by Buck's fascia. In lightskinned individuals a red rubber catheter may be inserted per meatus and the length of the relatively naked portion of the urethra may be appreciated.

The presence of a ventral curvature may be ascertained on physical examination at times just by examination of the penis from the lateral aspect. The examination is greatly facilitated if the penis becomes erect during the course of the examination. Again, inspection is carried out from a lateral aspect. Frequently, as the examination proceeds the penis will gain some turgidity which may be exaggerated by compression of the corpora cavernosa through the scrotal wall or the perineum. The resultant erection is rather refractory and may be difficult to reproduce immediately if the examiner desires a second look. A further technique to evaluate for ventral curvature is to simply retract the penile skin. If tethering ventrally is present, the penile tip will be flexed towards the shaft.

2.3. Special examinations

The evaluation for a ventral curvature of the penis may be inadequate if the penis is never examined in the erect state. A child may present for a surgical

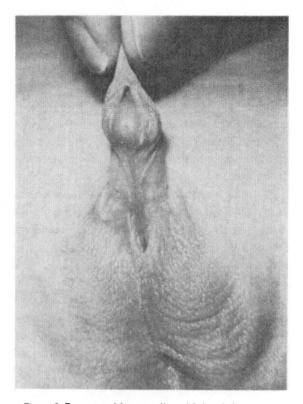

Figure 9. Penoscrotal hypospadias with hooded prepuce.

correction of the hypospadiac urethra and the operator may proceed with the surgery being unaware that the child also has a concomitant ventral curvature. To obviate the dilemna a diagnostic technique has been devised. A tourniquet, such as a rubber band, is placed around the base of the penis and held in place with a hemostatic clamp. Normal saline is injected via a scalp vein needle distally into the corpora spongiosa to produce erection. In older boys and adults this procedure may be done employing local anesthesia. Intraoperatively, this diagnostic technique may be employed multiple times to assess the adequacy of the penile straightening.

It is most important particularly in instances of very proximal hypospadias that the urethra be investigated by retrograde urethrography. The type of examination which is sometimes termed a genitogram is imperative if in addition to the hypospadias the testes are not present in the scrotum. The retrograde urethrogram is accomplished by placing the child in an oblique position and injecting the urethra with a radio-opaque contrast medium, such as an agent used for excretory urography. The meatus may be difficult to inject. The task is facilitated by the use of a beveled plastic cannula such as used for intravenous administrations. The cannula may be cut back until the caliber of the cannula approximates that of the meatus. The radiographic exposure is made with the maximum force of injection which should demonstrate, if present, Müllerian remnants emanating from the posterior urethra. Any meatus should be injected. Occasionally a distal meatus if present along with a hypospadiac meatus will be found to herald a rather long accessory urethra which at times may extend all the way to the bladder.

The need for excretory urography to determine the presence of concomitant upper urinary tract abnormalities has been the subject of numerous publications. The incidence of associated upper tract anomalies has varied from 5 to 25%. It is generally accepted that the more proximal the hypospadiac meatus the greater the yield of upper tract anomalies. Anomalies when found are generally nonconsequential. The admonition remains, however, that a screening excretory urogram should be done particularly with the more proximal hypospadiac meatus.

2.4. Therapeutic considerations

The discovery of hypospadias in the newborn nursery should be viewed as more than just the finding of a curiosity. Particularly with the more severe degrees of hypospadias, but not necessarily, the question of the presence of an intersex state exists (Allen, 1976). These diagnoses become even more frequent if associated with hypospadias in the absence of palpable gonads. A very distal hypospadiac meatus with descended testes may be viewed as male. Infants with penoscrotal, scrotal or proximally located urethral meati should undergo karyotyping since the incidence of an associated intersexual state approaches 25% (Aarskog, 1971). If an abnormal karyotype is found, surgical exploration and a gonadal biopsy should follow. The associated intersex state may include among others both male and female pseudohermaphroditism. An initial consideration with severe hypospadias is the assignment of sex (Jones and Scott, 1971). Although genitography, buccal smears, karyotyping and exploratory laparotomy will more accurately determine the child's sex, it has become apparent from the observation of these children's growth to adulthood that if the child's phallus is particularly small, the sex of rearing is best established early as a female. The studies of Money et al. (1955) well illustrate that the male with an extremely small phallus will be bedeviled by psychological problems and feelings of inadequacy for a lifetime. Serial serum sodium determinations are invaluable in severe hypospadias in the neonatal period to rule out the possibility of salt loss in a child with the adrenogenital syndrome. Failure to recognize this condition may well prove fatal in a newborn.

Circumcisions are not done in the newborn period but rather the prepuce is preserved for use in subsequent repair. Meatal stenosis is common and may be treated by meatotomy. The technique should be such that the incision in the meatus is distal and does not increase the degree of hypospadias. Reconstruction may begin at any age, but generally the age 18 months to 2 years is an appropriate time to start. Repair should be completed by the age 5-6, or at least prior to the child's starting of school.

REFERENCES

Aarskog D (1971) Intersex conditions masquerading as simple hypospadias. Birth Defects 7: 122.

Allen TD (1976) Disorders of sexual differentiation. Urol Suppl 7(4): 1.

Clain A (ed.) (1973) Hamilton Bailey's demonstrations of physical signs in clinical surgery, 15th edn. Baltimore: Williams & Wilkins.

Hardy JD (1977) Rhoades textbook of surgery. Principles and practice, 5th edn., Vol 2. Philadelphia: J.B. Lippincott.

Jones HW Jr, Scott WN (1971) Hermaphroditism, genital anomalies and related endocrine disorders, 2nd edn. Baltimore: Williams & Wilkins.

Koontz AR (1963) Hernia. New York: Appleton-Century-Crofts.

Lindsey D (1961) The sign of indirect inguinal hernia. Am Surg 2: 686.

Money J, Hampson JG, Hampson JL (1955) Hermaphroditism: recommendations concerning assignment of sex, change of sex, and psychologic management. Johns Hopkins Med J 97: 284.

Nyhus LM, Condon RE (1978) Hernia, 2nd edn. Philadelphia: J.B. Lippincott.

Zieman SA (1940) The diagnosis of hernia. JAMA 115: 1873.

Zimmerman LM, Anson BJ (1967) Anatomy and surgery of hernia, 2nd edn. Baltimore: Williams & Wilkins.

10. HYDROCELE, SPERMATOCELE AND VARICOCELE

S.D. GRAHAM, JR. and D.F. PAULSON

Accurate diagnosis of scrotal mass lesions may be difficult, even though the ease of access to the involved organs should make the physician more certain of the diagnosis than examination of most other anatomic areas. It is the purpose of this chapter to acquaint the physician with common non-neoplastic scrotal pathology and, in particular, to aid him in the diagnosis and treatment when necessary. The major topics considered will be hydroceles, spermatoceles and varicoceles, the three commonest lesions of the scrotal compartment.

1. HYDROCELE

Hydrocele is a pathologic state described in the earliest medical literature. It is a common finding in the general male population and only occasionally demands any medical attention. Its major importance to the clinician is that it may mimic, hide, or be the sign of a more serious disease.

A hydrocele is a cavity containing usually straw-colored fluid found in the scrotum. In the case of a simple hydrocele (Fig. 1), which is the commonest type of hydrocele found in adults, the defect is lymphatic obstruction and/or a portion of the processus vaginalis which has failed to obliterate, but does not communicate with the peritoneum. The usual simple hydrocele involves the tunica vaginalis surrounding the testicle, but rarer forms have been reported which involve the head of the epididymis (globus major), or the spermatic cord as a cyst. An even rarer form of hydrocele is the *hydrocele en bissac* which extends from the testicle along the spermatic cord, through the internal ring and into the abdominal cavity. Secondary hydroceles are formed in response to venereal infections, orchitis, epididymitis, tumors and other scrotal pathology.

1.1. Incidence

The incidence of hydroceles is between 2 and 4% of all urologic hospital admissions, and 0.2% of all male admissions (Campbell, 1927). For reasons which are so far unexplained, the incidence of hydrocele in the tropical climates is even higher – as much as 10% (Greene, 1937). Some series state that the commonest age group is among those over 40 (Greene, 1937) while others believe it to be over 20-30 years (Campbell, 1927). The lesion is bilateral in 4-8% of cases (Campbell, 1927; Greene, 1937). The incidence in infants is only 0.6% (Campbell, 1927). The hydrocele can occur on either side with equal incidence, although one series demonstrated a 50.2-44.1% predilection for the right side (Campbell, 1927).

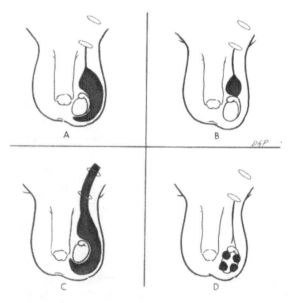

Figure 1. Differential diagnosis of benign scrotal masses. (a) Simple hydrocele, hematocele, chylocele; (b) hydrocele of the cord, spermatocele, tumor of the cord; (c) communicating hydrocele, *hydrocele en bissac*, hernia, varicocele; (d) benign testicular cyst; testicular tumor.

J. Bain and E.S.E. Hafez (eds.), Diagnosis in andrology, 121-134. All rights reserved.
Copyright © 1980 by Martinus Nijhoff Publishers bv, The Hague/Boston/London.

1.2. Anatomy

A hydrocele is a collection of fluid in the space between the visceral and parietal layers of the tunica vaginalis, which has failed embryologically to obliterate (Ratliff, 1953). Though the hydrocele usually involves only the testicle, it may less commonly be limited to the epididymis or the cord (Thomas and Thompson, 1924). An extreme, but rare, variation of the simple hydrocele is the *hydrocele en bissac*. This hydrocele involves the testicle and cord and extends into the abdominal cavity anteriorly to lie between the transversalis fascia and the peritoneum. It is occasionally, however, found retroperitoneally. While this is usually a single sac, there may be two separate sacs, one in the scrotum and one in the abdominal cavity (Sood and Aptekar, 1970; Tanzer, 1935).

Hydroceles do occur in women and are found in the canal of Nuck (Ariyan, 1973). The anatomy and pathology of this entity are completely analogous to the male counterpart with a patent processus vaginalis around the round ligament. These are more difficult to diagnose than male hydroceles due to the fact that they are covered by the fascia of the external oblique muscle and therefore may be mistaken for an incarcerated or strangulated hernia.

1.3. Pathology

Adult hydroceles can be classified as either acute or chronic. The acute hydrocele is almost always secondary to some other pathologic process, either infection, tumor or trauma. The chronic, idiopathic hydrocele is most often due to absorption defect and is called primary.

Hydrocele fluid is usually straw-colored, resembling a transudate (Clarke and Bamford, 1959). The specific gravity range is 1.020-1.026 (Campbell, 1927) and the quantity of fluid may vary from a few cubic centimeters to five gallons (Carforia, 1927). Aspirated hydrocele fluid shows very little cellularity, with up to 12 lymphocytes and up to 12 polymorphonuclear leukocytes per mm^3, scattered mesothelial cells, and occasional spermatozoa (Clarke and Bamford, 1959). Total protein in the hydrocele fluid is less than that of serum, with a higher proportion of albumin and β-globulin being

reported by some investigators (Cenciotti and Montella, 1970), but equal to serum percentages as reported by others (Sitadevi et al., 1970).

Grossly, the opened hydrocele sac shows a pale thinned-out tunica vaginalis in the idiopathic, chronic hydroceles. In some long-term hydroceles, particularly those resulting from previous infection or trauma, the sac wall may be thickened and even calcific. Histologically, the wall of the tunica vaginalis exhibits a lining of flattened mesothelial or low cuboidal cells. The wall itself is a dense layer of relatively avascular collagenous tissue with a few scattered elastic fibrils. The vascular supply of the lining membrane is chiefly from the outer zone (Clarke and Bamford, 1959). A loose avascular areolar tissue separates the tunica vaginalis from its covering cremasteric muscle fibers, which are usually splayed. The sac itself may contain villous growths (periorchitis prolifera) which may hyalinize to form free floating rice bodies, or may contain adhesions (periorchitis adhaesiva) which in turn may cause the hydrocele to become multilocular (Toulson, 1932).

1.4. Etiology

Primary idiopathic hydroceles constitute the largest group of hydroceles, over 50% in Campbell's series (Campbell, 1927). The reports and studies of the cause of this entity are few because, as Rinker and Allen (1951) point out, surgical management constitutes adequate treatment and no animal models are known to exist that embryologically have the same defect as man. However, the two studies that have been reported offer an adequate explanation. Huggins and Entz (1931) injected phenolsulfonphthalein into the cavity of the tunica vaginalis. In patients with hydroceles, the vital dye is resorbed across the tunica at a rate much slower than that of normal controls. Rinker and Allen (1951) further explored the problem by injecting India ink into the hydrocele cavity prior to surgical excision of the tunica. They noted a thickening of the parietal tunica vaginalis and an absence of the normal subserous lymphatic plexus, with few residual deep lymphatic plexuses.

The etiology of the obliterated lymphatics and resultant hydroceles is not known. Campbell (1927) postulates that idiopathic primary hydroceles are

actually subclinical secondary hydroceles. Trauma is a frequently cited cause, perhaps explained the higher incidence of hydroceles among circus riders and cowboys (Campbell, 1927; Greene, 1937), but most authors tend to agree that the most likely cause of idiopathic hydrocele is a subclinical epididymitis.

The etiology of secondary hydroceles is better explained. These are formed by a weeping of exudative fluid in response to infections, trauma, tumors or other pathological alterations. Infections may be bacterial, especially gonococcal, viral, such as mumps, or parasitic. Any bacterial infection of the testicle and epididymis may give rise to a reactive hydrocele which may or may not become infected. Tuberculosis and gonorrhea are the two most commonly cited agents (Campbell, 1927). Besides infection, secondary hydroceles may also accompany testicular tumors (Ewell et al., 1940). Hydroceles are reported to be associated in 2% of all testicular malignancies. Hydroceles may also accompany epididymal tumors (Glantz, 1966) and torsion of the testicle and its appendages (Skoglund et al., 1970).

Trauma is also known to be a cause of secondary hydroceles. In Campbell's series (1927), 6% of the patients attributed the hydrocele to a blow, fall or straining. Operative trauma is an often unrecognized cause of hydroceles. Hydrocele, as a postoperative complication, can occur in as many as 35% of varicocele cases, and is reported in 0.9-2.28% of cases following herniorraphy (Campbell, 1927; Obney, 1956). Hydroceles are also reported following transvesical prostatectomy (Schoenberg and Patterson, 1961), and have a reported incidence of up to 67% following renal transplantation (Nellans and Ravera, 1975; Penn et al., 1972). The etiology of these hydroceles is due to cord manipulation and interruption of the lymphatics.

Less common causes of secondary hydroceles are due to circulatory and lymphatic obstructions. These include cardiac and renal failure, hepatic disease and truss wearing. Rarely is a hydrocele associated with generalized ascites (Campbell, 1927).

1.5. Diagnosis

Uncomplicated primary hydroceles classically are asymptomatic except for the noticeable swelling. Few complain of pain, and where it exists, the pain is slight and continuous, being related to the tension on the cord as it is pulled by the mass. A few patients complain of either intermittent pain, severe pain, or nausea, vomiting and tenderness. Most patients complaining of symptoms other than pain are primarily bothered by a 'dragging sensation'. Occasionally, patients present with hydroceles so large that the penis is hidden from view, preventing coitus and causing voiding difficulties with excoriation due to uriniferous dermatitis.

The acute or secondary hydrocele, on the other hand, presents frequently with pain which may be quite severe. The severity of the pain is directly proportional to the tension of the hydrocele and rapidity with which it forms.

Physical examination of the patient will reveal a cystic, pear-shaped mass in the hemiscrotum with the apex towards the cord. The outline of the mass is smooth and regular. The mass is dull to percussion and on palpation is tense, yet resilient and compressible. The hydrocele is usually translucent. Hydrocles which are not translucent contain either turbid fluid or a thickened sac wall (Fig. 2). Secondary hydroceles of an acute onset may also have a reddened, indurated and shiny scrotum overlying them and are usually tender. However, in secondary hydroceles from tuberculosis and other nonbacterial causes, the hydrocele is frequently nontender.

The spermatic cord above the hydrocele is entirely normal and the testicle itself is not easily palpated due to its being enclosed in the hydrocele. In communicating hydroceles, *hydroceles en bissac*, and hydroceles associated with hernias, the spermatic cord is not normal to palpation. In hydroceles of the epididymis and cord, the testicle is palpable, but these conditions are uncommon. The hydrocele is freely mobile and cannot be reduced, unless associated with a hernia, in either men or women. No cough impulse is present in hydroceles. The differential diagnosis of a hydrocele is summarized in Table 1.

Methods other than physical examination have been advocated in the past by various authors to aid in the diagnosis of scrotal masses. Among these are radiography, using either contrast material (Dwoskin and Kuhn, 1973; Last, 1942) or ultrasound

(Gottesman et al., 1977). In the vast majority of cases, these methods add little more than physical examination to the diagnosis of a hydrocele.

Table 1. Differential diagnosis of hydroceles.

Diagnosis	Differentiating criteria
Hernia	Usually tympanitic
	Usually reducible
	Cough impulse
Spermatocele	Testicle palpable
	Aspirated fluid has spermatozoa
Hematocele	History of recent injury with acute onset of mass
	Solid, inelastic mass
	Does not transilluminate
	Superficial ecchymosis
Chylocele	Usually in the tropics
	Cloudy fluid which layers out to fatty and fluid
Gumma	Painless
	Hard, doughy
	Does not transilluminate
	Positive VDRL
Passive congestion	Fluid in scrotal skin
	Testicles, epididymis normal
Testicular neoplasm	Rapid growth with pain
	Hard mass
	Does not transilluminate

1.6. Treatment of hydrocele

Hydroceles are usually innocuous and treatment is indicated primarily for pain and large size. The patient complains of either a mild constant pain or a dragging sensation. Rarely, if ever, should a hydrocele be treated as an emergency.

Treatment of secondary hydroceles is accomplished by treating the primary disease. Many times, after the initiating pathology has been successfully treated, the hydrocele will resolve. Occasionally, however, the hydrocele may persist and may need treatment later.

Idiopathic hydroceles in children under the age of 1 year usually resolve spontaneously. In adults, they rarely resolve and gradually enlarge. However, patients have had hydroceles for as long as 60 years without needing surgery (Campbell, 1927).

1.7. Aspiration

This method has the attendant consequences of recurrent hydrocele and infection, although the infection is usually controllable. Despite the high

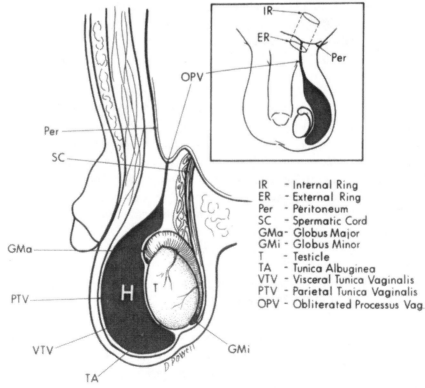

IR   – Internal Ring
ER – External Ring
Per – Peritoneum
SC – Spermatic Cord
GMa – Globus Major
GMi – Globus Minor
T   – Testicle
TA – Tunica Albuginea
VTV – Visceral Tunica Vaginalis
PTV – Parietal Tunica Vaginalis
OPV – Obliterated Processus Vag.

Figure 2. Anatomy of a hydrocele.

possibility of recurrence, aspiration of hydroceles does have its place in the treatment armamentarium (Veenema and Ehrlich, 1971). It is frequently curative in children. Treatment of hydroceles in adults by aspiration is indicated in patients unwilling to undergo an open procedure, debilitated patients, patients which severe cardio-respiratory disease, or patients with some other condition which may prevent any operation. Prior to aspirating a hydrocele, there are several facts the surgeon must realize, the most important of which is the high likelihood of recurrence. In a series of 502 patients, 25% had had at least one previous aspiration and nearly half of these had had two or more (Campbell, 1927). Aspiration of a hydrocele may cause formation of adhesions and thickening of the tunica, making follow-up surgery more difficult. There is the possibility of infection due to aspiration, which may necessitate an open procedure resulting in incision, drainage and possible orchiectomy.

A co-existent hernia is a contraindication to the aspiration of a hydrocele. Prior to aspirating the hydrocele, the surgeon must be absolutely sure that a hernia is not present. Other contraindications include the possible presence of co-existing pathology such as tumor or tuberculosis. If the hydrocele yields anything but clear yellow fluid, the surgeon should strongly consider an exploratory procedure. Communicating hydroceles and *hydroceles en bissac* are not amenable to aspiration. Chronic and acutely inflamed hydroceles are not usually treated in this fashion (Meyers, 1937).

The current therapy of hydroceles involves excision and/or imbrication of the hydrocele sac. Most operations done at present involve a modification of the original Jaboulay or Andrew's bottle-type operation. The procedure involves incision into the scrotum either transversally or longitudinally through the skin and dartos fascia, and the hydrocele is extruded through the wound. The layers are dissected off the hydrocele down to the sac itself in order to achieve better hemostasis (Young, 1940). The hydrocele is then entered and drained and the excessive hydrocele sac is excised. The remaining sac is then either closed with the free edges behind the testicle and epididymis so that the surface is exposed, or an alternative method requiring a placemat of a continuous hemostatic suture around the free edges is employed. The wound is then closed in layers consisting of the dartos fascia and muscle and the skin. A compressive dressing is usually applied.

Disadvantages of the surgical treatment include increased pain, length of hospital stay (9.4 days in Campbell's 1927 series), and the complications attendant upon any operative procedure. Hemorrhage is the most common complication, but if moderate it may produce no untoward results. However, if severe, it may produce a chronic mass in the scrotum that may require re-exploration. The degree of postoperative hemorrhage can be lessened by careful hemostasis and application of a tight scrotal bandage postoperatively. Infection is a second possible complication noted in 15% of Campbell's series. The risk of infection is increased if there is a postoperative hematocele. In Campbell's patients, of 18 hematoceles, 12 became secondarily infected and eight of these ended in orchiectomy. Other complications include scrotal edema and trauma to the testicle either by direct injury to the testicle or through vascular supply. Testicular atrophy from ischemia secondary to constriction of the vessels by the sac eversion has also been described.

1.8. Results of treatment

Results of therapy in patients with hydroceles show a very good prognosis. The results of aspiration of the hydrocele show a high rate of recurrence. If the hydrocele is aspirated and a sclerosing solution injected, there is a 6.1% incidence of recurrence (Campbell, 1927). Surgical treatment of hydroceles results in a 2.4% incidence of recurrence.

2. PEDIATRIC HYDROCELES

Hydrocele in the pediatric age group constitutes a different pathological entity from that found in adults. The hydrocele of the child and infant is usually congenital, implying a patent processus vaginalis. In the infant population, the hydrocele is almost always associated with a hernia and the hydrocele communicates with the peritoneal cavity. As the infant becomes older, the processus vaginalis becomes obliterated and, by the age of 1 year, most

infantile hydroceles have disappeared. Any hydrocele present after the age of 1 has a high likelihood of persisting (Allen, 1976). Though hydroceles in children are usually congenital, one should be careful to rule out those that are secondary to trauma, torsion, or tumor.

The treatment of pediatric hydroceles is surgical. By means of an inguinal incision, the surgeon is able to repair the hernia as well as resect the hydrocele. Postoperative hospitalization in this patient population is minimal and complications are relatively uncommon.

3. SPERMATOCELES

A spermatocele is a common cystic structure whose characteristic feature is that it contains spermatozoa. Its usual position is between the globus major (head) of the epididymis and the testicle. Though the spermatocele is a common finding in normal adults, it is usually more subtle than a hydrocele, and, therefore, more frequently missed in the physical examination.

3.1. Incidence

In an autopsy series of 332, Hochenegg discovered 27 patients with spermatoceles (Rolnick, 1928). Clinically, the incidence of spermatoceles in otherwise normal males is approximately 1/100 (Rolnick, 1928). The cyst is rarely noted by patients prior to the third decade, though it has been found in a patient age 14, and has a decreased incidence after age 50 (Campbell, 1928a).

3.2. Anatomy

Spermatoceles are usually found near the head of the epididymis and are extravaginal (Rolnick, 1928). The cyst itself is usually thin-walled and communicates with the seminiferous system. The size may vary from very small to larger than the testicle itself. Spermatoceles may be found singly or in clusters and may appear to be multilocular. Occasionally, they are found along the spermatic cord, but this is uncommon. Due to the close proximity of spermatoceles to hydroceles, an intravaginal spermatocele may on occasion rupture

into a hydrocele, thus accounting for the finding of spermatozoa in some hydroceles (Winslow, 1920).

3.3. Pathology

The *sine qua non* of a spermatocele is the presence of spermatozoa. The fluid of a spermatocele is clear to cloudy depending on the number of spermatozoa present. The cyst wall is lined with flattened epithelial cells and occasionally ciliated or cuboidal cells (Weisman, 1941). The wall itself is composed of connective tissue interspersed with smooth muscle fibers (Campbell, 1928a).

The fluid in spermatoceles is usually non-viscid with a pH approximating that of other body fluids (as compared to alkaline seminal fluid) (Weisman, 1941). Morphologic examination of spermatozoa in spermatoceles reveals varying types of immature forms, but nearly 50% are mature forms. Usually, most of the spermatozoa are alive, but quickly succumb following aspiration, rarely lasting 12 hours at room temperature (as compared to a life span of 24-48 hours for seminal spermatozoa). When spermatocele spermatozoa die, no crystallization occurs in the fluid to herald their death, probably due to the absence of spermine and other organic salts in the spermatocele fluid. Also, spermatocele spermatozoa lack the antigenic material found in seminal spermatozoa (Weil et al., 1961).

Compared to serum, spermatocele fluid is low in protein, sugar, cholesterol and phosphate, but high in calcium. The proteins present are electrophoretically similar to albumin and are immunologically comparable with serum proteins (Weil et al., 1961).

3.4. Etiology

Various hypotheses have been proposed as to the etiology of spermatoceles. Several unproven theories are: unsatisfied sexual desire, venereal infection, trauma and vascular or lymphatic abnormalities, and overlapping and sealing of the tunica vaginalis at the junction of the testicle and epididymis (Campbell, 1928a). Virchow first showed spermatoceles to be retention cysts (von Bergman, 1906). Dissections by Rolnick and others show that the spermatocele is a dilated cyst at the end of an aberrant tubule connected to the rete testes or seminal duct (Rolnick, 1928). Most of these tubules probably

represent Wolffian duct remnants, but it is thought that the larger cysts represent an aberrant vas deferens that is partially obliterated.

3.5. Diagnosis

The diagnosis of spermatocele, like that of hydroceles and other scrotal pathology, is made by physical examination. Typically, the patient will have a fluctuant mass near the head (globus major) of the epididymis. The mass is distinct from the testicle, non-tender unless infected, and unlike hydroceles, may or may not transilluminate. The size of the mass may vary from a few millimeters to several centimers and may be single or multiple, unilateral or bilateral.

Typically, the chief complaint in the patient with spermatocele is an asymptomatic testicular mass or, less frequently, a dragging sensation on the cord and testicle. Some patients will complain of pain which may be in the cord, testicle, or penis (Campbell, 1928a). The pain may be constant or, rarely, may follow intercourse. Some authors believe that pain in the testicle and scrotal swelling during sexual excitement is pathognomonic.

The absolute diagnosis of spermatocele is made by aspiration to demonstrate the presence of spermatozoa. Occasionally, a hydrocele may contain spermatozoa, but it is felt that this is due to a spermatocele having ruptured within it. Other methods of diagnosis have been tried including radiography with contrast (Last, 1938) or ultrasound (Gottesman et al., 1977), but as in the case of hydroceles, this is usually no more accurate than physical examination and, in general, is superfluous. The differential diagnosis of a spermatocele is the same as that of a hydrocele (Table 1).

3.6. Treatment

Treatment of spermatoceles is dependent upon the symptomatology. Obvious indications for treatment are debilitating pain, gross deformity, or signs of infection. Most patients, however, have either no symptoms, minimal pain and discomfort, or only a small mass. Usually, the clinician is wise to leave these latter patients untreated or treat them conservatively with scrotal support, sitz baths, or other nonsurgical therapy.

The definitive treatment of spermatocele, as in hydrocele, is surgical excision. The cyst is approached trans-scrotally and is usually extravaginal. It is dissected free of the epididymis by both sharp and blunt dissection to its narrow neck at its juncture with the epididymis. The neck is ligated with an absorbable suture and divided. It is not uncommon to find multiple cysts and/or multilocular cysts which are dealt with in a similar fashion. Complications are hematocele in 3.6% and infection in 7.2% (Campbell, 1928a).

Other methods of treatment of spermatocele have been tried, but none have had the success rate of open surgery. Aspiration alone is usually followed by recurrence and therefore is recommended only for diagnosis. Huggins and Noonan (1938) indicated that aspiration is not innocuous and described two patients who subsequently underwent orchiectomy for infected spermatoceles following aspiration. Aspiration with instillation of a sclerosing solution has also not proven to be successful.

Spermatocele in relation to fertility

Theoretically, in the patient who is subfertile, the spermatocele would provide the clinician with an easy access to spermatozoa for artificial insemination. Indeed, Wilhelm (1935) described a vasoorchidostomy procedure for the attempted creation of an artificial spermatocele. Unfortunately, the results of these attempts have been largely unsuccessful.

4. VARICOCELES

A varicocele is a scrotal mass consisting of multiple abnormally dilated veins within the spermatic cord which join to form the internal spermatic vein. Varicoceles are the commonest scrotal masses and are important to the clinician with respect to differential diagnosis. Varicoceles have also become clinically important because of their possible relationship to oligospermia. Resection of the varicocele may be an effective method of reversal of inferility.

4.1. Incidence

Primary or idiopathic varicoceles are found very frequently in young adults with a reported incidence ranging from 5 to 20% (Greene, 1937; Kiszka and Cowart, 1960). The age of peak incidence of idiopathic varicocele is from 15 to 35 years (Campbell, 1928b; Russell, 1954). Clarke (1966) showed an 8% overall incidence in patients aged 17-36 and 6% in those patients aged 37-57. The incidence of varicoceles may be as high as 39% in subfertile males (Dubin and Amelar, 1971). The incidence of varicoceles, however, has been noted to be dependent upon the persistence of the investigator in looking for them (Silvert, 1978a).

The incidence of secondary varicoceles is not known, but is probably very low. Even in patients with renal and ureteral tumors, a known cause of secondary varicoceles, the incidence is small, ranging from 14 of 2314 patients in one series (Riches et al., 1951) to 14 of 122 patients in another (Bates, 1927).

Idiopathic varicoceles are almost always confined to the left side. In one series of 500, 19 were bilateral, and two were right-sided (Campbell, 1928b). This is confirmed by Jordan (1965) who reports 98% left-sided and 2% bilateral, stating that primary right varicoceles do not exist. Other authors dispute this, but the number of right-sided idiopathic varicoceles is certainly quite small (Grillo-Lopez, 1971).

4.2. Pathology

A varicocele is an abnormal dilation of the veins of the pampiniform plexus. As noted above, in the idiopathic variety, this is more likely to be left-sided and occasionally bilateral. While initially the pathologic changes are solely tortuous, dilated veins, in the later stages, one may encounter testicular and cord changes.

The anatomy of the venous outflow of the testicle is divided into three groups of veins, the anterior, the middle, and the posterior. The anterior group drains the testicle, forming the internal spermatic vein which has a variable number of valves. On the right, the internal spermatic vein empties directly into the inferior vena cava caudal to the renal vein and at an acute angle. The left internal spermatic vein, however, empties directly into the renal vein in perpendicular fashion (Fig. 3). It is this anterior group which is the predominant venous component in the varicocele mass.

The other two groups of veins of the pampiniform plexus, the middle and posterior groups, are of less importance than the anterior group in the formation of varicoceles. The middle group drains the vas deferens, and the posterior group drains the epididymal tail. Though these groups are distinct anatomically, there are free anastomoses among all three groups which are thus all involved to some degree in the varicocele mass.

Connective tissue hyperplasia between the distended vessels accompanies the congestion (Campbell, 1928b). In the testicle, moderate varicosities in the cord do not seem to involve the testicular blood supply. However, more extensive vascular changes do tend to involve the testicular circulation, leading to atrophy in 1.6% of patients (Campbell, 1928b) and up to 11.5% in another series (Barney, 1910). Testicular atrophy is manifested by fatty degeneration and atrophic sclerosis (Campbell, 1928b). More recently, in testicular biopsies of subfertile males, even without gross signs of atrophy, the usual finding is primary spermatocytic arrest with varying degrees of tubular sloughing, focal necrosis, absence of germinal epithelium, and tubular hyalinization (Garduno and Mehan, 1970).

There may also be cord changes in varicoceles. These are either endophlebitis, phlebolith formation, or dilation of the perineural veins leading to a perineuritis. The latter is felt to be the cause of the testicular pain sometimes seen with varicocele (Campbell, 1928b).

Secondary varicoceles are those varicoceles which accompany another pathologic process and, therefore, are also referred to as symptomatic varicoceles (Bates, 1927). Classically, these varicoceles accompany renal and ureteral tumors, though uncommonly (Riches et al., 1951). These tumors occur with equal frequency on both sides, but a varicocele is more often found with left-sided rather than right-sided tumors. Aside from renal and ureteral tumors, secondary varicoceles have been reported to be associated with anomalies in renal vasculature, Pott's disease of the dorsal vertebrae, and pyonephrosis (Bates, 1927).

4.3. *Etiology*

The cause of varicoceles is not totally understood. The list of possible etiologies ranges from psychologic asthenia and sexual excess, to abnormal anatomic configuration or to hormonal causes. The commonest and most accepted explanation for the etiology of varicoceles, however, is anatomical malformation. The anatomical differences in the venous drainage from each side are represented in Fig. 3. In the case of the left spermatic vein, the largest valve is located at the area of the distal vein adjacent to or within the renal vein in normal subjects. In varicocele patients, cadaveric studies and phlebography demonstrate no valves allowing retrograde flow (Brown et al., 1967; Kohler, 1967). In support of this is the finding of retrograde flow in 12% of gonadal veins during aortography, which approaches the incidence of variococeles. Also, in the three cases of primary right-sided varicocele reported by Grillo-Lopez (1971), all had situs inversus totalis.

Hormonal theories of idiopathic varicoceles are linked to the anatomical theories. It has been proposed that adrenal hormones, including catecholamines from the left adrenal vein, interact with the valve of the internal spermatic vein, causing it to become incompetent and permitting retrograde flow (Silvert, 1978a).

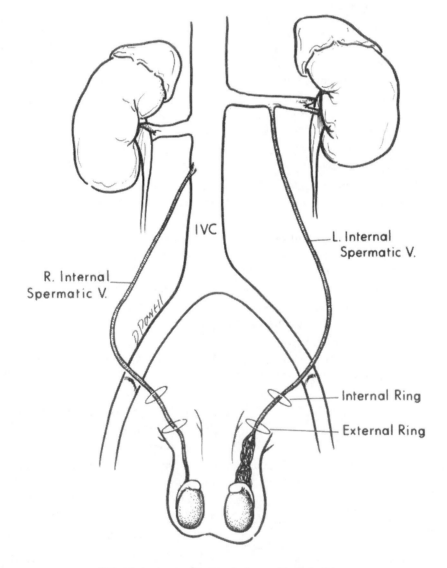

Figure 3. Anatomy of venous drainage of both testicles.

Secondary varicoceles are due to a pathologic process, usually a tumor, involving, compressing or obstructing the spermatic vessels. Two major points need be stressed, the first of which is that in one series of 14 symptomatic varicoceles in 122 patients with renal tumors, thrombosis of or tumor growth into the renal vein was present in two patients, neither of whom exhibited a varicocele (Bates, 1927). Thus, though tumor may be an important etiological factor, it is not a universal cause of varicocele. The second major point is that a varicocele in a young child is usually not idiopathic (Campbell, 1944). Only three cases in Campbell's (1928b) series were under 12 years old and he reported only one case of idiopathic varicocele in a child under 12.

4.4. Diagnosis

The diagnosis of varicocele is by physical examination. The patient should be examined in both the upright and the supine positions. Classically, a varicocele is a 'bag of worms', that is compressible and usually non-tender, and which may even by visible under the scrotal skin. Associated findings in varicoceles include a thickening of the cord (Fig. 1), scrotal varices (1%), testicular atrophy, and occasionally phleboliths in the varices. Some clinicians prefer to classify varicoceles according to degree (Silvert, 1978b). A simple system proposed divided the varicoceles into four grades (Table 2).

The differential diagnosis of varicoceles includes omental hernia which is usually reducible and hydrocele or hernia, both of which are readily distinguished (Glenn, 1965). Hernias were noted to be associated with varicoceles in 59 of Campbell's (1928b) 500 patients and hydroceles in five, which may make the diagnosis of varicoceles slightly more difficult.

Table 2. Grading of varicoceles.

Grade	Physical findings
I	Impulse felt in pampiniform plexus as patient performs Valsalva's maneuver
II	Varicocele evident to palpation with patient upright
III	Varicocele evident to palpation and visual inspection in upright patient
IV	Varicocele does not disappear when patient in supine position – usually secondary varicocele

Presenting symptoms found in varicocele patients include a dragging sensation (20%) often referred to the cord, groin, left lower quadrant, left lumbar region, epigastrium or along the penile shaft. Sixteen percent of patients notice swelling and 11% notice the mass composing the varicocele. Pain is present in 25% of cases ranging from low-grade ache in the testicle to severe pain (rare). Usually the pain is constant, but less often is apparent on exertion or standing. Lesser complaints include nausea, ruptured scrotal varices, scrotal burning following defecation, scrotal itching, and testicular burning. In 10% of patients with symptoms, the symptoms are aggravated by warm weather, probably due to vasodilation (Campbell, 1928b).

Further diagnostic procedures in adults such as phlebography are rarely needed or warranted for the diagnosis of varicocele (McLoughlin, 1977). In any child or adult suspected of having a secondary varicocele, or any adult with a right-sided varicocele, a more extensive urologic work-up is indicated. This should, at the minimum, include intravenous pyelography and urinalysis, and may also necessitate cystography or cystoscopy. There is evidence that in those patients with varicoceles and infertility problems, infertility does not depend on the size of the varicocele, but merely the presence of one (Dubin and Amelar, 1970). Therefore, there may be merit in undertaking thermography or Doppler studies in patients with infertility, as some improvement in fertility has been noted in patients with varicoceles discovered with these tools after varicocelectomy has been performed (Silvert, 1978b).

4.5. Varicocele and infertility

As reported by Greenberg (1977), Bennett was the first to note the relationship of fertility and varicocele. Wilhelm (1935) proposed surgical correction of varicocele as a method of treating infertility. Russell (1954) noted that in subfertile males with poor quality semen, there was a higher incidence of varicoceles than in fertile males and that this could not be accounted for by age alone. In his paper, he suggested a more aggressive approach to varicoceles. Tulloch (1955) reported that 30 patients surgically treated for infertility produced 10 pregnancies and sperm count in the others significantly improved. This was confirmed by Young (1956).

Since these early reports, interest in the relationship of varicoceles to subfertility has vastly expanded.

MacLeod (1969) noted that in patients with varicoceles, 50% showed abnormal semen analysis. These changes are primarily of the 'stress pattern' of oligospermia with increased numbers of tapered, amorphous and immature spermatozoa (McLeod, 1965). Changes in the testicle itself range from atrophy and sclerosis to primary spermatocytic arrest. It is now felt that the 'stress pattern' is, itself, due to the sloughing of immature spermatozoa into the semen (Garduno and Mehan, 1970).

Possible mechanisms by which the varicocele could cause the observed testicular changes are (1) thermal injury, (2) venous stasis with congestion, (3) decreased oxygen tension due to venous stasis, (4) retrograde flow of toxic metabolites, cortisol, or other substances to the testicle. The theory of thermal injury was one of the first proposed. It has been noted that the normal testicular temperature is at least $2°$ C lower than that of the body (Davidson, 1954). A varicocele, according to this theory, would cause injury by altering the thermoregulatory ability of the testicle by keeping the temperature of the testicle the same as that of the blood in the varicocele (Glover, 1955; Moore and Oslund, 1924). Further studies of this hypothesis, however, have tended to obscure rather than clarify the true relationship of temperature changes in varicoceles to testicular morphologic changes (Stephenson and O'Shaughnessy, 1968). The differences in data concerning intrascrotal temperature may be due to artifacts inherent in the test systems, making the data for this theory inconclusive (Zorgniotti and Mac-Leod, 1973).

The second theory for the cause of morphologic changes in the testicle seen in varicocele patients is that of venous stasis. Other than the pathologic observation of passive congestion, there is no experimental data at present proving or disproving this theory. Certainly, if this were the case, then the ligation of the veins would tend to aggravate rather than improve the testicular changes. To the contrary, however, the surgical treatment of varicoceles has a high rate of success in the treatment of subfertility.

The third major theory is that varicoceles cause venous stasis which lowers tissue oxygen tension and thus induces cellular hypoxic injury. Donohue

collected blood from the internal spermatic veins in 26 subfertile male patients undergoing varicocelectomy (Donohue and Brown, 1969). In no patient did he find a significant difference in PO_2 in the venous samples, concluding that hypoxia played a minimal role in testicular damage. Again, if the stasis caused hypoxia, one would expect increased hypoxia following varicocelectomy and thus an increase in testicular damage, the opposite of the usual postoperative observation.

The fourth major theory of testicular damage found in varicocele patients is the efflux of steroids, metabolites, or toxic substances down the internal spermatic vein via the renal and adrenal veins, as originally proposed by MacLeod (1965) and Baum (1968). Charny and Baum catheterized the internal spermatic veins of patients with varicoceles and found the renal vein cortisol to be 20.9 μg/dl, that of the femoral vein to be 10.1 μg/ml, and the internal spermatic vein to be approximately the same, 12.5 μg/dl. This was confirmed later by Koumans et al. (1969), who measured corticoids, dehydroepiandrostenedione, and androsterone levels and further by Agger (1971), who measured cortisol levels. The general conclusion from these authors was that since there was no demonstrable reflux of measurable metabolites, it was unlikely that any other toxic substances refluxed down the internal spermatic vein.

Comhaire and Vermeulen (1974) confirmed that there is no difference between spermatic vein and peripheral vein cortisol levels. However, they also found that in varicocele patients, there was an elevation in the mean catechol level when compared to normal patients. They postulated that it is the reflux of renal metabolites, and not adrenal, that is responsible for the testicular changes found in subfertile varicocele patients.

Other theories of testicular damage found in varicoceles include a systemic hormonal axis defect. Swerdloff and Walsh (1975) found that there was no difference between subfertile varicocele patients versus normal patients in levels of peripheral LH, FSH, testosterone or estradiol, and in levels of spermatic vein testosterone and estradiol. Schiff et al. (1976) found that serum LH, FSH and testosterone responses to LRF were identical in both pre- and postoperative subfertile varicocelectomy patients.

Results of surgical therapy of varicoceles in the infertile patient are somewhat encouraging. As many as 80% of patients have had elevation of the sperm count to fertile levels postoperatively with pregnancy rates ranging from 25 to 50% (Brown, 1976; Dubin and Amelar, 1970; Scott and Young, 1962; Tulloch, 1955). Patients with severe oligospermia or azoospermia have less of an improvement in semen quality post-varicocelectomy than those with mild oligospermia (Brown, 1976). Even more impressive than the change in numbers of sperm postoperatively is the change in motility and morphology. This is felt by some to be the reason patients with repaired varicoceles have a higher rate of pregnancy than anticipated from the percentage change in total numbers of sperm.

4.6. Therapy

Indications for surgical therapy in varicocele patients fall into two basic categories; infertility and symptomatic varicoceles. In those with infertility, varicocelectomy has been recommended either for any patient with a varicocele (Dubin and Amelar, 1970), or for only those patients exhibiting the 'stress pattern' semen analysis (Brown, 1976). There is evidence that in any patient who has a varicocele after age 20, there is a much higher risk of subfertility (Russell, 1954).

Surgical indications in symptomatic varicocels are much less clear. Campbell (1928b) divides all varicocele patients into three potential therapeutic groups. The first group consists of those patients who are asymptomatic, none of whom required any therapy. The second group consists of those patients with a large symptomatic varicocele in whom the chief symptoms are pain or a dragging sensation. These patients are usually first tried on scrotal supports and if no improvement is noted, surgery may be indicated. The third group is made up of those patients in whom there is a small varicocele and symptoms are out of proportion to the size of the varicocele. These are usually highly neurotic people and ones in whom no therapy should be contemplated other than psychological support (Campbell, 1928b). Occasionally, when all else has failed, the surgeon may be forced into definitive therapy. Other possible indications for

varicocele therapy may be either absence or disease of the opposite testicle, progressive testicular atrophy, existence of concomitant hydrocele or hernia, spontaneous rupture of the varicocele, or recurring phlebitis or thrombosis.

The definitive treatment of varicoceles is usually either ligation or excision of the spermatic vein or its tributaries. Occasionally, however, the clinician may resort to more conservative therapy. Among these are scrotal support, injection of sclerosing agents, and androgen therapy. Injection is rarely practiced (Greene, 1937). Androgen therapy has been proposed, but should be limited only to those patients with varicoceles with low or low normal serum testosterone levels (Check and Rakoff, 1977).

5. OTHER SCROTAL CYSTS

Aside from the three most common scrotal masses, hydroceles, spermatoceles and varicoceles, there are other scrotal cysts that the clinician may occasionally observe. Most are mere variations of the above entities, but have different etiologies and thus deserve mention.

5.1. Hematocele

A hematocele is a collection of blood within the confines of the tunica vaginalis, similar to a hydrocele. The two major etiologies of hematoceles are trauma and/or tumor. Hematoceles clinically resemble hydroceles except that they do not usually transilluminate and there may be external signs of trauma. Severe pain with a tensely swollen hematocele may follow trauma. A hematocele which follows minimal or no trauma should make the clinician suspicious of underlying pathology, especially the high likelihood of a neoplasm being present. If this is the presenting complaint, the testicle demands exploration via an inguinal approach whether a tumor is palpable or not. Also, a hematocele may tend to form an organized thrombus and later calcify to form a large calcific scrotal mass, or it may become infected requiring incision and drainage. Occasionally, a very large hematocele may become life-threatening from exsanguination (Cowdery et al., 1950).

5.2. Chyloceles

A chylocele is a collection of lymph fluid in the tunica vaginalis. This is again clinically similar to a hydrocele, but the fluid is cloudy with fat droplets present. The etiology of chyloceles is usually secondary to lymphatic obstruction as in microfilariasis.

5.3. Testicular cysts

There are few reported benign testicular cysts. There are several types, but most are very uncommon and thus the finding of a mass in the testicle should be assumed to be neoplastic. Benign simple congenital cysts are lined with cuboidal epithelium and are postulated to be due to ectopic epithelium within the testis (Schmidt, 1966). An epidermoid cyst is a second type found in the testicle. This cyst differs from the simple congenital cyst in that it is usually filled with an amorphous yellow laminated material and thus, unlike a simple cyst, does not usually transilluminate. Physical examination often reveals a firm marble-like mass attached to the tunica albuginea. Epidermoid cysts are thought to be the end-stage of benign teratomas with exclusive ectodermal development (Gilbaugh et al., 1967). Cysts of the tunica albuginea are a third type of testicular cyst (Arcadi, 1952). Theres are usually small and superficial to the testicle. The cause of these cysts is unknown but has been postulated to be secondary to infection or trauma with hematoma formation (Grater, 1929).

6. CONCLUSION

Presented in this chapter are the three major non-neoplastic scrotal masses: hydroceles, varicoceles and spermatoceles, as well as some less common benign scrotal masses. Keys to diagnosis lie in the recognition of the normal anatomy and etiology of the masses. Pathology is important in determining future therapy and while few, if any of these masses represent a need for emergent therapy, the definitive therapy for these masses is surgical and is based primarily upon symptomatic relief.

REFERENCES

Agger P (1971) Plasma cortisol in the left spermatic vein in patients with varicocele. Fertil Steril 22: 270.

Allen TD (1976) Disorders of the male genitalia. In: Kelalilis PP, King LR, eds. Clinical pediatric urology, p 662. Philadelphia: W.B. Saunders.

Arcadi JA (1952) Cysts of the tunica albuginea. J Urol 68: 631.

Ariyan S (1973) Hydrocele of the canal of Nuck. J Urol 110: 172.

Barney JD (1910) Publication Massachusetts General Hospital 3: 335. As quoted by Campbell (1928b).

Bates J (1927) Symptomatic varicocele. J Urol 18: 649.

Brown JS, Dubin L, Hotchkiss RS (1967) The varicocele as related to fertility. Fertil Steril 18: 46.

Brown JS (1976) Varicocelectomy in the subfertile male: a ten-year experience with 295 cases. Fertil Steril 27: 1046.

Campbell MF (1927) Hydrocele of the tunica vaginalis: a study of five hundred and two cases. Surg Gynecol Obstet 45: 192.

Campbell MF (1928a) Spermatocele. J Urol 20: 485.

Campbell MF (1928b) Varicocele: a study of 500 cases. Surg Gynecol Obstet 47: 448.

Campbell MF (1944) Varicocele due to anomalous renal vessel: an instance in a thirteen-year-old boy. J Urol 52: 502.

Carforia (1927) Sulla patogenesi dell'idrocele essenziale contribute alla diagnosi differenziale fra essudati e transudati. As quoted by Campbell (1927).

Cenciotti L, Montella G (1970) Sulla patogenesi del liquido dell'idrocele attraverso la ricerca elettroforetica sulle proteine. As quoted by Sitadeve et al. (1970).

Charny CW, Baum S (1968) Varicocele and infertility. JAMA 204: 1165.

Check JH, Rakoff AE (1977) Androgen therapy of a varicocele. J Urol 118: 494.

Clarke BG (1966) Incidence of varicocele in normal men and among men of different ages. JAMA 198: 1121.

Clarke BG, Bamford SB (1959) Hydrocele: studies of biochemical and histologic structure in relation to treatment. J Urol 82: 663.

Comhaire, F, Vermeulen A (1974) Varicocele sterility: cortisol and catecholamines. Fertil Steril 25: 88.

Cowdery JS, Gault ES, Conger KB (1950) Massive hydrocele threatening life by exsanguination. J Urol 61: 524.

Davidson HA (1954) Varicocele and male subfertility. Br Med J 1: 1378.

Donohue RE, Brown JS (1969) Blood gases and pH determination in the internal spermatic veins of subfertile men with varicocele. Fertil Steril 20: 365.

Dubin L, Amelar RD (1970) Varicocele size and results of varicocelectomy in selected subfertile men with varicocele. Fertil Steril 21: 606.

Dubin L, Amelar RD (1971) Etiologic factors in 1294 consecutive cases of male infertility. Fertil Steril 22: 469.

Dwoskin JY, Kuhn JP (1973) Herniagrams in undescended testes and hydroceles. J Urol 109: 520.

Ewell GH, Marquardt CR, Sargent JC (1940) End results of the injection treatment of hydrocele. J Urol 44: 741.

Garduno A, Mehan DS (1970) Testicular biopsy findings in patients with impaired fertility. J Urol 104: 871.

Gilbaugh JH, Kelalis PP, Dockerty MB (1967) Epidermoid cysts of the testis. J Urol 97: 876.

Glantz GM (1966) Adenomatoid tumors of the epididymis: a review of 5 new cases, including a case report associated with hydrocele. J Urol 95: 227.

Glover TD (1955) Some effects of scrotal insulation upon the semen of rams. Stud Fertil 7: 66.

Glenn JF (1965) Scrotal masses. Hosp Med 28 June: 32.

Gottesman JE, Sample WF, Skinner DG, Ehrlich RM (1977) Diagnostic ultrasound in the evaluation of scrotal masses. J Urol 118: 601.

Grater, K (1929) Cysts of the tunica albuginea (cysts of the testis). J Urol 21: 135.

Greenberg SH (1977) Varicocele and male fertility. Fertil Steril 28: 609.

Greene LB (1937) Hydrocele and varicocele: operative and injection treatment. Am J Surg 36: 204.

Grillo-Lopez AJ (1971) Primary right varicocele. J Urol 114: 540.

Huggins CB, Entz FH (1931) Absorption from normal tunical vaginalis, testis, hydrocele, and spermatocele. J Urol 25: 447.

Huggins CB, Noonan WJ (1938) Spermatocele, including its X-ray treatment. J Urol 39: 784.

Jordan WP (1965) Hydroceles and varicoceles. Surg Clin North Am 45: 1535.

Kiszka EF, Cowart GT (1960) Treatment of varicocele by high ligation. J Urol 83: 713.

Kohler FP (1967) On the etiology of varicocele. J Urol 97: 741.

Koumans J, Steeno O, Heyns W, Michelsen JP (1964) Dehydroepiandrosterone sulfate, androsterone sulfate, and corticoids in spermatic vein blood of patients with left varicocele. Andrologie 1: 87.

Last SJ (1938) Visulization of spermatocele. J Urol 40: 339.

Last SJ (1946) Radiograhpic demonstration of hydrocele. J Urol 48: 322.

MacLeod J (1969) Further observations on the role of varicocele in human male infertility. Fertil Steril 20: 545.

Mayers MM (1937) Treatment of hydrocele and similar scrotal cysts by the injection method. J Urol 37: 308.

McLeod J (1965) Seminal cytology in the presence of varicocele. Fertil Steril 16: 735.

McLoughlin MG (1977) Recurrent varicocele: radiographic documentation and surgical management. J Urol 117: 389.

Moore CR, Oslund R (1924) Experiments on sheep testes: cryptorchidism, vasectomy, and scrotal insulation. Am J Physiol 67: 595.

Nellans RE, Ravera J (1975) Seminoma in a renal transplant recipient. J Urol 113: 871.

Obney N (1956) Hydroceles of the testicle complicating inguinal hernias. Can Med Assoc J 75: 733.

Penn I, Mackie G, Halgrimson EG, Starzl TE (1972) Testicular complications following renal transplantation. Ann Surg 176: 697.

Ratliff RK (1953) Anatomy and technique of hydrocelectomy. J Urol 69: 181.

Riches EW, Griffiths IH, Thackeray AC (1951) New growths of the kidney and ureter. Br J Urol 23: 297.

Rinker JR, Allen L (1951) A lymphatic defect in hydrocele. Am Surg 17: 681.

Rolnick HC (1928) Etiology of spermatocele. J Urol 19: 613.

Russell JK (1954) Varicocele in groups of fertile and subfertile males. Br Med J 2: 1231.

Schiff I, Wilson E, Newton R, Shane J, Kates R, Ryan KJ, Naftolin R (1976) Serum luteinizing hormone, follicle stimulating hormone, and testosterone responses to gonadotropin-releasing factor in males with varicoceles. Fertil Steril 27: 1059.

Schmidt SS (1966) Congenital simple cyst of the testes: a hitherto undescribed lesion. J Urol 96: 236.

Schoenberg HW, Patterson L (1961) Acute hydrocele of the spermatic cord after transvesical prostatectomy. J Urol 85: 69.

Scott LS, Young D (1962) Variocele: a study of its effects on human spermatogenesis, and the results produced by spermatic vein ligation. Fertil Steril 13: 325.

Silvert MA (1978a) The role of varicocelectomy in the treatment of male infertility – Part I. Urol Times, May.

Silvert MA (1978b) The role of varicocelectomy in the treatment of male infertility – Part II. Urol Times, June.

Sitadevi C, Israel RP, Tarachand P, Reddy NV, Reddy RRM (1970) The study of electrophoretic pattern of hydrocele fluid in relation to pathologic changes in tunica vaginalis. J Urol 104: 298.

Skoglund RW, McRoberts JW, Ragde H (1970) Torsion of testicular appendages: presentation of 43 new cases and a collective review. J Urol 104: 498.

Sood ID, Aptekar S (1970) Co-existing abdominal and scrotal hydroceles. J Urol 104: 141.

Stephenson JD, O'Shaughnessy EJ (1968) Hypospermia and its relationship to varicocele and intrascrotal temperature. Fertil Steril 19: 110.

Swerdloff RS, Walsh PC (1975) Pituitary and gonadal hormones in patients with varicocele. Fertil Steril 26: 1006.

Tanzer RC (1935) Abdominoscrotal hydrocele. J Urol 34: 447.

Thomas BA, Thompson DC (1924) Hydrocele of the epididymis with report of a case. J Urol 12: 271.

Toulson WH (1932) The hyalinization of hydrocele sacs. J Urol 28: 247.

Tulloch WS (1955) Varicocele in subfertility: results of treatment. Br Med J 2: 356.

Veenema RJ, Ehrlich RM (1971) A new method for aspiration of hydroceles. J Urol 105: 112.

Von Bergman E (1906) A system of practical surgery, Vol 5, trans. by Bull WT. New York: Lea Bro.

Weil RJ, Herman JR, Goldbert AS, Rodenburg JM (1961) Immunologic and chemical studies of spermatocele fluid. J Urol 85: 665.

Weisman AI (1941) Studies of spermatocele fluid: a method of determining the source of the constituents of semen. J Urol 46: 423.

Wilhelm SF (1935) Vasa-orchidostomy with interposed spermatocele: procedure for treatment of sterility. Arch Surg 30: 967.

Winslow R (1920) Spermatoceles and hydroceles containing spermatozoa. Surg Gynecol Obstet 30: 568.

Young D (1956) The influence of varicocele on human spermatogenesis. Br J Urol 28: 426.

Young HH (1940) Radical cure of hydrocele by excision of serous layer of sac. Surg Gynecol Obstet 70: 807.

Zorgniotti AW, MacLeod J (1973) Studies in temperature, semen quality, and varicocele. Fertil Steril 24: 854.

11. TESTICULAR TUMORS AND CANCER OF THE PENIS

M.A.S. Jewett and J.L. Chin

1. TESTICULAR TUMORS

Testicular tumors are rare but the unusual histology which frequently reflects aberrations of normal development and the predominance in young men has always generated disproportionate attention. Recent developments in diagnosis and improvement in treatment of disseminated disease have refocused attention on these interesting tumors. It is important both to establish an accurate diagnosis of scrotal masses and to comprehend the implications of such diagnosis.

1.1. Classification and pathology

Neoplasms of the paratesticular tissues (epididymis, cord, tunicas) must also be considered in the differential diagnosis of a testis tumor but they will not be included in this chapter. Approximately 95% of primary testicular tumors are germinal, arising from the germ cell line. As with most tumors, they retain some of the characteristics of the normal tissues in which they arise. The normal germ cell line differentiates into mature spermatozoa, which upon fertilization grow and differentiate into an embryo containing tissues of endodermal, mesodermal and ectodermal origin. Neoplastic transformation interrupts this normal sequence and the first recognizable malignant cell has many of the characteristics of the morula inner mass cells (Fig. 1). Considerable experimental evidence (Jewett, 1977) suggests that this cell is toti-potential and that it is capable of differentiating along extra-embryonic lines to form *choriocarcinoma* and *yolk sac carcinoma*, or along embryonic lines to produce fully differentiated somatic cell types recognizable as endodermal, mesodermal or ectodermal derivatives (termed teratoma). These tumor types are collectively called non-seminomas and represent approximately 50% of the germinal tumors. The remainder are seminomas which may arise from a transformation of primary spermatocytes (Table 1). These elements can occur singly (60% of tumors) or together (remaining 40%) in each tumor.

Non-germinal testicular tumors are very rare and generally benign. Several of these may be functional and produce recognizable endocrine syndromes. Secondary tumors involving the testicle are rarely solitary secondaries although orchiectomy is frequently required to rule out a second primary or to make a histologic diagnosis.

1.2. Etiology

1.2.1. Histogenesis of germinal tumors. Current concepts of the histogenesis of germinal tumors is based on studies with a murine animal model (Stevens, 1973). The tumor incidence in the strain 129 mice is subject to genetic and environmental influences. The undifferentiated cells are embryonal carcinoma which progressively grow with gradual differentiation into somatic tissues, at which point they become self-limited. The differentiated cells of teratoma are, therefore, clinically benign. Occasionally growth is progressive due to incomplete differentiation producing transplantable embryonal carcinoma. Embryonal carcinoma cells are toti-potential (Kleinsmith and Pierce, 1964). Chemical induction of differentiation has been suggested as a form of therapy in view of these observations. Most recent advances in the characterization of embryonal carcinoma has been the preliminary definition of a cell surface antigen system (Artzt et al., 1973; Holden et al., 1977; Ostrand-Rosenberg et al., 1977). The antigen(s) appears to be a fetal antigen expressed on embryonal carcinoma tumor cells but

J. Bain and E.S.E. Hafez (eds.), Diagnosis in andrology, 135-149. All rights reserved.
Copyright © 1980 by Martinus Nijhoff Publishers bv, The Hague/Boston/London.

not on mature somatic cells. In fact a reciprocal expression with the major histocompatiblity complex antigens has been demonstrated in vitro. The antigen(s) has been linked with the mouse T-locus which is on the same chromosome as H-2 (Artzt and Bennett, 1975). It is tempting to speculate that a precursor of the H-2 antigen(s) controlled by a nearby genetic locus and present on murine embryonal carcinoma, early embryos and sperm might be a primal antigen system shared by other mammalian species, including man. Thus human sperm and human embryonal carcinoma may have similar surface properties expressed by a counterpart to the T-locus related to the histocompatibility complex that are important in surface recognition mechanisms of differentiation.

The embryonal carcinoma cell does not have any readily defined gene products apart from the above. However, when it differentiates into yolk sac carcinoma or choriocarcinoma, the markers alphafetoprotein and human chorionic gonadotropin (hCG) are elaborated. Alphafetoprotein (AFP) is a glyco-

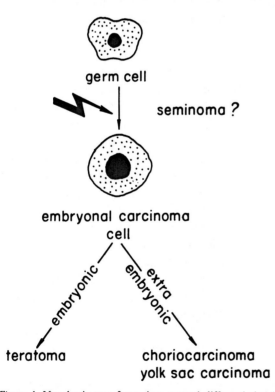

Figure 1. Neoplastic transformation: normal differentiation is interrupted and the first recognizable malignant cell, embryonal carcinoma, has many of the characteristics of morula inner cells. The embryonal carcinoma cell is totipotential and may differentiate along embryonic or extra embryonic lines. The origin of seminoma cells in uncertain.

Table 1. Classification of testicular tumors.

TESTICULAR
 PRIMARY
  Germinal
   1. Non-seminoma
    a) Embryonal carcinoma
    b) Teratoma
    c) (Teratocarcinoma)
    d) Choriocarcinoma
    e) Yolk sac carcinoma

   2. Seminoma

  Non-germinal
   1. Sertoli cell tumor
   2. Interstitial cell tumor (Leydig cell tumor)

 SECONDARY
  Lymphoma
  Metastases

PARATESTICULAR
 Adenomatoid tumor
 Fibroma, leiomyoma, lipoma
 Rhabdomyosarcoma, embryonic sarcoma, fibrosarcoma

protein normally present in fetal serum that rapidly falls to a very low level soon after birth. Detectable levels reappear with some liver and testicular tumors, presumably due to genetic derepression. The yolk sac elements and possibly embryonal carcinoma cells are responsible for this production. Similarly, choriocarcinoma cells secrete hCG. These provide useful diagnostic and staging aids and will be discussed below.

1.2.2. Extra-gonadal germinal tumors. Germinal tumors may occur in extra-testicular sites, including anterior mediastinum, retroperitoneal presacral area and pineal region (Luna, 1976). The histogenesis of these tumors is controversial. Occasionally scars or microscopic tumors are discovered in a testis suggesting a primary which has metastasized to extra-gonadal site. More frequently the testes are normal. There is general agreement, therefore, that germinal tumors can arise outside the testes. Embryologically germ cells originate in the yolk sac and migrate to the indifferent gonad. With further growth and differentiation the gonad migrates to the scrotum. Aberrations of this normal process could conceivably result in the presence of germ cells with the potential for malignant transformation in the mediastinum and/or retroperitoneum. Histologically these tumors are similar to testicular

germinal tumors although their detection is frequently late and the results of treatment adversely affected. Any abdominal or mediastinal tumor in a young man should immediately raise the possibility of a germinal neoplasm and prompt immediate examination of the scrotum.

1.2.3. Cryptorchidism and other factors. Approximately 10% of germinal testicular tumors occur with cryptorchidism or maldescent of the testis. About 20% of these tumors are in the normally descended testicle. Knowing the overall incidence of tumors and the incidence of cryptorchidism (which has been difficult to define accurately), the risk of developing a tumor in the presence of cryptorchidism is 50-100 times greater than in the general population. Orchidopexy does not reduce this incidence, except possibly when done at a very young age. The testicle only becomes more accessible for subsequent examination. The reason that cryptorchidism occurred is more likely to be the important etiologic factor than cryptorchidism per se.

No direct relationship between trauma and subsequent discovery of testicular tumor has been established although this frequently brings the tumor to the patient's attention. Occasional tumors are found in atrophic testes although again no specific cause and effect relationship has been substantiated statistically.

The differentiated testis migrates from the retroperitoneum to the scrotum. The blood supply and lymphatics therefore come from and drain to the retroperitoneum. This is the first echelon of nodal metastases rather than the inguinal lymph nodes which drain the scrotal skin area. This is of particular significance in early diagnosis as a transcrotal needle or open biopsy exposes a new lymphatic area to potential contamination. A high incidence of such tumor spillage has been reported (Markland et al., 1973).

1.3. Diagnosis

Every scrotal mass should be considered malignant until proven otherwise. However, with such a rare tumor it is not surprising that up to 50% are initially diagnosed incorrectly.

1.3.1. History. The most common presentation is a painless testicular enlargement, frequently with a sensation of heaviness. Discovery frequently occurs after minor trauma. Acute pain is rare although aching may be reported.

Other symptoms are related to metastases or endocrine effects of the primary tumor. All of the following may occur: abdominal pain, particularly in a patient with cryptorchidism, back pain, usually lumbar due to retroperitoneal lymph node metastases, non-specific gastro-intestinal complaints, vague malaise, and weight loss. Gynecomastia is a fascinating observation with testicular tumors, particularly choriocarcinoma. It is usually bilateral and fails to regress after orchiectomy. It is not simply due to excess production of hCG or other recognized tumor products but rather probably reflects an imbalance of androgen/estrogen metabolism.

1.3.2. Physical examination. The patient must be completely undressed and able to stand up as well as lie down for complete examination. The scrotum and contents are initially inspected and then palpated. Usually, the mass is not visible nor is there a consistently associated deformity. Large tumors distort the testicle or distend the scrotum and must be differentiated from hydroceles.

The second step of palpation should be done holding the testicle between the thumb and forefinger of one hand while holding the cord structures in the other. The normal testis provides a useful comparison and the peritesticular structures should be sought. Usually the epididymis and vas are identifiable. A mass that produces a heaviness of the testicle is usually discernible. Often the mass can be quite small and may elude identification if inadequate care is given. The exact site of the mass must be distinguished in order to exclude epididymal pathology. Often the mass is more accurately defined at this stage than after the testicle is exposed surgically. The thickness of the scrotal wall serves to amplify the topographical variation and gives a better clinical impression. Tumors are characteristically non-tender unless infarction has occurred and are associated with a small hydrocele in 5-10% of cases. A hydrocele in a young man presents a dilemma particularly if it is of acute onset. Customary aspiration may produce seeding of tumor cells into the scrotal skin of the tunica albuginia has been penetrated by the tumor. On the other hand

tumors are rarely of this size and tunicae are effective barriers to tumor penetration in most cases. These hydroceles should be aspirated when there is reasonable doubt of the diagnosis. Tumor marker measurement (AFP, hCG) from hydrocele fluid may be misleading due to slight elevations in the absence of tumor.

Examination of the scrotum is followed by a general physical examination which must include the head and neck for evidence of supraclavicular lymphadenopathy due to metastases via the retroperitoneum and thoracic duct. Pulmonary metastases are the usual first site of organ involvement and are best detected on chest X ray. Gynecomastia occurs inconsistently and elevations of hCG alone do not correlate in every case. Traditionally gynecomastia has been thought to reflect trophoblastic activity in the tumor but many exceptions to this can be seen. Examination of the abdomen is important to detect palpable lymphadenopathy. Hepatomegaly due to metastases is a relatively late event and extremely ominous. Even with the advances in chemotherapy, massive liver metastases are rarely cured. Superficial inguinal lymph nodes drain the scrotum. If a previous needle biopsy or scrotal incision has been made in the presence of tumor this lymphatic field may be contaminated and should be carefully inspected under these circumstances. Subsequent therapy must be modified to take this into account due to the high incidence of metastases.

1.3.3. Differential diagnosis. The differential diagnosis of testicular tumors can be extremely accurate but if there is any doubt, surgical exploration through an inguinal incision with proper control of the spermatic cord is preferable to a delay or error in diagnosis. Even experienced urologists may incorrectly diagnose a tumor as epididymitis, treat with a course of antibiotics and cause unnecessary delay.

The significant lesions to be differentiated from tumor include the following:
(a) *Epididymitis* with or without orchitis is the most frequent misdiagnosis. 5-15% of tumors are mistaken in this way. Acute swelling of the epididymis may obscure the landmarks of the testis making it difficult to establish a diagnosis by physical examination alone. Urine is fre-

quently sterile and microscopically clear in young men with epididymitis compounding the problem. An acute onset of pain with increase in blood flow as assessed by Doppler ultrasound is very suggestive of inflammation rather than tumor. The relative frequency of epididymitis contributes to the frequent error of initially treating a tumor as epididymitis.
(b) *Hydrocele* may be a particular problem when the hydrocele sac has become thickened or calcified. Even transillumination may not be useful and surgical exploration becomes necessary.
(c) *Inguinal hernia* can be generally excluded by careful physical examination.
(d) *Hematoma* is usually associated with a history of trauma although on palpation it may be very similar to tumor. Orchiectomy is preferable to leaving a tumor in situ if it is not possible under direct observation at surgical exploration to distinguish between the two.
(e) *Hematocele* is a rare condition which usually has an identifiable cause and is rarely due to rupture of a tumor.
(f) *Spermatocele* is usually not a problem due to its location at the head of the epididymis or in the cord, leaving a palpably normal testicle. The rare sarcoma of the cord may be mistaken for a spermatocele.
(g) *Gumma* of the testis is now becoming rare and is usually diagnosed by archiectomy.
(h) *Torsion* of the testicle can be diagnosed clinically by Doppler ultrasound. The absence of blood flow is conclusive evidence. Epididymitis is the most usual urgent differential diagnosis and this is associated with increased flow compounding the difference. The classical Prehn's sign is unreliable and has been superseded by the Doppler.
(i) *Varicocele* is common in the general population. It is rarely a significant problem in differential diagnosis from tumor as it is dilatation of the pampiniform plexus of the cord. In addition it enlarges with standing or Valsalva's maneuver.

1.4. Investigation

1.4.1. Laboratory. The majority of patients have

early stage disease and will therefore be apparently normal and healthy. However, advanced disease may produce anemia and disturbance of liver function. Baseline data on pulmonary and renal function are necessary if chemotherapy is to be instituted.

The markers AFP and hCG have revolutionized the laboratory investigation of these tumors. Their principal role is not so much in establishing diagnosis which must be done histologically, but rather in staging disease and following patients after initial treatment. Zondek (1937) originally reported the presence of urinary gonadotropins in patients with testis tumors. The bioassay system was relatively insensitive compared to the modern radio-immuno-assays and non-specific due to cross-reaction of the elevated pituitary gonadotropins (FSH and LH) following orchiectomy. The decrease in testicular androgen production following orchiectomy is responsible for the increase in pituitary secretion. The subsequent production of a specific antiserum to hCG has overcome many of these problems (Vaitukaitis et al., 1972). The polypeptide hormones FSH, LH and hCG are composed of α- and β-chains (Cochran et al., 1975). The α-chains are similar but the β-chains vary by secondary and probably tertiary structure creating potential antigenic specificity (Fig. 2). An antibody raised to the β-chain of hCG is relatively specific and by radio-immunoassay hCG alone is measurable. Tumors

may produce whole hCG molecules as well as whole or fragments of α- and/or β-chains. A good approximation of a tumor's function can be obtained by using an antiserum to the β-chain. False positives can be encountered with several other tumors but this is rarely a clinical problem. The cells responsible for hCG production have been identified by immunoperoxidase and immunofluorescent localization in tumors.

Syncitiotrophoblastic cells produce hCG but some embryonal and seminoma giant cells seem to have this capacity as well. The problem of elevated

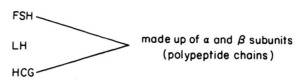

α subunit is identical for LH, FSH and HCG

β subunits differ

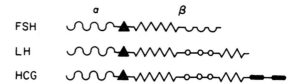

Figure 2. The polypeptide hormones FSH, LH, and hCG are composed of α and β subunits. The α-chains are similar but the β-chains vary by secondary and probably tertiary structure. This difference is the basis of a specific radioimmunoassay for β-hCG. (From Cochran et al., 1975).

Table 2. Primary germinal testicular tumors.

Type	Subtype	Clinical characteristics	Histological characteristics
Non-seminoma	Embryonal carcinoma	2nd and 3rd decade; rapidly growing; smaller at time of presentation; often metastasized by time of presentation	Anaplastic; frequent mitotic figures
	Teratoma	Clinically malignant in adults but benign in children; teratocarcinoma is a mixture of teratoma and embryonal carcinoma	Composed of fully differentiated somatic cells
	Choriocarcinoma	Younger patient; aggressive course	Similar to ovarian choriocarcinoma; contain both syncytiotrophoblastic giant cells and cytotrophoblastic cells
	Yolk sac tumor	Pure form in infants and children, mixed form in adults; secrete alphafetoprotein	Loose pattern of cells; resembles rat endodermal sinus
Seminoma	Classical	Peak incidence in 4th decade; radiosensitive; good prognosis; slow-growing smooth mass, larger at time of presentation	Homogeneous, smooth, sheets of uniform large cells with clear cytoplasm
	Anaplastic	More aggressive clinical course	Increased mitotic activity and anaplasia
	Spermatocytic	Older patients; better prognosis	

* (Johnson et al., 1976; Mostofi and Price, 1973; Pugh and Cameron, 1976; Rosai et al., 1969).

hCG with seminoma has yet to be clarified. Low levels are frequently encountered in classical seminomas that appear to behave normally, but high elevations often portend a poor outcome.

AFP is a normal constituent of human fetal serum but rapidly disappears after birth. Elevated levels were originally detected in mice with hepatoma leading to the discovery of elevated levels in humans with hepatoma. Screening of patients revealed that a number of nonseminomatous tumors are also associated with elevated levels. Yolk sac tumor cells and some embryonal cells are responsible for AFP production. Pure seminomas do not produce AFP and an elevated level indicates occult non-seminomatous elements (Lange et al., 1976).

Approximately 80% of tumors produce one or both markers. The presence of a marker reflects a clone of producing cells within the tumor which may subsequently be altered or eradicated by therapy. The presence of tumor in the absence of marker or the elevation of one but not the other marker is therefore possible.

An example of the usefulness of these markers is illustrated in Fig. 3. A 17-year-old man presented with a testicular mass that was diagnosed as an embryonal carcinoma by inguinal orchiectomy. Subsequent investigations did not demonstrate metastases and he underwent a retroperitoneal lymphadenectomy. The lymph nodes contained a focus of microscopic embryonal carcinoma. During these procedures the AFP was normal but the hCG was elevated at 20 mIU/ml at the time of diagnosis which had remained essentially unchanged at the time of surgery. Following the node dissection the hCG dropped to two, which is still slightly elevated but at which level false positives are frequently seen. Subsequent determinations at intervals demonstrated a persistent and, in fact, rising level of hCG, which was associated with the appearance for the first time of AFP 3½ months later. Despite reinvestigation, no evidence of disease could be discovered until 5 months after surgery, when a chest X ray revealed pulmonary metastases. Chemotherapy was initiated and both markers dropped to the normal range. The patient remains free of disease. This case illustrates the clinical usefulness of the markers as a more sensitive indicator of residual disease. Chemotherapy would now be initiated at an earlier stage even with normal investigations.

1.4.2. Radiology. In order of priority the following radiological investigations are clinically useful:
(a) Chest X ray. A chest X ray will detect pulmonary metastases which are often the first sign of metastic disease. Rarely, chest tomograms will detect lesions in the face of a normal X ray but this procedure is reserved for the situation in which exclusion of metastases above the diaphragm is required, e.g. retroperitoneal lymphadenectomy.
(b) *Intravenous pyelogram.* Retroperitoneal lymphadenopathy may displace ureters or kidneys even with a normal lymphangiogram. The lymphatic drainage of the testis may reach lymph nodes that are in the renal hilum and lateral to the nodal chain normally opacified by the bipedal lymphangiogram.
(c) *Lymphangiography.* Bipedal lymphangiograms are useful in detecting small metastases although there is a significant false positive and false negative rate. Lymphangiography via the spermatic cord lymphatics has been undertaken

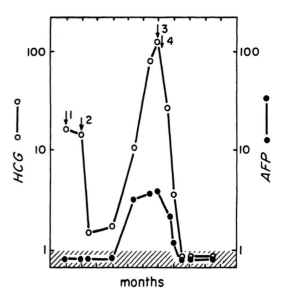

months

Figure 3. Case of 17-year-old man with testicular tumor. The radioimmunoassay results of the β-subunit of human chorionic gonadotropin (hCG in mIU/ml) and α-fetoprotein (AFP in ng/ml) are plotted during his clinical course. At the time of orchiectomy for embryonal carcinoma (1) his AFP was normal but his hCG was greater than 10. Following retroperitoneal lymphadenectomy (2) the AFP remained normal and his hCG dropped to near normal. The hCG gradually rose however, as did the AFP until finally his chest X ray revealed pulmonary metastases (3). Chemotherapy was instituted (4) with a drop of both markers to normal where they have remained.

but is time consuming and may compromise an otherwise clean cancer procedure at the time of orchiectomy.

(d) *Scanning*. Ultrasound or the more recent CT scan are gaining in popularity as means of assessing the retroperitoneum accurately, although even here false positives and negatives have been encountered. Generally, retroperitoneal disease that is not palpable and that does not displace ureters can be excised surgically so that scans and lymphangiograms are not being as widely used at present. However, follow-up of patients on chemotherapy may be aided by these techniques.

(e) *Inferior venacavogram*. Inferior venacavography can be done at the time of the intravenous pyelogram or independently. Enlarged retroperitoneal nodes may indent the outline of the inferior vena cava.

(f) *Percutaneous biopsy of retroperitoneal lymph nodes*. Recent interest in transabdominal percutaneous biopsies of the lymphangiographically opacified lymph nodes suggest that this can be uncomplicated despite inserting the needle through hollow or solid viscera. This may find application in testicular tumors (Wallace et al., 1977).

1.5. Clinical staging

Using the information obtained by the above diagnostic investigations, a clinical stage of disease is established to determine subsequent therapy.

Stage I   Tumor clinically limited to the testis.
Stage II   Clinical or radiographic evidence of tumor beyond the testic but limited to the regional lymphatics below the diaphragm. Massive retroperitoneal disease should be distinguished and is frequently referred to as 'bulky II'.
Stage III Extension beyond the diaphragm or to involve viscera.

1.6. Treatment

Management of the primary tumor consists of any inguinal orchiectomy which is both therapeutic and diagnostic (Markland et al., 1973). For the reasons discussed above, a scrotal incision risks contaminating a new lymphatic field.

The first level of metastases, if present, is the regional nodes in the retroperitoneum which are treated by lymphadenectomy, radiation or both (Donahue, 1977; Maier et al., 1969; Maier and Lee, 1977; Skinner, 1976; Staubitz et al., 1973; Van der Werf-Messing, 1976; Whitmore, 1973).

Stage I and non-bulky II seminomas should be managed by external irradiation of the retroperitoneal nodes (Smithers et al., 1972). The majority of seminomas present as stage I and do not appear to have metastasized. However, obvious stage II tumors are usually radiosensitive. Stage III and possibly bulky II seminomas require more aggressive therapy as cures of disease with pulmonary metastases are rare with radiotherapy alone. The best combination of drugs or drugs plus radiotherapy are not yet known. An elevated hCG may be an ominous sign, also suggesting more aggressive therapy (Lange et al., 1976).

Stage III non-seminomatous disease was uniformly fatal until the early 60's when combination chemotherapy was introduced (Li et al., 1960). Intense combination chemotherapy now achieves an overall complete response rate of greater than 70% (Cvitkovic et al., 1977; Einhorn, 1979; Samuels et al., 1975). At least 50% of the complete responders remain in long-term remission and may be cured.

A significant complication of retroperitoneal lymphadenectomy is the loss of ejaculation. This results from sympathectomy performed in conjunction with removal of the lymph nodes, causing loss of semen emission from the seminal vesicles into the posterior urethra. This is frequently mistaken for retrograde ejaculation. Sympathomimetic agents have been used without much success although more selective drugs may become available. It is therefore advisable to discuss sperm banking with prospective surgical candidates, particularly in the face of improved survival figures. More than 75% of patients with testicular tumors can now be expected to survive as potential parents.

A final point of andrological interest is when patients should consider having a family following therapy. It is rare for a patient to develop recurrent disease more than two years after surgical therapy. Although follow-up is short on the patients treated by chemotherapy alone, similar observations are now being made. Certainly five years is a safe time period.

2. CARCINOMA OF THE PENIS

Carcinoma of the penis is theoretically readily accessible for early diagnosis and treatment. However, early symptoms are usually neglected by the patient either through fear or ignorance. Often even after consultation with a physician, different modalities of treatment are tried before the correct diagnosis is made. There is an average delay of 6-9 months between the initial symptoms and the initiation of treatment. A multitude of benign, pre-malignant and malignant lesions of the penis may mimic penile carcinoma in clinical and histological findings. Early diagnosis is essential for this potentially mutilating disease.

2.1. Pathology

More than 90% of cancer of the penis is squamous cell carcinoma. Basal cell carcinoma, malignant melanoma and mesenchymal tumors account for the remainder. The presenting lesion occurs on the glans (38-58%), prepuce (20-35%), coronal sulcus (4-32%), corpus (less than 5%) or frenulum (1%) (Ekstrom and Elsmyr, 1958; Marcial et al., 1962). Metastases via the regional lymphatics may occur with infiltration through the basement membrane so that even small tumors are at risk. The inguinal lymph nodes are the first regional nodes and metastases may be bilateral. Distant metastases are relatively late.

2.2. Epidemiology

Carcinoma of the penis is estimated to constitute 0.5% of all malignancies in male patients and 2.5% of all cancers of the genitourinary tract (Hanash et al., 1970). The incidence varies geographically with a high of 12% in Uganda. The incidence increases with age with few reported cases below 30 years. Most series show a mean of slightly over 60 years.

2.3. Etiology

Poor penile hygiene is a definite contributing factor to carcinogenesis. It is a rare disease in Jews who are circumcised shortly after birth and in India, the incidence is much lower in Moslems, as compared to Hindus, presumably for the same reason. Smegma is carcinogenic (Persky and deKernion, 1976) and specific carcinogenic agents have been isolated from decomposed smegma. Improvements in the standard of hygiene reduces the incidence of penile carcinoma (Templeton et al., 1972). Although patients frequently have a positive VDRL, this has not been shown to be causally related. The role of trauma is controversial. A number of benign penile lesions of various etiologies may undergo malignant transformation and are therefore considered pre-malignant from a therapeutic view (Table 3).

2.4. Diagnosis

Systemic symptoms for early penile carcinoma are rare and therefore most patients present with local complaints. Circumcised patients may have a painless excoriated lesion that is readily visible. More frequently, patients have phimosis or are uncircumcised and develop foul discharge with ulceration. Pain, hemorrhage and micturitional problems are rare, although urinary fistulas and urethral obstruction may develop in advanced disease.

In the presence of phimosis, a circumcision or dorsal slit may be necessary to expose the lesion, taking care not to incise the tumor itself. Endophytic tumors will appear as superficial round ulcers with indurated edges whereas exophytic tumors are wart-like masses. Palpable lymphadenopathy may occur in the inguinal area secondary to metastases or in response to a necrotic infected primary lesion.

Table 3. Epidemiology.

Overall incidence	2.5/100,000 males/year (Mostofi and Price, 1973), second most common male malignancy (after leukemia) between ages 20 and 35
Histological distribution	Varies with pathological interpretation in different reported series
Age distribution	Seminomas in slightly older age group (peak in 4th decade)
Racial distribution	Infrequent in Asiatics and extremely rare in blacks
Site distribution	Right-sided slightly more common, bilateral in 2% of cases
Familial distribution	No recognized increased incidence

There are many benign and malignant penile lesions which may mimic carcinoma of the penis.

2.4.1. Benign lesions

(a) *Cysts*. These smooth round, skin-coloured lesions occur commonly at the corona beneath the skin. They typically enlarge slowly and often are asymptomatic except when traumatized. Treatment is by excision.

(b) *Benign papillomas*. These are small, grayish papules found along the coronal sulcus. The majority occur in young adults. They are usually asymptomatic and require no treatment. They are only of diagnostic significance because they may resemble condylomata acuminata and must be distinguished from these lesions.

(c) *Condyloma acuminata*. Also known as venereal warts, these are soft, papillary epithelial growths occurring in the coronal sulcus and on the mucosa of the prepuce. They are not painful. Similar lesions may be found in the perianal area, urethral meatus or the genital areas of the sexual partner. The absence of adjacent tissue destruction is an important distinguishing feature from Buschke-Lowenstein tumors (to be discussed below).

(d) *Chancre*. This is the primary lesion of syphilis and it usually appears on the glans or the corona of the penis. It is a hard, solitary ulcer, with an elevated firm edge, an eroded base and a scant serious exudate. It is usually painless and is always associated with hard, nontender, non-suppurative inguinal lymphadenopathy. Diagnosis is made by identifying spirochetes on dark field examination of a smear from the ulcer base. Biopsy of the lesion will also confirm the diagnosis.

(e) *Condylomata lata*. These are the lesions of secondary syphilis which occasionally occur in the coronal sulcus. They are flat, broad-based growths with a moist surface in contrast to condylomata acuminata which are usually asymptomatic. The patient may have other manifestations of secondary syphilis although diagnosis is established by finding *Treponema pallida* in the secretion from the lesions. Serological tests for syphilis are strongly positive.

(f) *Gumma*. The lesion of syphilis of the penis is exceedingly rare. The lesion is a painless ulcer or nodule, resembling chronic granulomatous inflammation histologically and other features of tertiary syphilis are usually present.

(g) *Chancroid*. The most frequent locations for this infection ulcer is the preputial cavity and the frenulum. The infective agent is *Hemophilus ducrey*. The soft penile ulcers are shallow and non-indurated, with a necrotic exudate in the base and irregular 'moth-eaten' edges. The initial painful papule or pustule ulcerates within 3-5 days. Inguinal nodes are acutely painful and tender and if untreated, they may become matted and ulcerated. The diagnosis is suggested by the history and clinical picture, but is often dependent upon exclusion of herpes progentalia, lymphogranuloma venerum, etc. Isolation of *H. ducrey* from stained smear of the ulcer is difficult.

(h) *Lymphogranuloma venereum*. This venereal disease is characterized by a small, painless vesicle or papule on the penis followed in a few weeks by markedly painful inguinal nodes that soon coalesce with inflammation of the overlying skin and suppuration. The most sensitive method of diagnosis is by counterimmunoelectrophoresis using chlamydia antigen (Caldwell and Kuo, 1977). The Frei skin test is not reliable.

(i) *Granuloma inguinale*. This chronic indolent venereal disease involves the groin and genitalia. The initial lesions are papules which ulcerate, with formation of irregular friable granulation tissue in the base and edges. Secondary infection gives rise to mucopurulent exudate and pain. The differential diagnosis from carcinoma of the penis may be difficult because histological studies show pseudoepitheliomatous hyperplasia and acanthosis. Diagnosis is best made by punch biopsy of a lesion stained with Wright-Giemsa stain which reveals the causative agent, the 'Donovan Body', a Gram-negative coccobacillus found in mononuclear cells. Dark field examination should also be performed to rule out syphilis.

(j) *Herpes progenitalis*. Following itching and irritation, multiple vesicles develop on the penis or prepuce. The vesicles rupture, producing moist superficial ulcerations. Scrapings from the vesicles may show eosinophilic intranuclear

inclusions and immunofluorescence and electron microscopic examination reveal herpes antigen and herpes virus respectively.

(k) *Scabies.* Infestation by *Sarcoptes scabiei* may present as red and edematous papules on the shaft or glans of the penis which are characteristically pruritic and excoriated. Mites demonstrated microscopically from skin scraping are pathognomonic.

2.4.2. Premalignant lesions

(a) *Penile horns.* These are warty projections characterized microscopically by excess keratinization of hyperplastic epithelium. Penile cutaneous horns should be considered premalignant (Raghavaiah et al., 1977) because up to one third of these lesions undergo malignant changes. Metastases have been reported which show epidermoid carcinoma.

(b) *Leukoplakia.* These irregular grayish-white hypertrophic or atrophic plaques on the mucosal surfaces of the penis often occur at sites of chronic irritation. The histologic hyperkerotosis and parakerotosis have definite malignant potential and leukoplakia is found with 17% of specimens of squamous cell carcinomas of the penis (Hanash et al., 1970).

(c) *Erythroplasia of Queyrat.* These lesions present as moist, well-defined, red, velvet plaques on the dorsum of the penis, the urethral meatus or preputial cavity. Characteristic microscopic interpapillary acanthosis and hyperplasia of the strata corneum and granulosum establish the diagnosis (Persky and deKernion, 1976). The histological appearance can be classified as carcinoma in situ and frequent progression to invasive squamous cell carcinoma has been reported (Hanash et al., 1970).

(d) *Bowen's Disease.* This lesion is histologically similar to erythoplasia of Queyrat as an intraepithelial carcinoma of the penis.

(e) *Balanitis xerotica obliterans.* This is a form of lichen sclerosus et atrophicus localized to the penis. The thin atrophic scaly patches on the glans may ulcerate and fissure. If the urethral meatus is involved urinary symptoms often develop. Microscopically, the epidermis is atrophic with loss of rete pegs and homogenization of the collagen. Diagnosis is made by the

characteristic clinical picture and confirmed by biopsy. Malignant degeneration rarely occurs.

(f) *Buschke-Lowenstein tumor (condylomata acuminata giganticum).* This exophytic lesion is clinically similar to condylomata acuminata except for its larger size and evidence of local extension and destruction of adjacent tissues. Histologically, the lesions show expansive compressive downgrowth into underlying tissues rather than invasion. These giant condylomata can be classified as well-differentiated squamous cell tumors. Often within the same lesion, there is a wide spectrum of growth patterns and degrees of differentiation ranging from benign condyloma to squamous cell carcinoma, sometimes necessitating multiple biopsies to arrive at the diagnosis.

2.4.3. Malignant lesions

(a) *Basal cell carcinoma and melanoma.* Both tumors are extremely rare in the penis with 10 and 50 cases reported respectively. The penile lesions are very similar to those of other skin sites.

(b) *Malignant mesenchymal tumors.* These are cancers arising from stromal and connective tissues of the penis, occurring most commonly in the shaft. The most frequent presentation is a palpable mass in the penis. Diagnosis should be made by biopsy, preferably by needle biopsy (Persky and deKernion, 1976).

(c) *Metastatic disease of the penis.* Metastases to the penis are late manifestations of malignant disease elsewhere. Over two-thirds of the primary tumors are from the genitourinary tract (Abeshouse and Abeshouse, 1961). In order of frequency, the primary sites are bladder, rectum, prostate, kidney, testes, lung. There is usually little problem with diagnosis because of manifestations of the primary disease.

2.5. Staging and treatment

Biopsy is essential to establish the diagnosis. Multiple biopsies with extensive sectioning may be necessary to show malignant elements (Goldstein et al., 1977). The biopsy may be excisional and will therefore also be therapeutic. Once the histologic diagnosis has been obtained, the extent of

disease must be established to determine management and prognosis.

The Jackson (1966) staging system for penile cancer is generally accepted in North America:

Stage 1 – Tumor limited to the glans penis and/or prepuce.

Stage 2 – Invasion into shaft or corpora but without nodal or distant metastases.

Stage 3 – Primary tumor confined to the shaft with proven regional node metastases.

Stage 4 – Invasion from the shaft, with inoperable regional node involvement or distant metastases.

There is considerable discrepancy between clinical and histologic staging. More than 50% of palpable nodes are in fact benign and biopsy reveals lymphadenitis. Conversely, small benign nodes may show occult metastases. Cabanas (1977) demonstrated the 'sentinel lymph node' which appears to be the first site of metastases and may be the only positive nodes in early stage disease. Biopsy of this node at the time of treatment for the primary tumor produces little morbidity and can accurately differentiate inflammatory from malignant enlargement.

For small tumors confined to the prepuce, local excision by circumcision appears to be sufficient therapy in the face of a negative sentinel node. Partial or total penectomy may be necessary for the lesions on the glans or shaft with at least a 2 cm margin of normal tissue. If the simultaneous sentinel node biopsy is negative, no further surgical therapy is required. If positive, regional metastases can be managed by *en bloc* ileoinguinal node dissection, although this is controversial. The precise role of radiotherapy is not well defined either. The primary tumor may be managed by radiation alone. The 5 year survival rates for stage I and stage II disease are approximately 90% and 65% respectively (Jensen, 1977; Persky and deKernion, 1976). Nodal involvement decreases survival appreciably.

Table 4. Benign and pre-malignant penile lesions.

Lesion	Appearance, characteristics	diagnosis
Cyst	Asymptomatic, smooth skincolored	Clinical
Papilloma	Asymptomatic, gray papules	Clinical, biopsy
Condylomata acuminata	Asymptomatic multiple, papillary cauliflower-like warts	Clinical
Chancre	Hard, solitary, painless ulcer with inguinal lymphadenopathy	Darkfield identification of spirochetes, biopsy
Condylomata lata	Asymptomatic, broad-based papilla with other secondary syphilis manifestations	Serology, *Treponema* isolation
Gumma	Painless nodule	Serology
Chancroid	Painful necrotic ulcer and suppurative inguinal nodes	Clinical, stained smear isolation of *H. ducrey*
Lymphogranuloma venereum	Small, painless vesicle or papule with painful matted inguinal nodes	Counterimmunoelectrophoresis of chlamydia antigen
Granuloma inguinale	Ulcerating papules with secondary infection	Biopsy Wright-Giemsa stain to isolate Donovan's bodies
Herpes progenitalia	Prodromal irritation, multiple vesicles	Clinical, immunofluorescence, e.m.
Scabies	Pruritic, excoriated red papules	Identification of mite from skin scrapings
Tuberculosis	Painless ulcer, subcutaneous nodules and associated tuberculosis infection	Biopsy, identify tubercle bacilli from ulcer
Amebiasis	Rapid growing, painful ulcer	Biopsy, wet preparation
Penile horns	Warty projection	Biopsy
Leukoplakia	Irregular, grayish-white plaques frequently on sites of chronic irritation	Biopsy
Erythroplasia of Queyrat	Moist, velvety, red plaque	Biopsy
Bowen's disease	Moist, velvety, red plaque	Biopsy
Balanitis xerotica obliterans	Thin atrophic scaly patches	Biopsy
Buschke-Lowenstein tumor (condylomata acuminata giganticum)	Exophytic condylomata with local extension and destruction of adjacent tissues	Biopsy

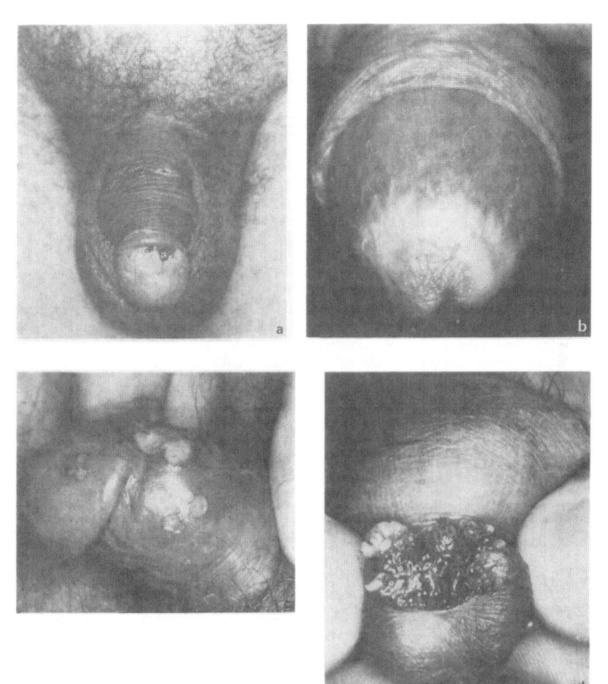

Figure 4. Some common lesions of the penis. (a) Syphilis: primary chancre on glans penis and secondary rash on thighs; (b) balanitis xerotica obliterans; (c) herpes progenitalis; (d) condyloma acuminata.

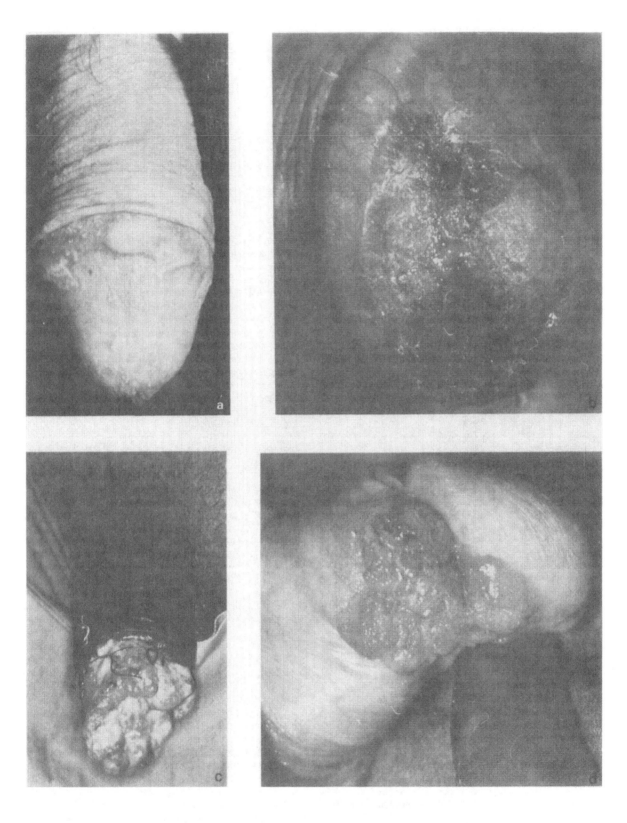

Figure 5. Lichen planus (a) and carcinoma of the penis (b, c and d).

3. CONCLUDING REMARKS

Lesions of the testis and penis will come to the andrologist's attention often as incidental findings. It is important to recognize the neoplastic lesions and seek appropriate urological consultation for definitive treatment. The results with testicular cancer have dramatically improved recently but prompt diagnosis is still imperative to achieve optimal results. Malignant lesions of the penis tend to be in an older age group but may still confront the andrologist.

ACKNOWLEDGEMENTS

The authors gratefully acknowledge the help of the Ontario Cancer Treatment and Research Foundation no. 382, Ontario Ministry óf Health PR630C, and the Wellesley Hospital Research Foundation; our thanks are also due to Ms Joan MacDonald, Mrs Barbara Naglie (manuscript) and Ms Frances Key (illustrations).

REFERENCES

Abeshouse BS, Abeshouse GA (1961) Metastatic tumors of the penis: a review of the literature and a report of 2 cases. J Urol 86: 99.

Artzt K, Bennett D (1975) Analogies between embryonic (T/t) antigens and adult major histocompatability (H-2) antigens. Nature 256: 545.

Artzt K, Dubois P, Bennett D, Condamine H, Babinet C, Jacob F (1973) Surface antigens common to mouse cleavage embryos and primitive teratocarcinoma cells in culture. Proc Natl Acad Sci USA 70: 2988.

Cabanas RM (1977) An approach for the treatment of penile carcinoma. Cancer 39: 456.

Caldwell HD, Kuo C-c (1977) Serological diagnosis of lymphogranuloma venereum by counterimmunoelectrophoresis with a *Chlamydia trachomatis* protein antigen. J Immun 118: 442.

Cochran US, Walsh PC, Porter JC, Nicholson TC, Madden JD, Peter PC (1975) The endocrinology of human chrorionic gonadotropin-secreting testicular tumors: new methods in diagnosis. J Urol 114: 549.

Cvitkovic E, Cheng E, Whitmore WF, Golbey RB (1977) Germ cell tumor chemotherapy update. Proc Assoc Cancer Res 18: 324.

Donahue JP (1977) Retroperitoneal lymphadenectomy: the anterior approach including bilateral suprarenal-hilar dissection. Urol Clin North Am 4: 509.

Einhorn LH (1979) Combination chemotherapy with cis-Dichlorodiammine platinum (II) in disseminated testicular cancer. Cancer Treat Rep 63: 1659.

Ekstrom T, Elsmyr F (1958) Cancer of the penis: a clinical study of 229 cases. Acta Chir Scand 115: 25.

Goldstein AMB, Reynolds WF, Terry R (1977) Diagnostic problems of epithelial tumors of the penis. Urology 9: 79.

Hanash KA, Furlow WL, Utz DC, Harrison EG (1970) Carcinoma of the penis: a clinicopathological study. J Urol 104: 291.

Holden S, Bernard O, Artzt K, Whitmore WF Jr, Bennett D (1977) Human and mouse embryonal carcinoma cells in culture share an embryonic antigen (F9). Nature 270: 518.

Jackson SM (1966) The treatment of carcinoma of the penis. Br J Surg 53: 35.

Jensen MO (1977) Cancer of the penis in Denmark 1942-1962. Dan Med Bull 24: 66.

Jewett MAS (1977) Biology of testicular tumors. Urol Clin North Am 4: 495.

Johnson DE, Gemez JJ, Ayala AG (1976) Histologic factors affecting prognosis of pure seminoma of the testis. South Med J 69: 1173.

Kleinsmith LJ, Pierce GB (1964) Multipotentiality of single embryonal carcinoma cells. Cancer Res 24: 1544.

Lange PH, McIntire KR, Waldmann TA, Hakala TR, Fraley EE (1976) Serum alphafetoprotein and human chorionic gonadotropin in the diagnosis and management of nonseminomatous germ cell testicular cancer. N Engl J Med 295: 1237.

Li MC, Whitmore WF, Golbey R, Grabstald H (1960) Effects of combined drug therapy on metastatic cancer of the testis. JAMA 174: 1291.

Luna MA (1976) Extragonadal germ cell tumors. In: Johnson DE, ed. Testicular tumors, pp 261-265. Flushing, NY: Medical Examination Publications.

Maier JG, Lee SN (1977) Radiation therapy for nonseminomatous germ cell testicular cancer in adults. Urol Clin North Am 4: 447.

Maier JG, Van Buskirk KE, Sulak MH, Schamber DT (1969) An evaluatuon of lymphadenectomy in the treatment of malignant testicular germ cell neoplasms. J Urol 101: 356.

Marcial VA, Figueroa-Colen J, Marcial-Rojas RA, Colon JE (1962) Carcinoma of the penis. Radiology 79: 209.

Markland C, Kedias K, Fraley EE (1973) Inadequate orchiectomy for patients with testicular tumors. JAMA 224: 1025.

Mostofi FK, Price EB Jr (1973) Tumors of the male genital system. In: Atlas of tumor pathology, 2nd ser., Fasc. 8. Washington, DC: Armed Forces Institute of Pathology.

Ostrand-Rosenberg S, Edidin M, Jewett MAS (1977) Human teratoma cells share antigens with mouse teratoma cells. Dev. Biol 61: 11.

Persky L, deKernion J (1976) Carcinoma of the penis. CA 26: 130.

Pugh RCB, Cameron JM (1976) Teratoma. In: Pugh RCB, ed. Pathology of the testis, pp 199-243. Oxford: Blackwell Scientific.

Raghavaiah MV, Soloway MS, Murphy WM (1977) Malignant penile horns. J Urol 118: 1068.

Rosai J, Silber I, Khodadoust K (1969) Spermatocytic seminoma. I. Clinicopathologic study of six cases and review of the literature. Cancer 24: 92.

Samuels ML, Johnson DE, Hologe PY (1975) Continuous intravenous Bleomycin therapy with vinblastine in stage III testicular neoplasia. Cancer Chemother Rep 59: 570.

Skinner DG (1976) Non-seminomatous testis tumors: a plan of management based on 96 patients to improve survival in all stages by combined therapeutic modalities. J Urol 115: 65.

Smither D, Wallace ENK, Wallace DM (1972) Radiotherapy for patients with tumours of the testicle. Br J Urol 44: 217.

Staubitz WJ, Early KS, Magoss IV, Murphy GP (1973) Surgical treatment of nonseminomatous germinal testis tumors. Cancer 32: 1206.

Stevens LC (1973) A new subline of mice (129/terSu) with a high incidence of spontaneous congenital testicular teratomas. J Natl Cancer Inst 50: 235.

Templeton AC, Buxton E, Bianchi A (1972) Cancer in Kyandonuo County, Uganda 1968-70. J Natl Cancer Inst 48: 865.

Vaitukaitis JL, Braunstein GD, Ross GT (1972) A radioimmunoassay which specifically measures human chorionic gonadotropin in the presence of human luteinizing hormone.

Am J Obstet Gynecol 113: 751.

Van der Werf-Messing B (1976) Radiotherapeutic treatment of testicular tumors. Int J Radiat Oncol Biol Phys 1: 235.

Wallace S, Jing B, Zornoza J (1977) Lymphangiography in the determination of the extent of metastatic carcinoma: the potential value of percutaneous lymph node biopsy. Cancer 39: 706.

Whitmore WF Jr (1973) Germinal testis tumors in adults. In: Proc 7 Natl Cancer Conf, p 793. Philadelphia: J.B. Lippincott.

Zondek B (1937) Gonadotropic hormone in the diagnosis of chorioepithelioma. JAMA 108: 607.

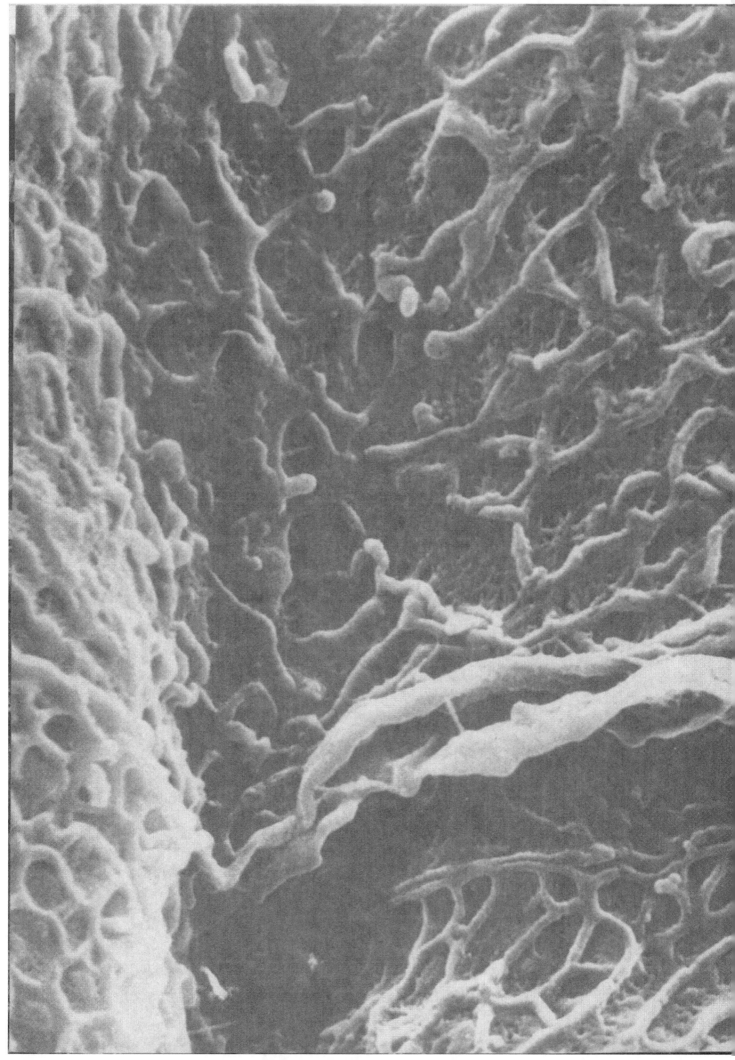

III. RADIOLOGICAL TECHNIQUES

12. DIAGNOSTIC RADIOLOGY IN ANDROLOGY

W.A. CUMMING and J.E. CAMPBELL

Radiological examinations along with other medical investigations have increased in complexity and number over the years until we sometimes have trouble deciding which should be done or if any should be done at all. Any examination being considered must have a reasonable likelihood of providing information that will affect the patient's management. If such information is considered a benefit, then it must be weighed against whatever risk is involved to the patient and against the financial cost. A statistical evaluation of benefits and risks of cystourethrography suggests that the benefits significantly exceed the risks, particularly in boys (Saenger et al., 1976). The difficulty in attempting to analyze the risk of any radiological examination lies in the multiplicity of factors involved: psychological trauma, anesthetic hazards, contrast reactions, arterial or venous thrombosis, and potential radiation-induced malignancy. Since most of these factors cannot be evaluated quantitatively, a calculation of risk is just an approximation. A radiologist, in consultation with a referring physician, is reponsible for deciding on the most rewarding and least hazardous course of radiological investigation in each clinical situation. If one assumes all X-radiation to be potentially harmful in a biological sense, then one is obliged to submit a patient to the least amount consistent with an adequate investigation for diagnosis and management. Since disorders of the male genital system provide a variety of opportunities for the application of radiological techniques, we will discuss the indications, methods and complications of the techniques in Part 1 and their application to various clinical conditions in Part 2 of this chapter.

1. RADIOLOGICAL EXAMINATIONS

1.1. Examinations without contrast media

1.1.1. Genital region. Indications. Radiographs of the genital area are an incidental part of abdominal or pelvic radiography being done for various reasons. For instance, a film taken as part of an excretory urogram may show calcification of the vas deferens (Fig. 1). Occasionally, films of the penis or scrotum are taken specifically to search for calcifications in Peyronie's disease or to evaluate a penile prosthesis.

Method. Sand-like penile calcification may be seen in the indurated nodules of Peyronie's disease. The method of examination involves the use of amplification fluoroscopy and spot films in A.P. and oblique projections. In each of these positions, one film is taken of the penis and a second is taken with the patient placing the tip of his index finger on top of the nodule. The films can then be examined under magnification in search of the calcification. The patient's finger localizes the area to be examined closely.

Penile radiographs may be helpful in the examination of complications of penile prostheses. Fluoroscopy and spot films can be helpful in assessing the function of an inflatable prosthesis filled with radiopaque contrast medium.

When the gonadal area is included in radiographs, as it frequently is in urography, testicular shielding should be used for most films, but at least one must be taken without the shield so soft tissue findings in the scrotum are not obscured.

Findings. Gas, in soft tissue, shows as a radiolucent area radiographically. It may be seen outlining the

J. Bain and E.S.E. Hafez (eds.), Diagnosis in andrology, 153-169. All rights reserved.
Copyright © 1980 by Martinus Nijhoff Publishers bv, The Hague/Boston/London.

154 CUMMING, CAMPBELL

bladder in diabetics with *E. coli* infection or enlarging the scrotum and extending up the abdominal wall in patients with scrotal gangrene. Gas is occasionally seen in the genital area in patients with suppurative peritonitis or retroperitoneal infections or in patients with accidental or surgical trauma. Bowel gas in the scrotum occasionally allows a serendipitous diagnosis of inguinal hernia.

In infants, calcification of the tunica vaginalis in the scrotum is evidence of meconium peritonitis, probably due to antenatal intestinal perforation, and usually associated with peritoneal calcification in the abdomen. Calcification of the testes is seen in some gonadal tumors, dysplastic testes, and in testicular microlithiasis.

Calcification in the distal part of the vas deferens and its ampulla is seen in patients with long-standing diabetes (Fig. 1a) (Hafiz and Melnick, 1968). It is also seen in patients with granulomatous infections such as tuberculosis when it is patchy and plaque-like and may be associated with sacroiliac tuberculosis (Fig. 1b). Sometimes calcification of the vas is seen in healthy men. Minute prostatic calculi occur in 14% of men over 50 year of age (Fox, 1960). Larger calculi are less common, occurring in males under 50 with lower urinary tract infections and prostatitis. In a detailed study of these calculi, *E. coli* was found to be the infecting agent, lying in the middle of the calculi and protected from the action of anti-microbial agents (Eykyn et al., 1974).

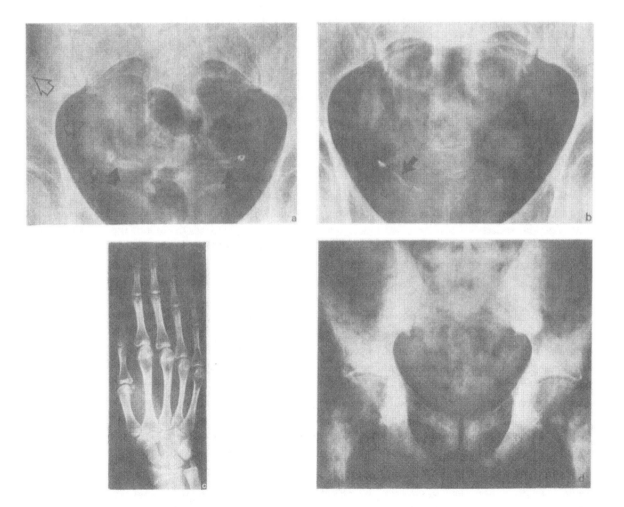

Figure 1. (a) Diabetic calcification of the vasa deferentia. There is symmetrical smooth, tubular calcification of the vasa of this 47-year-old diabetic (solid arrows). Note also the faint calcification of iliac arteries (open arrows). (b) Tuberculous calcification of the vas deferens. There is a symmetrical dense, irregular calcification of the right vas in this patient who had genitourinary tuberculosis (arrow). (c) Arachnodactyly in myotonia dystrophica. Metacarpal index is 11.5. (d) Osteoblastic skeletal metastases in prostatic carcinoma.

These stones sometimes grow in size despite treatment of the associated infection. Giant calculi, replacing virtually the entire prostate gland, are sometimes found in patients with tuberculosis. Calculi in the seminal vesicles are easy to diagnose because of the characteristic anatomy. They are usually asymptomatic but may be palpable on rectal examination, tend to occur in older males, and may or may not be associated with inflammation. Occasionally they cause hematospermia, painful intercourse, or pain on urination.

1.1.2. Skeletal surveys. Radiographic surveys of the entire body can be carried out in a search for features of various syndromes which have genital abnormalities as a prominent feature (Taybi, 1975). Although such a survey must be tailored to the suspected condition, a typical skeletal examination would include A.P. and lateral skull, P.A. chest, P.A. hand and wrist, A.P. pelvis, lateral lumbar spine and possibly A.P. upper and lower limbs if they seem abnormal clinically.

A common indication for a skeletal survey is the identification of metastatic malignancies. Such a survey should include a lateral view of the skull, an overpenetrated chest including shoulders and ribs, a lateral cervical spine, lateral lumbar spine, A.P. pelvis, and a routine P.A. and lateral chest. Other areas may be examined as indicated by pain or findings of survey. Most tumors cause osteolytic lesions in the skeleton but prostatic carcinoma is a well-known cause of osteoblastic metastases. Nuclear medicine scans are, in general more sensitive and more easily performed than skeletal surveys for malignancy. In children, they should be done in preference to radiographic examinations.

1.1.3. Bone age. The skeleton of healthy children matures by ossification of cartilage in a predictable fashion from birth to adulthood. This process is mostly due to estrogenic activity although thyroxine is important in early childhood and testosterone plays an indirect role through its metabolic product, estradiol. This maturation is independent of growth in size which depends on growth hormone and testosterone. Estimation of skeletal maturation of bone age is, therefore, an indirect measure of sex hormone activity in a child. Precocious sexual development is accompanied by accelerated skeletal maturation and delayed sexual development is accompanied by retarded skeletal maturation.

Our method of bone age estimation is based on the Greulich and Pyle Atlas (1959) which presents a series of hand and wrist radiographs of a group of white children in Cleveland arranged as a series of age standards. To estimate a child's bone age, a P.A. radiograph of the hand and wrist is compared with the standard of the same age and sex in the atlas, and with the standards above and below this. until the standard most resembling the subject is determined. The age of this standard is then the bone age of the child. The atlas also provides tables of standard deviations at various ages and tables that allow adult height prediction. If some ossification centers in the hand and the wrist are of a much different age from the others, the difference should be noted since the difference may be significant (Poznanski et al., 1971). In infants, it is difficult to assign significant bone ages, but the knee is more useful than the hand and wrist and an atlas of standard knee radiographs is available (Pyle and Hoerr, 1969).

1.2. Cystourethrography

Cystourethrography is a radiographic recording of an image of a contrast-filled bladder and urethra. A voiding examination is a study of the dynamic process of bladder emptying. A dynamic retrograde examination is a functional study of the urethra during the injection of contrast via the penile urethra (McCallum and Colapinto, 1976).

Indications. Cystourethrography is usually carried out to investigate urinary infections and vesico-ureteral reflux. It is also important in the investigation of suspected urethral obstruction, assessment of congenital abnormalities including sexual ambiguity and in evaluation of early and late results of trauma. Cystourethrography may be helpful in assessing the urethra when problems arise following prostatic surgery.

Method. The contrast agents used in cystourethrography are aqueous solutions of from 15 to 50% sodium or methylglucamine, diatrizoate or iothalomate. There are three different techniques in

general use. The urethra can be visualized when a patient voids at the conclusion of an excretory urogram when the bladder is filled with contrast medium that has been excreted by the kidneys. This method avoids catheterization, but the concentration of contrast may be inadequate for visualization of the anatomy and the patient, particularly if he is young, may be unable to void voluntarily.

The usual cystourethrogram in an adult is carried out after the introduction of a Foley catheter into the bladder through the urethra. The contrast medium runs in by gravity until the patient feels the desire to void (usually about 500 ml in an adult). The patient then turns to the right posterior oblique projection with the left leg out of the way as much as possible. The catheter is removed and the patient holds a plastic urinal in his right hand into which he voids. Under fluoroscopic control, radiographs and

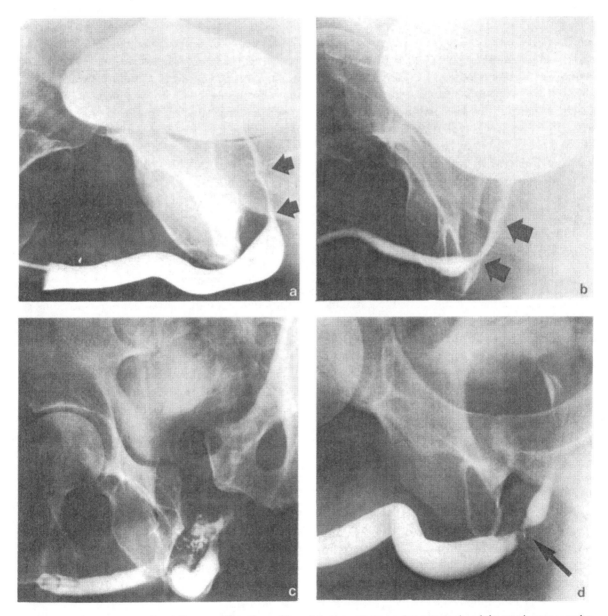

Figure 2. (a) Normal retrograde urethrogram. Note the position of the verumontanum (upper arrow) and the membranous urethra (lower arrow). The posterior urethra is always poorly filled in a retrograde study. (b) Normal voiding cystourethrogram. Note the positions of the verumontanum and membranous urethra (arrows). (c) Urethral trauma. A retrograde urethrogram after pelvic trauma shows extravasation of contrast and obstruction at the level of urogenital diaphragm where the urethra was divided. (d) A retrograde urethrogram shows a tight stricture of the bulbous urethra, close to the membranous urethra (arrow).

a video-tape recording of the urethra, bladder, and lower ureters are made during voiding.

A retrograde urethrogram combined with a voiding cystourethrogram is most apt to be rewarding in an andrological study. To do this, a Foley catheter under sterile conditions is introduced with its balloon in the fossa navicularis, the balloon is inflated with 1 or 2 ml of sterile water or air, and a slight tug is put on the catheter to straighten the bulbar and penile urethra. The patient is turned 45° to the right with the left leg well out of the way. Under image amplification fluoroscopy, contrast medium is slowly injected into the urethra through the catheter. As the contrast arrives at the membranous urethra, there is a natural tendency for the patient to contract his pelvic muscles which results in obstruction of the urethra at the urogenital diaphragm. To avoid this, the patient should be instructed to breathe slowly in and out through his mouth throughout the entire examination and under no circumstances to suddenly hold his breath. The contrast will pass the urogenital diaphragm through the prostatic urethra, and flow into the bladder. The proces is recorded on films and video-tape if available. The bladder is filled until the patient has the desire to void. The catheter is then removed and an antegrade voiding study is performed as already described.

Retrograde filling of the urethra does not allow proper visualization of the prostatic urethra or bladder neck, although one can usually see the verumontanum as the contrast trickles through the clamped-down prostatic urethra (Fig. 2a). The antegrade or voiding study provides the reverse (Fig. 3b). The degree, length, site and possibly the etiology of any obstruction are verified by combining the retrograde and voiding studies. With obstruction, the antegrade study will demonstrate dilatation of the proximal urethra and the retrograde study will demonstrate the urethra distal to the point of obstruction.

In a normal subject, on the retrograde examination, the point of tapering of the anterior urethra (the urethral cone), marks the site of the membranous urethra. With voiding, the membranous urethra is marked by the proximal end of the slightly ballooned bulbous urethra. Further, during voiding, a command to stop voiding will localize the membranous urethra. It is the site of the external sphincter and usually when it closes, all contrast distal to it is voided and that proximal to it goes retrogradely back into the bladder. Thus, sphincter localization and control can be assessed. The pelvic floor is contracted during the retrograde injection and completely relaxed during the voiding urethrogram. If two measurements are taken on the film one will find that between the retrograde and voiding studies, the position of the membranous urethra descends from any bony landmarks by 2-3 cm. Thus, techniques that attempt to relate its site to the symphysis pubis have to be looked upon with a certain amount of suspicion.

In children the bladder is usually filled by a soft rubber transurethral catheter, although some prefer a suprapubic injection. We use size 8 or 10 French rubber catheters or size 3 or 5 French plastic feeding tubes after urethral anesthesia with topical lidocaine. The catheter is introduced, the bladder is filled until voiding starts, the catheter is pulled out and voiding usually continues with the event recorded on video-tape and spot films. There is little to choose between the various spot film devices available and we use conventional fluoroscopic films, 70 mm films and 105 mm films interchangeably. Retrograde urethrography in infants and small children is done with a catheter of appropriate size to fit snugly in the urethral meatus. In older children we use a small Foley catheter and inflate its balloon in the fossa navicularis as would be done in an adult.

Findings. The findings in cystourethrography include obstructing lesions, such as strictures and valves and congenital anomalies such as Müllerian derivatives.

Complications. Proper technique will generally avoid complications. Traumatic catheterization or examination too soon following urethroscopy may result in reflux of contrast material into the venous system. A minimum of two weeks delay after cystoscopy is essential. Reflux into prostatic ducts, Cowper's glands, ejaculatory ducts, seminal vesicles and vas deferens generally does not cause trouble. Very rarely, reactions to contrast medium can occur during cystourethrography (McAllister et al., 1974; Redman and Robinson, 1977).

Radiation dose. Radiation to the testes is a concern in this examination. The testes are partly out of the field of view and can be shielded using metal foil or commercially available shields. The gonad dose has been estimated to be in the neighbourhood of 100-200 mrads, but the actual amount of radiation absorbed varies with the fluoroscopy technique, time and the number and type of spot films taken. It is probably more important to consider radiation dose in young people than in old men (Ardran et al., 1978; Hertz and Werner, 1977; Kaude et al., 1969; Pratt et al., 1973).

1.3. Excretory urography

Excretory urography, a sophisticated name for what has been called intravenous pyelography is used, to examine the kidneys and their collecting systems.

Indications. It is carried out in andrological investigation when there is evidence of infection, obstruction, or an anomaly such as anal atresia which is known to be associated with renal abnormalities.

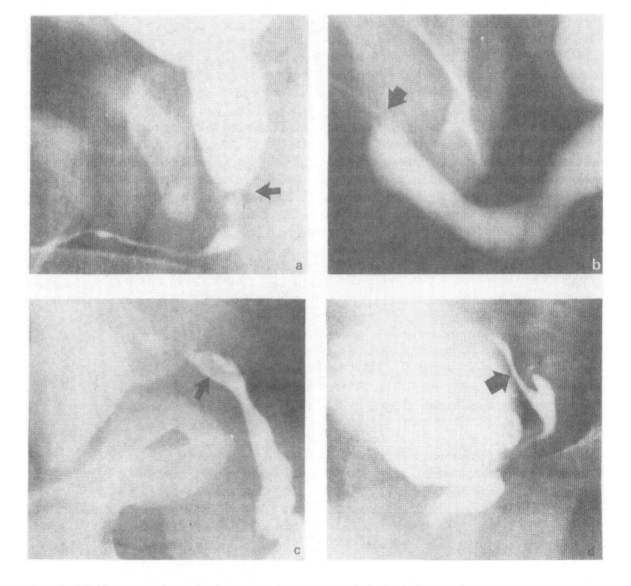

Figure 3. (a) Voiding cystourethrography shows obstructing posterior urethral valves in the usual site (arrow). (b) Anterior urethral valve. Note the abrupt narrowing of the penile urethra (arrow) during voiding cystourethrography. (c) Retrograde urethrography shows the calculus in the lumen of the urethra (arrow) of a patient with repaired hypospadias. (d) A uterus and fallopian tube (arrow filling from a Müllerian structure entering the posterior urethra of a boy with hypospadias).

Method. Following a plain film of the abdomen, the examination is performed after the intravenous injection of 50-60% diatrizoate or iothalomate by taking further films over an appropriate time period. Compression of the ureters may be used to promote filling of the calyces and pelves. Tomography can be used to get more information about renal parenchyma. Excreted contrast can sometimes be used to outline the urethra.

Complications. A small number of patients will have serious shock-like reactions to contrast medium but a considerable number will have minor reactions such as hives. The cause of these reactions remains obscure (Lieberman et al., 1978).

Radiation dose. The testicular radiation dose in excretory urography depends on the number of films taken and the size of the patient among other things, but probably averages in the neighbourhood of 500 mrads per examination.

1.4. Vasography (vasoseminal vesiculography)

Vasography is the opacification of the vasa deferentia and related structures with radiopaque contrast material.

Indications. The major indication is the investigation of male sterility. Uncommon indications include primary or secondary tumors in the region of the ampulla of the vas deferens, seminal vesicles or the ejaculatory duct, or evaluation of the vas following vasectomy or other surgery affecting the ejaculatory ducts. Rarely it may be necessary to prove the site of vesicular calcification.

Method. Under local anesthesia, a scrotal incision is made to expose the vas and a 23 or 25 gauge needle is inserted directly into its lumen. Injecting first toward the epididymis and then toward the seminal vesicle, 2-3 ml of contrast are introduced. Radiographs are taken in the A.P. projection angled 30-35° toward the feet. A lateral view is often helpful. A second film may be taken after ejaculation to insure patency of the ducts. With normal filling, contrast will not go further down the urethra than the urogenital diaphragm and will take the easier route back into the bladder. Catheterization

of the ejaculatory ducts has been done with a special catheter via the urethra using a panendoscope. It can also be used therapeutically for dilatation of the ejaculatory duct. This method however is difficult to perform and there is a definite risk of introducing infection (Hebert et al., 1971).

Findings. The vas deferens is a narrow tube of constant diameter of 1-1.5 mm (Fig. 4b). The epididymis appears as a relatively dense string folded upon itself. The ampulla of the vas appears as a dilatation which becomes tortuous until it ends at a short and narrow duct at the neck of the seminal vesicle. The seminal vesicle itself may have various appearances. It may be a rather uniform tube or it may have ramifications or segmentary dilatations and may have a bifid appearance. The ampullary portion of the vas deferens may have numerous folds which look like diverticula, but this is a normal appearance. Changes due to infection are not often seen although tuberculosis may be destructive and produce abscess cavities. Calcification of the distal part of the vas can be characteristic of this lesion. Masses may invade or impress themselves upon the seminal vesicles. Seminal vesicle cysts, myomas, and prostatic carcinoma are primary tumors that may deform the vesicles. Secondary cancer from the bladder, rectum or the testes may also distort or invade the vesicles.

1.5. Corpus cavernosography

This is the visualization of the corpora cavernosa of the penis by direct injection of contrast medium.

Indications. Corpus cavernosagraphy is usually carried out as part of the investigation of Peyronie's disease to delineate the extent of involvement and to evaluate treatment. It is sometimes used to search for metastatic malignancy such as carcinoma of the penis (Ney et al., 1976). Other indications include priapism, impotence, penile atrophy and fibrosis, trauma, and the assessment of a patient for installation of penile prosthesis.

Method. The penis is maintained in an extended position by means of adhesive straps attached to the glans. Local anesthetic is injected into the skin and subcutaneous tissue on one side of the midline just

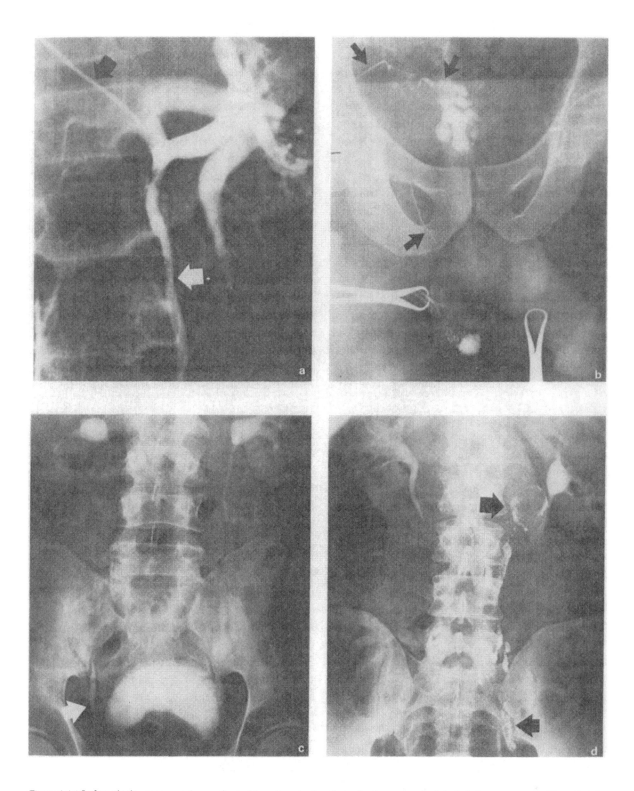

Figure 4. (a) Left testicular venogram in a patient with varicocele. A catheter has been passed up the inferior vena cava and into the left renal vein (black arrow). Injection of contrast opacifies the testicular vein which has no valves (white arrow). (b) A normal right vasogram in a 40-year-old male with azoospermia. (c) Benign prostatic hyperplasia causes a smooth filling defect in the bladder at excretory urography. Note fishhook ureters (white arrow). (d) Metastatic testicular seminoma from left testis. Note the large node medial to the left kidney (arrow) deflecting the upper ureter laterally and other affected nodes deflecting the lower ureter medially (arrow).

behind the glans. In order to prevent leakage, the needle injecting the local anesthetic is not permitted to enter the corpus cavernosum. A No. 22 or 23 needle is then injected directly into the corpus cavernosum at the site of the anesthetic. A flexible plastic tube is interposed between the needle and the syringe and 10 ml of contrast material are injected under fluoroscopic control. Because there are venous connections across the midline, only one corpus need be injected. When both are filled, films are taken in the A.P. and oblique projections and lateral films are taken at intervals until all of the contrast material has disappeared. By this method, the emptying time of the corpora can be estimated. Some perform the examination by putting rubber tubing around the base of the penis to impede drainage from the corpora cavernosa. They get better filling of the corpora and avoid diagnosing narrowings that do not exist. With this modification however, the emptying time cannot be assessed (Bystrom et al., 1974).

In the normal examination, the outline of the corpora is wide in the middle and tapers to a convex termination at the distal end impinging on the glans. The boundaries are smooth and regular. The septum is represented by a thin regular radiolucent line with some widening at the distal portion. The corpora themselves are homogeneously filled. There are many intercommunicating veins passing through the septum from one side to the other. Normal emptying time is about 1½ hr. There are superficial and deep dorsal venous systems in the corpora and intricate circumflex venous systems and intercommunicative network of vessels within the draining system (Fitzpatrick, 1975).

1.6. Angiography

1.6.1. *Arteriography.* Arteriography of the male genitalia involves selective opacification of the appropriate arteries supplying the area.

Indications. It is an uncommon procedure in the genital region although it may be helpful in investigation of tumors which are bing considered for surgery and it has been used to search for clinically undetectable testes.

Method. Using the Seldinger technique, an intra-arterial catheter is introduced into a femoral artery and its tip is manipulated into the appropriate branches (Nordmark, 1977). The testes receive their arterial blood supply from the anterior aspect of the aorta just below the renal arteries, the penis is supplied by the internal pudendal branch of the internal iliac artery, while the scrotum is supplied by both the internal pudendal and the external pudendal, which is a branch of the femoral artery. Other small sources of arterial supply are the cremasteric branch of the inferior epigastric artery and branches of the inferior vesical artery, another branch of the internal iliac. In practice then, arteriography of the area would include injections into the testicular arteries arising from the aorta and into the internal and external iliac arteries in the pelvis. Although arteriography of the testicular artery will show the presence or absence of a testicle and its location, it may be difficult to carry out.

Complications. Complications of arteriography include trauma to the femoral artery at the injection site, arterial thrombosis and reactions to contrast medium.

1.6.2. Venography
Indications. Venography is used to locate hidden testes, and to investigate varicoceles.

Method. The testicular veins drain to the inferior vena cava on the right and into the renal vein on the left. They can be catheterized using a Seldinger technique similar to that used for the arteries, but the femoral vein is punctured and catheterized (Weiss et al., 1977). Venography of the cremasteric vein and the internal and external pudendal veins is usually carried out at the time of operation when the veins are exposed and directly injected with contrast medium (Hill and Green, 1977). Testicular venography is technically easier than arteriography.

Findings. In cryptorchidism, visualization of the testicular vein can identify the presence or absence and the location of a hidden testis. In varicocele, venography can demonstrate the presence and adequacy of valves in the testicular vein and the anastomoses with the internal and external pudendal veins (Fig. 4a).

1.6.3. Lymphography. Indications. Lymphography has been used to investigate the spread of testicular malignancies. Testicular lymphatics terminate in sentinel lymph nodes at the level of L1 and L2 on the left side and L2 and L3 on the right side (Busch and Sayegh, 1963, 1965). These sentinel nodes are better demonstrated by testicular than by pedal lymphography, but fear of accelerating the spread of testicular malignancy contradicts it. From the right sentinel node there may be immediate cross-over to the contralateral lymph nodes. Then spread takes place caudally in the periaortic nodes filled by pedal lymphography. This helps explain why nodes may be positive at the time of radical resection despite being negative on lymphography. However, a positive lymphogram by the pedal route is significant and reliable.

Method. Pedal lymphography is carried out by injecting lymphatic vessels in the dorsum of the foot with oily contrast material after locating them with the help of methylene blue. The passage of the medium up the lymphatics is followed and when it reaches the abdomen, delayed films are taken.

Complications. Complications include rare infections at the operative site in the dorsum of the foot and more commonly pulmonary complications from pulmonary embolism of the oily contrast material. This can usually be avoided by restricting the amount of contrast used.

1.7. Herniography

Indications. Herniography allows the visualization of an inguinal hernia that may or may not be evident on clinical examination. Its chief indication is the identification of a second inguinal hernia when one has been found and is being considered for surgical repair. A herniogram can be helpful in deciding if the contralateral side needs repair. Herniography has also been used to search for a hidden testicle. Although many competent and experienced pediatric surgeons do not believe the herniogram is helpful to them, others find that the knowledge gained allows them to plan their surgery more rationally.

Method. The technique is simple, consisting of a peritoneal puncture and injection of urographic contrast medium in about the same amounts as would be used in an excretory urogram. The patient is then positioned to allow the medium to run down to the hernial sites and one or two P.A. films are taken. A delayed film at 45 minutes should give a useful excretory urogram as a bonus if desired. This appears to be a safe and reliable diagnostic technique that was first described in 1967 but has not achieved general utilization (Ducharme et al., 1967; Shakelford and McAlister, 1972).

1.8. Pelvic pneumography

An uncommon procedure for investigating pelvic structures is pelvic pneumography which has been called andrography (Lunderquist and Rafstedt, 1967). It requires the intraperitoneal injection of nitrous oxide to outline the pelvic structures and to search for an undescended testes.

1.9. Computerized tomography

This addition to the diagnostic armamentarium provides information about pelvic masses that is available in no other way. It also provides a means of assessing retroperitoneal lymph nodes in the investigation of the spread of testicular tumors (Boldt and Reilly, 1977; Kreel, 1976; Lee et al., 1978).

2. CLINICAL APPLICATIONS OF RADIO-GRAPHIC TECHNIQUES

2.1. Trauma

Fifteen percent of pelvic trauma sufficient to cause fracture is associated with disruption of either the bladder or the urethra (Clarke and Prudencio, 1972). The usual cause is a motor vehicle accident. When the pubic bones break, great strain is placed on the urogenital diaphragm which may be disrupted, tearing the membranous urethra within it and the proximal bulbous urethra below it. Associated with this there may be disruption of the periprostatic venous plexus resulting in a large hematoma which will displace the prostatic gland upward and posteriorly. Injury to the spongy por-

tion of the urethra is most likely from a straddle injury, surgical instrumentation, or a knife or gunshot wound. Of all injuries to the lower urinary tract, 60% involve the urethra and 40% involve the bladder.

Whenever significant trauma to the bladder or urethra is suspected, a retrograde urethrogram should be the first radiological procedure (Fig. 2c). Physical examination of the injured patient may demonstrate prominence in the suprapubic region or peritoneal irritation caused by blood or a distended bladder. There may be discoloration and swelling of the perineum, scrotum and penis if there has been extensive extravasation of blood and urine extraperitoneally. Rectal examination may reveal injuries in the anus and rectum and allows evaluation of the prostate gland. Hematuria throughout urination usually indicates bleeding from a site higher than the urethra while hematuria which clears during urination indicates a urethral lesion. There is no correlation between the seriousness of the injury and the amount of bleeding. The inability of the conscious patient to urinate in the presence of a distended bladder or blood extruding from the external meatus are diagnostic signs of an injured urethra.

The injudicious use of a diagnostic catheter is to be avoided. Careless catheterization can infect a perivesical hematoma by introducing bacteria. Blood issuing from a catheter passed into a hematoma may be misinterpreted as blood from the bladder. These errors may all be avoided by performing a retrograde urethrogram as the first diagnostic procedure. It is carried out as described earlier. If the contrast flows freely into the bladder, the urethra is intact and the catheter can be advanced to fill the bladder with contrast to rule out its rupture. The catheter can be left in place at the end of the examination to avoid subsequent catheterization. Intraperitoneal extravasation of the contrast is shown by the contrast outlining loops of bowel; extraperitoneal extravasation is recognized as irregular collections of contrast, like tear drops above the bladder.

An intravenous urogram should be performed at this time to rule out injury of the upper tract. Anyone suffering an injury severe enough to have hematuria should be suspected of having a renal injury as well. The examination should be done with an infusion with a large amount of contrast medium and tomography if possible in the nephrogram phase. By this method renal lacerations can be diagnosed.

2.2. Peyronie's disease and priapism

Peyronie's disease is usually of unknown etiology, and is characterized by fibrous plaques developing in the corpora cavernosa (Thomas and Rose, 1972). Sometimes it is secondary to trauma to the penis. The patient complains of painful erections or impotence. Hard plaques can be palpated along the shaft of the penis although palpation seldom reveals the full extent of the lesion. Soft tissue radiographs may reveal areas of calcification which usually indicate that surgery will be required. When there is no calcification, cortisone is used in the treatment. Corpus cavernosography is useful to determine the extent of the plaques and the induration around the septum which cannot be detected by palpation. Response to treatment with corticosteroids can be followed with repeated examinations. The drainage time of the corpora is often delayed to $1\frac{3}{4}$ hr but with treatment this may return to the normal $1-1\frac{1}{2}$ hr.

Priapism is a state of sustained penile erection. Local changes in the corpora cavernosa may cause slowing of the drainage via the deep dorsal veins of the penis. Priapism is usually of unknown etiology but may be associated with sickle cell anemia, or prostatitis. It only occurs proximal to the suspensory ligament where a congenital membrane is found in each corpus at the peno-scrotal junction separating turgid proximal from flaccid distal erectile tissue. Cavernosography is best performed during a quiescent stage when the penis is flaccid.

2.3. Penile prostheses

Penile prostheses are devices which are inserted surgically into the corpora cavernosa to achieve erection. A corpus cavernosogram could be done prior to insertion to determine the patency of the corporal tubes in patients in whom corporal fibrosis is a possibility. Fibrosis from previous priapism would change the surgical approach to the prosthesis. Inflatable prostheses are usually filled with radiopaque fluid so that function of the device can be checked fluoroscopically.

2.4. Glands, ducts, cysts and structures impressing themselves on the urethra

Cowper's glands are two accessory male sex glands the size of peas lying at the level of the membranous urethra between the two layers of the urogenital diaphragm. Each is drained by a duct about one inch long which passes distally alongside the urethra to enter the bulbous urethra. These glands discharge a clear fluid which acts as a lubricant and vehicle for the sperm. These structures may be opacified as an incidental finding at cystourethrography. They are much more frequently filled when there is a distal stricture or a urethral infection, or if they are dilated. Cowper's glands rarely cause symptoms unless they are infected or obstructed, or if there are stones in their ducts. Most so-called 'diverticula' originating from the ventral surface of the proximal bulbous urethra probably represent congenitally dilated Cowper's ducts and glands. The glands themselves are far less frequently visualized than the ducts. If the Cowper's ducts are blocked, retention cysts form and these may cause dysuria frequency or even urinary retention. Their cystic dilatation shows up as smooth rounded defects in the posterior wall of the urethra during urethrography. After surgical drainage of a Cowper's duct cyst, urethrography may show reflux into a dilated duct.

Cystic structures may impress themselves upon the posterior urethra or communicate with it. A Müllerian duct cyst, the result of incomplete Müllerian inhibition, is a midline cyst in the region of the prostate. It may present as a mass palpable on rectal examination. It tends to be large, may be associated with urinary tract infections, and may contain calculi. It does not contain sperm. A Müllerian duct cyst may rarely be associated with renal agenesis. Seminal vesicle cysts tend to be located laterally. They may contain sperm but do not contain stones. They are often associated with renal agenesis and ectopic hypoplastic ureter. They can be demonstrated by vasography, urethrography or injection during endoscopy. Ejaculatory duct cysts and prostatic cysts are smaller, laterally placed, and do not contain stones or sperm. Rare cysts are hydatid cysts of the prostate. In all these cases vasography may be worth undertaking to show patency of the epididymis, vas deferens, seminal vesicles, ejaculatory duct and verumontanum prior to surgery. A seminal vesicle cyst which does not communicate with the urethra may be injected through the rectum and filled with contrast material as part of the investigation. Patients with these lesions should all have excretory urograms to assess their ureters and kidneys (Levisay et al., 1975).

2.5. Duplication of the urethra

A rare anomaly of the tissues forming the abdominal wall and external genitalia is an accessory or duplicated urethra. The duplication may be complete or incomplete and is usually associated with obvious penile or scrotal anomalies. It is important to inspect the genital area carefully to find tiny orifices that may be seen to pass urine. These can be injected with contrast material using sialography catheters to outline their anatomy. There are several various categories of urethral duplication: the blind accessory urethra with the meatus opening externally to the skin or internally to the urethra, a Y-shaped duplication in which one end communicates with the skin surface of the penis and the other joins the urethra, complete duplication of the two parallel channels passing from the bladder, and an accessory channel conveying seminal fluid which is independent of the urethra. This is really an ectopic ejaculatory duct. A double urethra is generally asymptomatic but attention is drawn because of an abnormal penile and genital appearance, double urinary stream, infection of incontinence.

2.6. Sexual ambiguity and hypospadias

The sex of an infant is usually assigned immediately upon delivery. Although this is normally easily done after examining the external genitalia which are clearly male or female, a few children have genital abnormalities such as hypospadias, micropenis, or clitoral enlargement that raise the question of which sex should be assigned. These children should be investigated immediately and the investigation should include urethrography. Not everyone agrees on the importance of radiological investigation (Dewhurst, 1975; Shopfner, 1964), but the knowledge of internal anatomy gained with relative ease and safety by urethrography justifies

the procedure. Even when surgical exploration is intended, pre-operative knowledge of Müllerian derivatives will help the surgeon decide whether to leave gonads in place or to remove them. As in other situations, the more information available, the more likely is management to be appropriate. Genitography consists of injecting contrast medium into the urethral or vaginal openings by means of a small catheter. Soft rubber catheters, feeding tubes or cut-off plastic intravenous catheters are suitable methods of introducing contrast. Filling the urethra will usually fill urogenital sinus remnants or Müllerian structures if these are present and connecting with the urethra (Fig. 3d). Occasionally however these do not fill and are only later discovered at operation. At operation, injection of the lumen of Müllerian structures may show a communication with the urethra which could not be shown previously at urethrography. Similarly, at operation, Wolffian duct derivatives (vasa deferentia) can be injected to determine their connection with the urethra.

The presence of a urogenital sinus remnant indicates incomplete masculinization of the sinus by dihydrotestosterone and is usually associated with hypospadias. The presence of Müllerian structures indicates failure of Müllerian inhibiting substance (MIS) to act. It may indicate that no testes are present or that the testes are incapable of producing MIS. Since both MIS action on the Müllerian duct and testosterone action on the Wolffian duct occur only on the same side as the functioning testis, there can be unilateral Müllerian structures. A vaginal introitus in the perineum may lead to a normal vagina, uterus and tubes or it may just be a urogenital sinus remnant. Vaginography by injection of contrast medium provides an easy way to determine the size of the vagina and the presence of a cervix as indicators of Müllerian development.

Most children with sexual ambiguity other than those with adrenal hyperplasia will have an exploratory laparotomy for gonadal localization and biopsy. In general, the role of genitography is to detect urogenital sinus remnants and Müllerian structures. This will usually be possible pre-operatively but contrast injection at the time of operation should be considered when ambiguous structures are encountered. Since the majority of children with ambiguous genitalia will be assigned a female sex of rearing, it will usually be advantageous to retain

those structures of Müllerian origin.

Hypospadias is usually treated surgically to create a longer penile urethra. Following such a repair, the urethra will be irregular in outline, and may develop a stricture, or occasionally a urethral calculus (Fig. 3c).

2.7. Posterior urethral valves

Posterior urethral valves are exaggerated epithelial folds which obstruct the posterior urethra just below the verumontanum (Fig. 3a). The degree of obstruction is variable. The posterior urethra is invariably dilated in boys with valves. The bladder is usually thick-walled and sacculated and there is often vesico-ureteral reflux into dilated ureters and hydronephrotic upper tracts.

Boys with posterior urethral valves have a poor urinary stream and their kidneys are at risk because of the obstruction. In the newborn, any child with an enlarged bladder, bilateral renal masses or any evidence or urinary obstruction should have a voiding cystourethrogram and an excretory urogram. It is easy to pass a catheter through these valves but the valves will not be seen until the catheter is removed and the patient voids. These valves are said to occur in patients with the prune-belly syndrome but because almost everyone with the syndrome has a dilated posterior urethra and poor bladder emptying, it is impossible to diagnose valves radiologically. They all look as if they might have valves. In any patient, the differential diagnosis of a dilated posterior urethra includes valves, stricture, neurogenic bladder and ectopic ureterocele prolapsing into the urethra. The thick-walled bladder of a patient with valves may have a prominent neck but this is unlikely to cause obstruction.

Most patients with posterior urethral valves present early in life but a few have been diagnosed in adults. Patients with valves sometimes survive unrecognized and untreated into their adult years. They may be entirely asymptomatic or only mildly symptomatic with enuresis, frequency, urgency or occasional bouts of dysuria. They may on questioning, state that they have had a weak small stream all their life. Intravenous urograms are usually normal, but secondary reflux of urine into the seminal vesicles and vas may occur on voiding. In a group of 26 adults with valves, 15 had voiding

cystourethrograms and only two were normal. However, the findings tended to be relatively non-specific with either an abnormal bladder neck configuration or evidence of diminished flow with poor filling of the posterior urethra (Mahony and Laferte, 1974).

2.8. Anterior urethral valves

Anterior urethral valves are really diverticula in the wall of the urethra that fill during voiding to obstruct the lumen of the urethra. In general, anterior urethral valves usually present as swellings of the penis and dribbling of the urinary stream. The diverticulum is usually ventral to the penile urethra. Diagnosis is accomplished by cystourethrography (Fig. 3b). Early diagnosis and treatment is essential to prevent infection and obstruction of perforation. Diverticula or pseudodiverticula seen in patients with paraplegia or other severe neurological disease are the result of traumatic catheterization.

2.9. Imperforate anus

Boys with ano-rectal atresia almost always have communication between the rectum and the urethra. The exceptions are those with low atresias who have a communication between the rectum and skin and those with very high atresias who have a fistula from colon to bladder. Children born with ano-rectal atresia should have urethrography and they should also have excretory urograms or renal scans early in life because over 25% will have some urological anomaly (Parrott, 1977). After surgery to correct their rectal abnormality, cystourethrography will be helpful to assess the integrity of the urethra. Some of these post-operative patients will have posterior urethral diverticula. The origin of these diverticula is obscure but they may be remnants of rectourethral fistulae.

2.10. Cryptorchidism

How much radiographic investigation is reasonable in cryptorchidism? Some would say none, but others would insist on complicated procedures, even those requiring anesthesia. This is a common anomaly and the financial cost and the radiation

dose of investigation are appreciable. If we believe that any unnecessary radiography is a disservice to the patient, then we should be prepared to justify our procedure. A review of 400 intravenous urograms in asymptomatic cryptorchid boys showed that unless there were urinary infections or other significant anomalies then intravenous urography was not indicated in the routine investigation of cryptorchidism (Watson et al., 1974). Many unnecessary urograms would be avoided if that advice were heeded.

Testicular venography is advocated by some to locate undescended and ectopic testes (Weiss et al., 1977). Others prefer arteriography for the same purpose (Nordmark, 1977). Intraperitoneal nitrous oxide can be used to search for testes (Lunderquist and Rafstedt, 1967). Another method uses intraperitoneal urographic contrast material. Since none of these investigations obviates the need for surgical exploration, we question whether any should be considered necessary. On the other hand if a surgeon finds pre-operative localization a significant help to his operation, then whatever means is used, the result justifies the procedure.

2.11. Various syndromes with genital abnormalities (Taybi, 1975)

A patient with adrenogenital syndrome may show advanced skeletal maturation, excessive pneumatization of the skull, advanced dentition, and premature calcification of costal and thyroid cartilages. Radiographs of a patient with myotonic dystrophy, presenting with gonadal atrophy and frontal baldness, may show a thick calvarium, a small sella turcica, large frontal sinuses, hypotelorism, a large mandible, temporo-mandibular dislocation, fatty infiltration of atrophic muscles, diaphragmatic elevation, arachnodactyly or a deformed sternum (Fig. 1c). An obese retarded boy with hypogonadism due to Prader-Willi syndrome may have retarded skeletal maturation, microcranium, sutural bones in the skull, small sella turcica, absent sinuses, scoliosis, coxa valga, syndactyly, dislocated hips and osteoporosis. A skeletal survey of a patient with Laurence-Moon-Biedl syndrome may show polydactyly, syndactyly, clinodactyly of the 5th finger, skull defects and hip dysplasia. An excretory urogram may reveal renal abnormalities. Patients

with total lipodystrophy may present with hirsutism or penile enlargement early in life and a skeletal survey may show advanced skeletal maturation, excessive skull pneumatization, dense transverse lines in the vertebrae and calcification of the falx. Excretory urography will show large kidneys. The kidneys will not be visible on plain films because there is no fat surrounding them and it is only the fat around a kidney that makes it visible without the addition of contrast medium. Noonan's syndrome presenting as delayed puberty, may show hypertelorism, parietal foramina in the skull, a large head or a small head, steeply-sloped anterior fossae, retarded skeletal maturation, deformed sternum, vertebral anomalies, radial head dislocations, and clinodactyly of the 5th finger. Patients with Klinefelter's syndrome are tall thin eunuchoid males who may show radio-ulnar synostosis, long phalanges, narrow metacarpals and delayed skeletal maturation.

2.12. Urethral stricture

Urethral strictures are often the result of trauma, either accidental or iatrogenic (Fig. 2d). They may result from infections or for no known reason. Penoscrotal junction strictures are often the result of previous catheterizations. Strictures of the bulbous portion may occur with straddle injuries. They may be multiple following gonococcal infections and may occur following prostatectomies or resection of posterior urethral valves. It is essential to evaluate the degree of narrowing, the site, and the length of the stricture before the patient goes into retention and prior to instrumentation of the urethra. This involves a dynamic retrograde urethrogram and a voiding cystourethrogram. The two combined will delineate the exact anatomical degree of stricture and the length of the stricture. This will allow a decision to be made regarding dilatations or surgical repair. With strictures distal to the verumontanum there is frequently reflux of the contrast, not only into Cowper's ducts but also into ejaculatory ducts, seminal vesicles, and vas deferens right down to the epididymis. Similarly trabeculation of the bladder and vesico-ureteral reflux may occur. These can all be radiologically demonstrated on a voiding cystourethrogram.

2.13. Varicocele

A varicocele is a tortuous, dilated complex collection of veins involving the pampiniform plexus around the testis and epididymis in the scrotum. The condition is usually unilateral, left-sided and appears in young men after childhood. A painful varicocele or a varicocele in a patient with sterility may deserve surgical treatment. A recurrent varicocele, a varicocele on the right side, or one in a boy may deserve pre-operative investigation by venography (Diamond and Ravitz, 1975). Venography may be carried out pre-operatively via the testicular veins which normally show one to three valves between the inguinal ring and the insertion into the renal vein or the inferior vena cava. Other venous connections to the internal and external iliac veins may be shown by venography at the time of operation if indicated. The usual cause of a varicocele is absence of the valves in the testicular veins. Other causes which sometimes must be excluded include renal vein thrombosis, hydronephrosis and retroperitoneal tumor obstructing the testicular vein.

2.14. Prostatic enlargement

Prostatic enlargement causing urethral obstruction is a common problem. It may be due to benign hyperplasia or to carcinoma. Radiological investigation should include an excretory urogram, but cystourethrography is only necessary if a stricture is suspected. Long-standing obstruction of the urethra may cause bladder wall thickening and trabeculation. The lower ends of the ureters are typically elevated into a fish-hook shape as the trigone is pushed upward by the enlarging gland (Fig. 4c). The ureters may be dilated and there may be vesicoureteral reflux. The prostatic urethra is elongated or spread posteriorly and if the median lobe is enlarged, the proximal urethra is displaced anteriorly.

Benign hyperplasia causes smooth symmetrical filling defects in the base of the bladder while carcinoma tends to cause asymmetrical irregular filling defects which may mimic a bladder tumor. Rarely, carcinoma spreads along the urethra. Dilatation of one urether in a patient with prostatic

symptoms suggests carcinoma invading a seminal vesicle.

Osteoblastic skeletal metastases are characteristic of prostatic carcinoma (Fig. 1d). The earliest lesions are often in the iliac bones near the sacro-iliac joints where they may be mistaken for signs of rheumatoid arthritis or even benign bone islands. However they soon spread around the pelvis, sacrum, lumbar spine and upper femora to reveal their true nature. Occasionally prostatic metastases are difficult to differentiate from the lesions of myelofibrosis or Paget's disease. A patient can have both prostatic carcinoma and Paget's disease. The best mean of searching for skeletal metastases is the nuclear bone scan. If it shows one or two areas of increased bone metabolism, then those areas should be radiographed. If it shows many areas, no radiographic investigation is necessary because the diagnosis is self-evident. Similarly, if an abdominal film taken as part of an excretory urogram shows multiple osteoblastic lesions in the spine and pelvis, no bone scan is necessary.

2.15. Male sterility

The investigation of male sterility consists primarily of history, physical examination and laboratory tests. On rare occasions, intravenous urography, retrograde cystourethrography and vasography will be necessary. If an intravenous urogram demonstrates an ectopic kidney or agenesis of a kidney on one side, this suggests congenital anomalies of the Wolffian duct as a cause of the sterility. In such cases, vasograms should be performed to show patency of the epididymis, vas, seminal vesicles, ejaculatory duct and verumontanum. If a patient has azoospermia and a normal testicular biopsy, an obstructed vas deferens should be suspected. If he has arrested germinal cell maturation on biopsy, he probably has a patent vas.

2.16. Testicular neoplasms

Radiological investigation is not important in the primary diagnosis of testicular neoplasm, but plays an important role in the investigation and treatment of secondary disease. Recent advances in the detection of biochemical tumor markers which predict metastatic disease somewhere in the body, the availability of powerful chemotherapeutic agents, and the possibility of aggressive radical and complete lymph node dissection of the retroperitoneal spaces put the onus on the various imaging devices of radiological sciences to localize correctly and to find the recurrent disease. This information will influence the type of therapy and allow evaluation of response to therapy.

The retroperitoneal space is examined by intravenous urography, computerized tomography (CT), lymphography and ultrasonography (Fig. 4d). Metastases in nodes can be discovered and their response to the treatment monitored by CT or ultrasonography. Needle biopsy of retroperitoneal nodes which have previously been opacified at lymphography can be carried out under fluoroscopic control. After surgical dissection of retroperitoneal nodes, alternate lymphatic pathways develop and metastases may be found in unusual sites such as the omentum or mesentery (Pollack et al., 1978).

3. CONCLUDING REMARKS

Because of the multiplicity of radiological techniques available, clinicians and radiologists must collaborate to decide what should be done for a patient. If such collaboration does not take place, and if the clinician and radiologist work in isolation, then unnecessary examinations will be done and necessary ones will be omitted. The patient suffers when the best use is not made of available equipment and professional talent. Cystourethrography and excretory urography will remain the main means of investigating the genital system but computerized tomography will be of increasing importance in the pelvis and retroperitoneum. Knowledge and common sense will always be the most important tools of all.

REFERENCES

Ardran GM, Dixon-Brown A, Fursdon PS (1978) Gonad dose in cineurethrocystography. Br J Radiol 51: 210.

Boldt DW, Reilly BJ (1977) Computed tomography of abdominal mass lesions in children: initial experience. Radiology 124(2): 371.

Busch FM, Sayegh ES (1963) Roentgenographic visualization of human testicular lymphatics: a preliminary report. J Urol 89: 106.

Busch FM, Sayegh ES, Chenault OW (1965) Some uses of lymphangiography in the management of testicular tumors. J Urol 93: 490.

Bystrom J, Johansson B, Edgren J, Alfthan O, Kohler R (1974) Induratio penis plastica (Peyronie's disease). Cavernosography in assessment of the disease process. Scand J Urol Nephrol 8: 155.

Clark SS, Prudencio RF (1972) Lower urinary tract injuries associated with pelvic fractures. Diagnosis and management. Surg Clin North Am 52: 183.

Dewhurst CJ (1975) The Aetiology and management of intersexuality. Clin Endocrinol 4: 625.

Diamond A, Ravitz G (1975) Venographic demonstration of a varicocele in a boy. J Urol 114: 640.

Ducharme JC, Bertrand R, Chacar R (1967) Is it possible to diagnose inguinal hernia by X-ray? J Can Assoc Radiol 18: 448.

Eykyn S, Bultitude MI, Mayo ME, Lloyd-Davies RW (1974) Prostatic calculi as a source of recurrent bacteriuria in the male. Br J Urol 46: 527.

Fitzpatrick T (1975) The corpus cavernosum intercommunicating venous drainage system. J Urol 113: 494.

Fox M (1960) The association of stones in the upper urinary tract with prostatic calculi. Br J Urol 32: 458.

Greulich WW, Pyle SI (1959) Radiographic atlas of skeletal development of the hand and wrist, 2nd ed. Stanford: Stanford University Press.

Hafiz A, Melnick JC (1968) Calcification of the vas deferens. J Can Assoc Radiol 19: 56.

Hebert G, Bouchard R, Charron J (1971) Vasoseminal vesiculography. Am J Roentgenol 113: 735.

Hertz M, Werner A (1977) Radiation dose to the gonads during cystourethrography in children. Israel J Med Sci 13: 614.

Hill JT, Green NA (1977) Varicocele: a review of radiological and anatomical features in relation to surgical treatment. Br J Surg 64: 747.

Kaude JV, Lorenz E, Reed JM (1969) Gonad dose to children in voiding urethrocystography performed with 70 mm image-intensifier fluorography. Radiology 92: 771.

Kreel L (1976) The EMI whole body scanner in the demonstration of lymph node enlargement. Clin Radiol 27: 421.

Lee JKT, Stanley RJ, Sagel SS, McClennan BL (1978) Accuracy of CT in detecting intra-abdominal and pelvic lymph node metastases from pelvic cancers. Am J Roentgenol 131: 675.

Levisay GL, Holder J, Weigel JW (1975) Ureteral ectopia associated with seminal vesicle cyst and ipsilateral renal agenesis. Radiology 114(3): 571.

Lieberman P, Siegle RL, Taylor WW (1978) Anaphylactoid reactions to iodinated contrast material. J Allergy Clin Immunol 62(3): 174.

Lundequist A, Rafstedt S (1967) Roentgenologic diagnosis of cryptorchidism. J Urol 98: 219.

Mahony DT, Laferte RO (1974) Congenital posterior urethral valves in adult males. Urology 3: 724.

McAllister WH, Cacciarelli A, Shackelford GD (1974) Complications associated with cystography in children. Radiology 111: 167.

McCallum RW, Colapinto V (1976) Urological radiology of the adult male lower urinary tract. Springfield: Charles C. Thomas.

Ney C, Miller HL, Friedenberg RM (1976) Various applications of corpus cavernosography. Radiology 119: 69.

Nordmark L (1977) Angiography of the testicular artery. Acta Radiol Diag 18: 25.

Parrott TS (1977) Urologic implications of imperforate anus. Urology 10(5): 407.

Pollack HM, Banner MP, Ring EJ, Wein AJ (in press) Applications of thin needle aspiration biopsy in uroradiology.

Poznanski AK, Garn SM, Kuhns LR, Sandusky ST (1971) Dysharmonic maturation of the hand in the congenital malformation syndromes. Am J Phys Anthropol 35: 417.

Pratt AV, Galbraith RH, Kereiakes JG (1973) Evaluation of 16 mm cine cystourethrography in children: method and dosimetry. Radiology 106: 183.

Pyle SI, Hoerr NL (1969) A radiographic standard of reference for the growing knee. Springfield: Charles C Thomas.

Redman JF, Robinson CM (1977) Allergic reaction secondary to voiding cystourethrography. J Urol 9: 560.

Saenger EL, Kereiakes JG, Cavanaugh DJ, Hall JL, Eiseman W (1976) Cystourethrography procedures in children: evaluation of benefits vs dose. Radiology 118: 123.

Shackelford GD, McAlister WH (1972) Inguinal herniography. Am J Roentgenol, Radiat Ther Nucl Med 115(2): 399.

Shehadi WH (1975) Adverse reactions to intravenous administered contrast media. A comprehensive study based on a prospective survey. Am J Roentgenol 124: 145.

Shopfner CE (1964) Genitography in intersexual states. Radiology 82: 664.

Taybi H (1975) Radiology of syndromes. Chicago: Year Book Medical Publishers.

Thomas ML, Rose DH (1972) Peyronie's disease demonstrated by cavernosography. Acta Radiol Diag 12: 221.

Watson RA, Lennox KW, Gangai MP (1974) Simple cryptorchidism: the value of the excretory urogram as a screening method. J Urol 111: 789.

Weiss RM, Glickman MG, Lytton B (1977) Venographic localization of the non-palpable undescended testis in children. J Urol 117: 513.

13. NUCLEAR MEDICINE IN ANDROLOGY

N.D. GREYSON

Nuclear medicine is a diagnostic modality which utilizes a wide variety of pharmaceuticals with specific organ-localizing properties. These pharmaceuticals are labeled with a radioisotope which is detectable by means of external monitors, such as a gamma camera or rectilinear scanner.

The images obtained by these recording devices are of poor resolution when compared with conventional radiographs, computerized tomograms or ultrasound, but have the unique property of being 'functional images'. Following the administration of the radiopharmaceutical, the rate of accumulation, pattern of distribution within the organ, and rate of excretion are related to the physiological activity of the organ and thus reflect function as well as morphology.

While the slower rectilinear scanners are still useful the gamma camera has virtually replaced them for all new installations. The gamma camera permits very rapid imaging and thus rapidly changing patterns of distribution of radioactivity may be recorded. Such studies as radionuclide angiography of the scrotum demonstrate the blood flow to scrotal masses, differentiating vascular from non-vascular lesions.

A variety of pharmaceuticals, appropriately labeled with a radioactive tracer, have been developed to localize in a specific organ, such as bone, liver, etc. The localization in the organ usually requires an active metabolic interaction between the organ and the radiopharmaceutical. Some radiopharmaceuticals such as gallium-67 (^{67}Ga) citrate have the property of localizing in actively metabolizing tissues and have been useful for imaging soft tissue tumors and sites of inflammation. Difficulties in obtaining the optimal combination of pharmaceutical and safe radioactive label have not always been resolved. Thus, prostate imaging, while theoretically feasible, has not been clinically successful, and adrenal scanning, while successful, is expensive and results in a moderately high radiation exposure to the patient. The details of these radiopharmaceuticals will be dealt with in the specific sections.

1. RADIONUCLIDE SCROTAL IMAGING

Radionuclide scrotal imaging with ^{99m} Technetium (^{99m}Tc) pertechnetate and diagnostic ultrasound complement physical examination of the scrotal contents by palpation and transillumination (Winston et al., 1978). Diagnostic ultrasound applications are dealt with elsewhere in this book. Radionuclide imaging was 94% accurate in the diagnosis of a variety of intrascrotal lesions, while clinical assessment was only 48% accurate (Riley et al., 1976). The radionuclide scrotal image demonstrates the initial perfusion, and distribution of vascularity within the scrotum, producing a more specific diagnosis (Holder et al., 1977; Mishkin, 1977).

1.1. Method

The patient is placed supine with the gamma camera positioned over the scrotal area. The penis is taped up to the abdomen so that penile blood flow will not obscure scrotal contents. A lead shield, cut from lead impregnated rubber, or an old X ray apron is draped over the thighs with the scrotum resting on top of the shield. This provides a 'cold' non-radioactive background to assess the radioactivity within the scrotum.

An intravenous injection of 10 mCi of ^{99m}Tc-pertechnetate is injected rapidly into an antecubital vein and within 15 sec the bolus of activity is demonstrated in the iliac arteries and entering the scrotum. A series of six images taken at 3-sec intervals are obtained to show the arterial inflow, capillary phase, and venous return.

Following recirculation, within 1-5 min, a static image of the scrotum and contents is made, collecting 250,000-500,000 counts. Detail in the image may be enhanced by using a converging or pinhole collimator. This image demonstrates the blood pool and is a reflection of the volume of the vascular space.

1.2. Indications

Acute testicular torsion is a surgical emergency requiring immediate diagnosis and treatment to prevent complications of testicular infarction. However, the clinical symptoms of testicular pain, swelling, and tenderness may resemble orchitis or epididymitis. In children particularly, where untreated torsion may result in loss of testicular function, accurate diagnosis as early as possible is desirable. In adults, inflammatory conditions are more common and these do not require diagnosis as urgently, but diagnoses such as testicular hemorrhage, hydrocele, inguinal hernia and tumor may be made pre-operatively (Lutzker et al., 1977).

1.3. Results

The initial dynamic sequence is analogous to a low resolution angiogram and demonstrates the major arterial inflow. Hot areas on the 'flow study' are indicative of highly vascularized areas and usually represent regions of marked inflammation. Testicular tumors may have increased arterial blood flow, as will testicular arteriovenous malformations; varicoceles usually have a less rapid arterial inflow but will show increased blood pool on the venous phase of the study.

Areas of diminished arterial inflow are not as well delineated in the dynamic phase of the examination, but are best seen in the equilibration static image. This image is obtained within 5 min of injection and shows the composite arterial, capillary, and venous pools. Normally there is a uniform blush of activity

within the scrotum with slight accentuation of the testes. Inflammation or vascular lesions show activity considerably above background while areas of infarction, hemorrhage, and cystic changes are cold on the scan. Acute inflammatory lesions are initially diffusely hot, but with abscess formation a central cold area may be noted.

Untreated testicular torsion eventually produces an inflammatory response and appearance simulating an abscess. Thus, the test is most useful when performed as soon as possible after the onset of symptoms in order to produce an uncomplicated image for accurate diagnosis.

Typical findings in radionuclide scrotal imaging are summarized in Table 1. Examples are illustrated in Fig 1-5.

Gamma camera images may be quantified and flow curves, giving a semi-quantitative assessment of vascularity, can be generated from the dynamic flow study. It is possible that in the assessment of impotence and infertility, the measurement of testicular and penile blood flow may have some diagnostic applications.

The demonstration of avascularity of the testis in acute torsion is not of value in predicting the outcome of surgery, but persisting avascularity following correction of the torsion suggests nonviability of the testis.

2. TESTICULAR TUMOR IMAGING

The diagnosis of testicular lesions by scrotal scanning depends on the relative blood pool of the scrotal contents. There is no radiopharmaceutical available which specifically localizes in the testis. However, ^{67}Ga citrate has been found to localize in a wide variety of tumors and acute inflammatory conditions. This has been applied to imaging of testicular neoplasms and soft tissue metastases (Bailey et al., 1973; Jackson et al., 1976).

When injected intravenously, gallium binds to plasma proteins, particularly transferrin, lactoferrin, albumin and haptoglobins. The protein bound gallium is carried to the tumor site by the increased blood flow to the area and passes into the extracapillary space where it exchanges its binding protein for the cell membrane. It then localizes intracellularly where it is bound to organelles called 'Gal-

Table 1. Diagnosis by ^{99m}Tc scrotal scanning.

Lesion	Radionuclide angiogram	Blood pool	Comment
Normal	Symmetrical faint scrotal blush	Faint symmetrical scrotal activity, testis slightly visible	
Acute torsion of testis	↓ flow	Cold on affected side	
Subacute torsion	↓ flow to testis, ↑ flow to rim	Cold testis, hyperemic rim	Simulates abscess
Torsion of appendix testis	Normal	Normal	
Acute epididymo-orchitis	↑ flow	Hyperemic testis and cord	
Abscess	↓ flow central, ↑ flow peripheral	Cold center, hyperemic rim	
Hematoma	↓ or normal	Hematoma cold ± hyperemic rim	Inflammatory response to trauma
Hernia	↓ or normal	Avascular mass, both testes seen	
Hydrocele	↓ or normal	Avascular mass surrounds normal testis	
Varicocele	Normal or ↑ venous phase	Vascular mass	
Neoplasm	Slight ↑ or normal	Large testis, slight hyperemic but often irregular	Variable depends on type and presence of necrosis
Atrophy	↓ flow	Small scrotum and testes	
Non-descended testis	↓ flow	Non-visualized testis	

lium Binding Granules' which are similar to lysosomes. Not all tumors have a propensity for concentrating ^{67}Ga citrate, but various of the lymphomas, melanoma, hepatoma, primary brain tumors, and lung malignancies may be demonstrated on a gallium scan. There has been moderate success in the use of gallium scanning in the presence of testicular neoplasms, and the detection of metastases.

Three to five millicuries of ^{67}Ga citrate is administered intravenously and imaging is begun approximately 48 hr after the injection, during which time the non-localized radioactivity in the body background is diminishing. A normal gallium image shows moderate uptake in the liver and spleen, the nasopharyngeal region, lacrimal glands, estrogen stimulated breasts (see 'Gynecomastia', below), and diffuse skeletal uptake. A large percentage of the gallium is excreted via the colon and meticulous bowel cleansing prior to imaging is necessary to prevent confusion of fecal activity with intra-abdominal metastases. Repeat scanning following a further bowel purge is often required to confirm the positive finding. The diagnosis of metastases is made by the demonstration of a persisting focal accumulation of gallium outside the sites of normal uptake (Fig. 6).

As gallium also concentrates in active inflammatory sites and healing operative incisions, false positive diagnoses due to these causes should be excluded.

Gallium may also be concentrated in the lungs following lymphangiography because of the inflammatory reaction of the lungs to iodinated oily contrast administered via the lymphatic route. Thus, if both gallium scanning and abdominal lymphangiography are considered at the time of tumor staging, the gallium scan should precede the lymphangiogram. Jackson et al. (1976) compared the results of gallium scanning with staging via lymphangiography, radiography, surgery, and autopsy. In 13 patients five had confirmed gallium positive metastases with one false negative study. Seven patients with normal gallium scans had no other evidence for tumor.

Paterson et al. (1976) found that 13 of 15 seminomas demonstrated true positive scans with two false negative studies. Eight teratomas in the series showed no abnormal uptake.

As a non-invasive means of detecting testicular metastases, particularly in areas not amenable to conventional lymphangiography, gallium scanning should be included in the diagnostic evaluation of these patients. It may also be useful in pre-operative diagnosis of seminoma in adult patients with untreated non-descended testes.

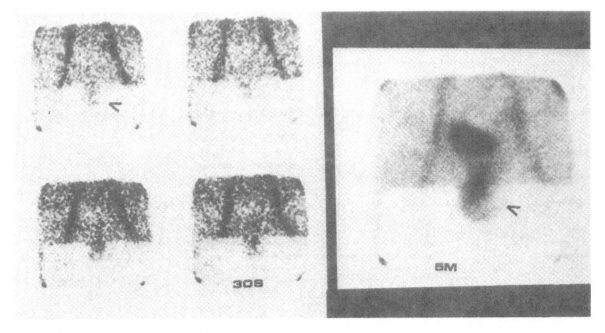

Figure 1. Scrotal scan in 7-year-old boy with 6-hr history of severe pain in the left testis. Sequential flow images show diminished perfusion to the left hemiscrotum, and blood pool images at 5 min shows diminished vascularity in the area of the left testis (arrows).

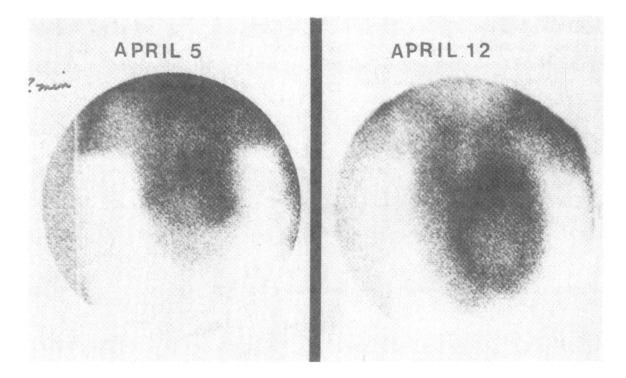

Figure 2. Scrotal scans in a 17-year-old boy with left testicular pain. History suggested similar episodes previously. The first scan of 5 April shows slight hyperemia in the area of the left testis and ultrasound examination also showed good blood supply. An inflammatory process was diagnosed and the patient was treated conservatively with antibiotics. However, over the next week the pain intensified and the testis enlarged. The repeat scan on 12 April shows a large cold center with a hyperemic rim surrounding the left testis. This was interpreted as either a necrotic testis with an inflammatory reaction or an abscess. At surgery the testis was hypermobile and necrotic, without evidence of pus. The revised diagnosis was recurrent torsion of the testis which, at the scan of 5 April had spontaneously corrected and showed mild inflammatory response. Probable re-torsion produced testicular infarction. (Figures 1 and 2 through the courtesy of Doctors J.M. Ash and D.L. Gilday, Hospital for Sick Children, Toronto.)

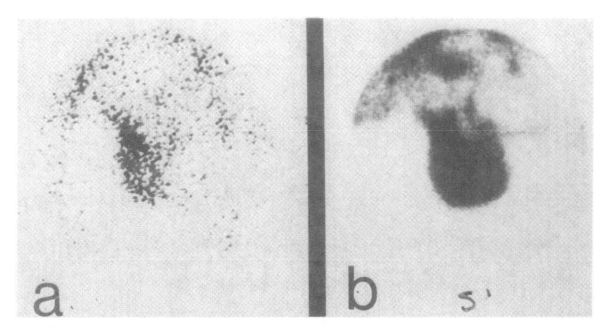

Figure 3. Scrotal scan in 38-year-old man with pain in the right testis. The flow image (a) shows intense hyperemia to the right scrotum, particularly in the area of the epididymis and cord. Equilibration blood pool image (b) shows generalized hyperemia of the scrotum, more marked on the right side. Diagnosis of epididymo-orchitis was made and the patient was treated conservatively.

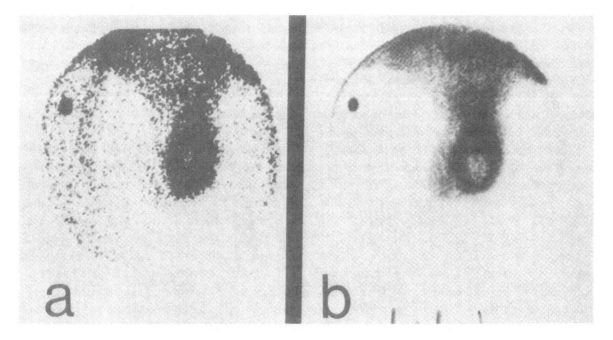

Figure 4. Scrotal scan in 25-year-old male with 2-week history of swelling and pain in the left testis. The flow phase (a) shows intense increased blood flow to the left scrotum, accentuating a hyperemic rim surrounding the left testis. The equilibration blood pool image (b) shows diminished blood pool in the left testis with marked hyperemia surrounding. The right testis appears normal. At surgery the left testis was necrotic and a pus-filled abscess sac was drained.

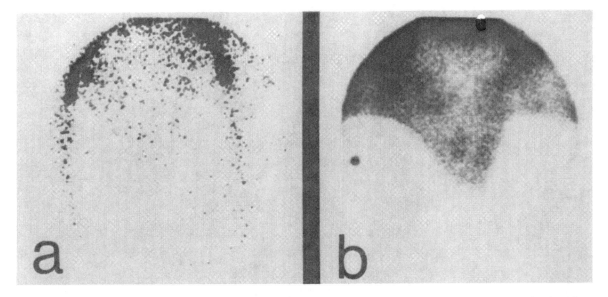

Figure 5. Scrotal scan in a 52-year-old alcoholic with long standing liver disease, gynecomastia and testicular atrophy. The blood flow phase (a) shows generally reduced blood flow to the scrotum. The equilibration blood pool image (b) shows a small scrotum with faint visualization of the testes.

3. PROSTATE IMAGING WITH RADIOISOTOPES OF ZINC

High concentrations of the trace element, zinc, were detected in the prostate, seminal vesicles, kidneys, liver, and pancreas (Siegel et al., 1961; Wakeley et al., 1960). It was suspected that this might provide a means of imaging the prostate and differentiating benign from malignant diseases (Verrelli et al., 1962). Gold and Lorber (1970) demonstrated localization of zinc in prostates of dogs and showed good uptake of zinc in normal and hypertrophied prostates with poor uptake in carcinomatous organs.

In the human, research has been handicapped by the physical properties of the radioisotopes of zinc available. Zinc-69m has a 13.8-hr half-life and is relatively safe for use in humans in low doses, but is not generally available. It does, however, contain an impurity of zinc-65 which has a 245-day half-life. This contaminant gives a relatively high radiation burden to the patient. Thus, only small amounts of radio-zinc may be administered and imaging has proved disappointing (Chisholm et al., 1974).

More specific localization using zinc-62 amino acid chelate (Yano and Budinger, 1977) has been partly successful. Iodinated estradiol and diethylstiboestrol localize in normal and hypertrophied prostates, but poorly in carcinoma (Szendroi et al.,

1973). The high radiation dose of the iodine-131 label has been reduced by the use of the short-lived, but not readily available, iodine-123 (Ghanadian et al., 1976).

It is likely that eventually a suitable prostate localizing pharmaceutical may be developed, but at present, prostate scanning is not a clinically useful procedure.

4. BONE SCANNING FOR PROSTATIC METASTASES

The development of ^{99m}Tc labeled organic phosphates and diphosphonates has permitted the widespread safe use of radionuclide scanning in a variety of benign and malignant conditions. These radiopharmaceuticals are avid bone localizers and high quality bone images are readily obtained following an intravenous injection of 15 mCi of ^{99m}Tc labeled methylene diphosphonate or one of the many other available phosphate derivatives.

Roughly 50% of the administered dose is localized in the bone and the remainder is excreted in 2-6 hr. Thus, a bone scan performed 2 or more hours after injection shows good visualization of the normal skeleton with areas of increased uptake in regions of increased bone metabolism. As an in-

cidental finding, the urinary tract and bladder are outlined, and obstruction, renal abnormalities and bladder lesions are demonstrated on the bone scan.

Increased uptake is noted in any focal bone lesion producing osteoblastic activity and in metabolic bone diseases producing rapid calcium turnover. The bone scan seems particularly well suited to the detection of metastases from carcinoma of the

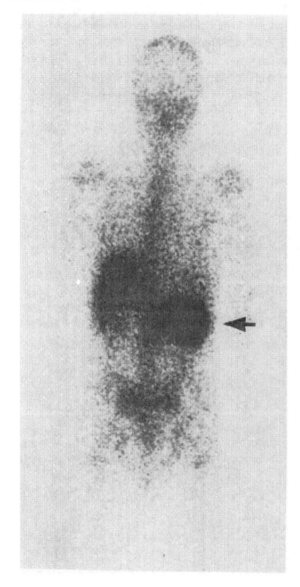

Figure 6. Gallium-67 citrate scan, posterior view, in a 27-year-old male with recent orchiectomy for seminoma of the testis. X-ray lymphangiography was negative. The gallium scan shows the normal distribution of gallium in the skeleton and liver. There is a large area of intense uptake in the left abdomen (arrow) which is not a normal site of gallium accumulation. Laparotomy confirmed the presence of metastatic seminoma in this area. (This case courtesy of the Department of Nuclear Medicine, Cross Cancer Institute, Edmonton, Alberta.)

prostate because of the relatively high osteoblastic response to these lesions.

Conventional radiographs have been used as the traditional skeletal metastatic survey, but a 30-50% alteration in bone calcium content is required to be detected has altered density on the radiograph. The bone scan is able to detect altered bone metabolism at a much earlier stage. The bone scan is also able to detect lesions in areas difficult to visualize on plain X rays, such as rib ends, scapula, and base of skull. It is easier to perform on a patient complaining of bone pain than a metastatic survey. The whole body may be imaged with the patient remaining supine on the scanning table for 20-40 min.

Many studies confirm the sensitivity of the bone scan in the early detection of prostatic metastases. Pistenma et al. (1975) showed 64% agreement between radiographs and the scan, while in 28,5% of 200 patients, the X ray was unable to detect metastases when the scan was positive. There were only 1.5% of patients in whom the X ray was positive when the scan was negative. Lentle et al. (1974) found 34 abnormal scans in 100 newly diagnosed patients with carcinoma of the prostate, while the radiographs were positive in only 18 patients. Eleven of the 16 patients had positive radiographs on later studies or on re-interpretation of the initial X ray.

Even combinations of radiographs and serum enzymes are not as reliable as the bone scan (Schaffer and Pendergrass, 1976). Shafer and Reinke (1977) compared bone scans with radiographs and blood enzymes in 110 newly diagnosed patients. Thirty-seven had positive bone scans, 25 had abnormal radiographs, 20 had abnormal alkaline phosphatase, and 18 had abnormal acid phosphatase. The alkaline phosphatase was abnormal in 18 patients with normal bone scans and the acid phosphatase abnormal in 12 patients without other evidence of metastases.

Our current routine recommends bone scans on all newly diagnosed patients with tumors of the prostate. Any abnormal areas detected are specifically radiographed to exclude benign causes such as fracture, Paget's disease, etc. Any area of focal bone pain should also be radiographed. The course of therapy is then followed with sequential bone scans (Fig. 7). It is noted that during estrogen therapy the bone scan might revert back to normal even though

the radiograph still shows an osteoblastic lesion. The scan demonstrates that the hormone therapy has suppressed the activity of the metastatic deposit, although the radiographs still reflect the former osteoblastic nature of the lesion (Fig. 8).

5. ADDITIONAL METASTATIC STAGING TECHNIQUES

5.1. Liver scanning

The sinusoids of the liver are lined with Kupfer cells which are part of the reticuloendothelial system (R.E.S.). The cells remove particulate matter from the sinusoids which are perfused by the portal vein.

Approximately 80% of the reticuloendothelial function resides in the liver, with smaller percentages in the spleen, bone marrow, and diffusely throughout the body. Following the injection of 3-5 mCi of ^{99m}Tc labeled sulfur colloid particles, there is rapid localization within the liver and spleen, outlining the distribution of functioning R.E.S. in these organs. Any lesions displacing or replacing the R.E.S. cells will fail to accumulate the radioactivity and result in a cold area on the scan. The limit of resolution is approximately 2 cm and thus very tiny solitary deposits are not visible. Liver scanning has roughly 85% accuracy in detecting metastases and is more sensitive than serum enzyme determinations of liver disease.

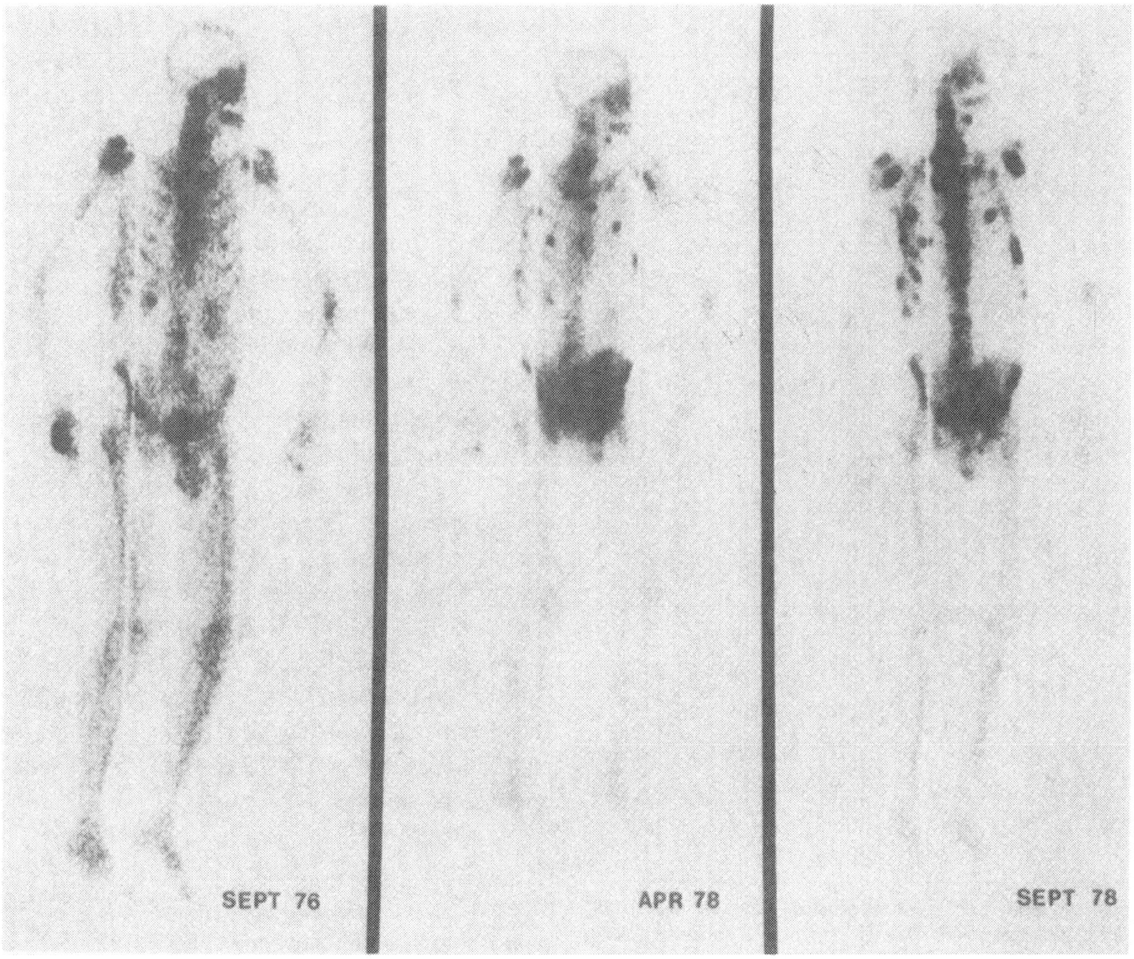

SEPT 76   APR 78   SEPT 78

Figure 7. Technetium-99-methylene diphosphonate bone scans in a 62-year-old man with carcinoma of the prostate. The initital scan, taken in September 1976, shows uptake in the right shoulder which may be due to metastatic or degenerative joint disease. The scan taken in May 1978 shows multiple metastatic deposits in the ribs, spine and pelvis and both shoulders. Although the patient was complaining of bone pain, radiographs were normal at that time. The follow-up scan (September 1978) shows further progression of the metastases. Radiographs now show osteoblastic changes in some of the involved areas.

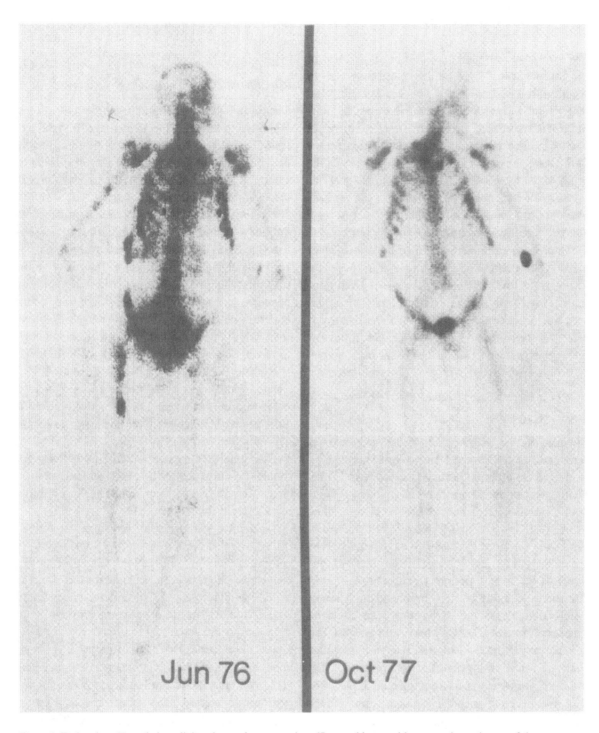

Figure 8. Technetium-99-methylene diphosphonate bone scans in a 67-year-old man with metastatic carcinoma of the prostate. The scan of June 1976 shows multiple metastatic deposits throughout the ribs, spine, pelvis, and long bones. The patient was treated with orchidectomy and estrogens and the follow-up scan (October 1977) shows marked improvement with overall diminution of activity, indicating suppression of the metastases, although radiographs were unchanged.

5.2. Brain scanning

Following the intravenous injection of 15 mCi of the ionized salt, ^{99m}Tc sodium pertechnetate, an equilibration is established between the intravascular and extravascular distribution of this radiopharmaceutical. However, the blood-brain barrier is impermeable to this material and images of the head show the extracerebral tissues, while the brain remains non-radioactive. Lesions such as primary or secondary brain tumors, as well as cerebral infarcts and infalmmatory lesions have altered capillary permeability which permits the diffusion of the radioactivity into the lesion. Brain scans in these cases will show the area of the lesion to be radioactive, surrounded by the normal non-radioactive brain substance. Although the brain scan is non-specific, it is a sensitive means of detecting intracranial metastases, and following their progress. The role of brain scanning in the detection of perisellar lesions is discussed below.

5.3. Lung scanning

The distribution of pulmonary artery perfusion is demonstrated following the intravenous injection of human serum albumin particles labeled with ^{99m}Tc. These particles are larger than the capillary bed and thus diffusely microembolize the lungs and show patency of the pulmonary artery circulation. Lesions with a tendency to metastasize to lung, such as testicular tumors, may be evident on the scan, but as the scan has a poorer resolution than conventional radiographs, any peripheral lung lesion which could be diagnosed by lung scan could be diagnosed much earlier on chest radiographs. The possible exception is the presence of a perihilar metastasis obstructing the pulmonary artery. This situation, however, is uncommon and lung scanning is not recommended to detect pulmonary metastases.

6. NUCLEAR ASSESSMENT OF OTHER ENDOCRINE ORGANS

As many of the patients brought to the attention of the andrologist have complex endocrinological problems, a brief review of the nuclear medicine applications in related endocrine organs may be useful.

6.1. Thyroid uptake and scan

The thyroid gland traps and organifies a portion of the dietary iodides. The percentage trapped and oganified is one of the measures of thyroid function and this is easily determined by the oral administration of a small quantity of radioactive iodine-131 in the sodium iodide form.

The initial radioactivity of the capsule is determined, and the concentration of the radioactivity over the thyroid gland is detected at intervals. The early accumulation reflects the thyroid trapping function while the 24-hr uptake by the gland is a measure of the organified and stored radioiodinated thyroid hormones. The percentage of radioactivity within the gland compared with the administered dose is a reflection of the activity of the gland. Clinicians should be aware that the normal range of iodine uptake has been decreasing as there is increased use of iodized salt in many food stuffs. Normal ranges vary, but in our locality, the normal 24-hr uptake is 6-25%.

This is but one measure of thyroid activity and should be correlated with other indices, such as circulating T3 and T4 hormone levels in establishing a thyroid function profile.

Technetium-99m pertechnetate ion is also trapped by the thyroid gland, although it is not organified and intravenous administration of the sodium pertechnetate salt results in accumulation of activity within the thyroid gland. The gland may be imaged within 20 min after intravenous administration of the pertechnetate ion, or 24 hr after the administration of radioiodine. There is a disparity of findings: good visualization of the pertechnetate image with very low iodine uptake indicates good trapping but poor organification. This might result from an enzyme defect of organification or occult painless thyroiditis (Fig. 9). The gland as imaged by either ^{131}I or ^{99m}Tc shows the morphology of the thyroid and may define nodules within the gland substance. Comparison of the scan image with the palpation findings may characterize a nodule as being functioning (shows uptake on the scan) or nonfunctioning ('cold').

6.2. Pituitary gland

As indicated in the section on brain scanning above, brain tumors are associated with an abnormality of the blood-brain barrier which permits the diffusion of the radioisotope into the lesion. Solid pituitary tumors such as chromophilic or chromophobic adenomas may be visualized on the brain scan as a focal area of increased uptake in the sellar region. The brain scan normally has a high level of activity in the cranial floor and this frequently obscures lesions at the base of the brain. Pituitary lesions are thus not generally appreciated on the brain scan until they are large enough to rise up out of the sella. By this time, however, the lesions are associated with erosions of the clinoids and are readily demonstrated on plain skull films before they are large enough to be visualized on a brain scan. Craniopharyngiomas, despite their large size are often not visualized on the brain scan, particularly if they are cystic in nature (Penning and Front, 1975). An example of a mixed solid and cystic craniopharyngioma is illustrated in Fig. 10.

Thus, brain scanning is an insensitive means of detecting pituitary lesions and assessment by other means such as computerized tomography of the base of the skull is a more valuable modality (Alderson et al., 1977).

6.3. Adrenal gland

In 1971, radioiodinated 19-iodocholesterol was synthesized (Counsell et al., 1970) and this radiopharmaceutical was used successfully as an adrenal cortex scanning agent (Beierwaltes et al., 1974; Blair et al., 1971). Subsequently, other labeled steroids have demonstrated improved adrenal localizing properties (Sarkar et al., 1975).

Images of the adrenal gland are of poor resolution, but demonstrate cortical function of the adrenals and are able to demonstrate functioning neoplasms, hyperplasia, and adrenal insufficiency. Imaging may be done with and without suppression for differential diagnosis of hyperplasia versus adenomas.

The radiopharmaceutical is regrettably expensive and the iodine-131 label results in a moderately high patient radiation dose. It does, however, provide non-invasive assessment and directs the clinician to the site of the lesion and may indicate bilateral adrenal disease when a unilateral lesion is suspected.

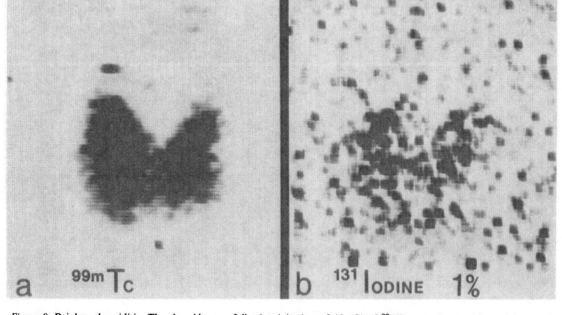

Figure 9. Painless thyroiditis. The thyroid scan, following injection of 10mCi of ^{99m}Tc-pertechnetate shows very good visualization of the gland. The iodine-131 scan, taken on the same day, shows poor visualization due to only 1% iodine uptake. The disparity between pertechnetate trapping and 24-hr iodine uptake (organification) helps confirm the diagnosis of asymptomatic subacute thyroiditis, suspected only because of elevated serum hormone levels.

7. GYNECOMASTIA

Physical examination is sufficient to diagnose gyne-comastia, but it may be demonstrated on a bone scan or gallium scan as an incidental finding. As mentioned in the section on gallium scanning, gallium binds to lactoferrin (Hoffer et al., 1977) which has a high concentration in the breast, particularly under estrogen stimulation. In bone scanning of patients on estrogen therapy, increased male breast tissue may be demonstrated as diffuse increased soft tissue activity overlying the ribs.

8. SUMMARY

Nuclear medicine techniques provide physiological images which have some use in diagnosing diseases

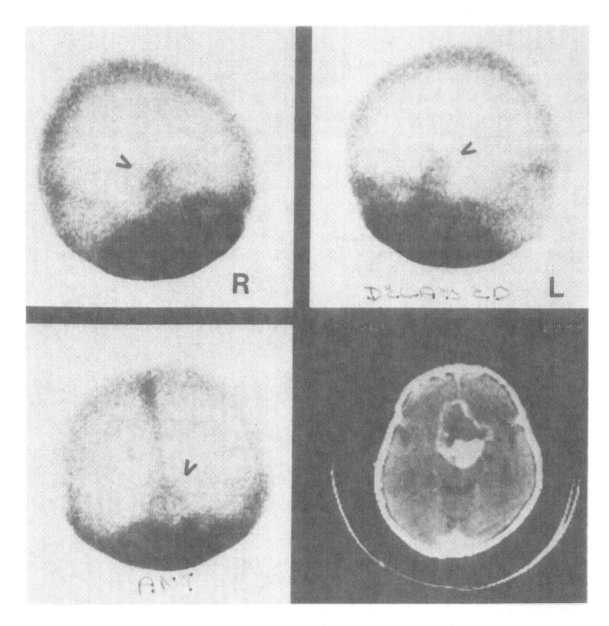

Figure 10. Static brain images in a 24-year-old with panhypopituitarism due to recurrent craniopharyngioma. Right and left lateral and anterior scans show uptake in the posterior portion of the tumor (arrows) which correspond to the densely calcified area seen on the computerized tomographic section through the skull. There is a faint rim-like uptake in the anterior portion of the tumor, which corresponds to a cyst wall anteriorly.

of male sex organs and endocrine disorders. Scrotal imaging permits early differentiation between torsion and inflammation of the testis as well as assessment of testicular masses. Soft tissue testicular metastases may be demonstrated by tumor-seeking radiopharmaceuticals such as ^{67}Ga citrate. Prostate imaging, per se, is not satisfactory, but assessment of skeletal metastases by bone scanning is of great clinical significance. Adrenal function and thyroid function and morphology are demonstrable by concentration of radionuclides relative to their physiological activity. Brain scanning demonstrates primary intracranial neoplasms in the region of the pituitary fossa as well as metastatic deposits from remote tumors. Liver scanning is a vital step in all metastatic surveys.

REFERENCES

Alderson PO, Gato MH, Siegel BA (1977) Computerized cranial tomography and radionuclide imaging in the detection of intracranial mass lesions. Semin Nucl Med 7: 161.

Bailey TB, Pinsky SM, Mittenmeyer BT et al. (1973) New adjuvant in testis tumor staging: gallium-67 citrate. J Urol 111: 307.

Beierwaltes WH, Sturman MF, Ryo U et al. (1974) Imaging functional nodules of the adrenal glands with ^{131}I-19-iodocholesterol. J Nucl Med 15: 246.

Blair RJ, Beierwaltes WH, Lieberman LM et al. (1971) Radiolabeled cholesterol as an adrenal scanning agent. J Nucl Med 12: 176.

Chisholm GD, Short MD, Ghanadian R, McRae CU, Glass HI (1974) Radiozinc uptake and scanning in prostatic disease. J Nucl Med 15: 739.

Counsell RE, Ranade VV, Blair RJ et al. (1970) Tumor localizing agents. IX. Radioiodinated cholesterol. Steroids 16: 317.

Ghanadian R, Waters SL, Williams G et al. (1976) The use of ^{123}I labelled oestradiol in detecting the human prostate using a gamma camera. Eur J Nucl Med 1: 159.

Gold FM, Lorber SA (1970) Radioisotope ^{69m}Zn chloride prostate gland scan: I^{69m}Zn organ distribution studies and gamma camera scan in canine subjects. Invest Urol 8: 231.

Hoffer PB, Huberty J, Kayam-Bashi H (1977) The association of Ga-67 and lactoferrin. J Nucl Med 18: 713.

Holder LE, Martire JR, Holmes ER III, Wagner HN Jr (1977) Testicular radionuclide angiography and static imaging: anatomy, scintigraphic interpretation, and clinical indications. Radiology 125: 739.

Jackson FI, Dierich HC, Lentle BC (1976) Gallium-67 citrate scintiscanning in testicular neoplasia. J Can Assoc Radiol 27: 84.

Lentle BC, McGowen DG, Dierick H (1974) Technetium-99m-polyphosphate bone scanning in carcinoma of the prostate. Br J Urol 46: 543.

Lutzker LG, Novich I, Perez LA, Freeman LM (1977) Radionuclide scrotal imaging. Appl Radiol/NM, Jan-Feb: 187.

Mishkin FS (1977) Differential diagnostic features of the radionuclide scrotal image. Am J Roentgenol 128: 127.

Paterson AHG, Peckham MJ, McCreedy VR (1976) Value of gallium scanning in seminoma of the testis. Br Med J 1: 1118.

Penning L, Front D (1975) Brain scintigraphy, a neuroradiological approach, pp 79-81. Amsterdam: Excerpta Medica.

Pistenma DA, McDougall JR, Kriss JP (1975) Screening for bone metastases: are only scans necessary? JAMA 231: 46.

Riley TW, Mosbaugh PG, Coles JL et al. (1976) Use of radioisotope scan in evaluation of intrascrotal lesions. J Urol 116: 472.

Sarkar SD, Beierwaltes WH, Ice RD, Basmadjian GP, Hetzel KR, Kennedy WP, Mason MM (1975) A new and superior adrenal scanning agent, NP-59. J Nucl Med 16: 1038.

Schaffer DL, Pendergrass HP (1976) Comparison of enzyme, clinical, radiographic, and radionuclide methods of detecting bone metastases from carcinoma of the prostate. Radiology 121: 431.

Shafer RB, Reinke DB (1977) Contribution of the bone scan, serum acid and alkaline phosphatase, and the radiographic bone survey to the management of newly-diagnosed carcinoma of the prostate (Abst.). J Nucl Med 18: 605.

Siegel E, Graig, FA Crystal MM (1961) Distribution of ^{65}Zn in the prostate and the organs of man. Br J Cancer 15: 647.

Szendroi Z, Kocsar L, Karika Z, Eckhardt S (1973) Isotope scanning of the prostate. Lancet i: 1252.

Verrelli RA, Brady LW, Croll MN et al. (1962) Zinc-65 uptake by the prostate. J Urol 88: 664.

Wakeley JCN, Moffat B, Crook A et al. (1960) The distribution and radiation dosimetry of zinc-65 in the rat. Int J Appl Radiat Isot 7: 225.

Winston MA, Handler SJ, Pritchard JH (1978) Ultrasonography of the testis – correlation with radiotracer perfusion. J Nucl Med 19: 615.

Yano Y, Budinger TF (1977) Cyclotron-produced Zn-62: its possible use in prostate and pancreas scanning as Zn-62 amino acid chelate. J Nucl Med 18: 815.

14. ULTRASONIC TECHNIQUES IN ANDROLOGY

M. MISKIN

This chapter will concern itself with the ultrasonic investigation of the endocrine system in the male. Although the testes play the major role in male reproductive capacity, diseases of other endocrine organs may have a greater or lesser bearing on androgenization and fertility and will, therefore, also be considered.

1. PRINCIPLES AND TECHNIQUES OF ULTRASOUND

Ultrasonography is a diagnostic modality which employs high frequency sound waves to make images of various parts of the body. At the present time, there are three main types of diagnostic ultrasound which are of concern to us and which will be mentioned in this chapter – A-mode, Grey scale cross-sectional sonograms and real time scanning.

In the A-mode presentation, diagnostic information is obtained from study of an oscilloscope screen which has an electronic base line across it. When an ultrasound transducer is placed on a patient's body, the observer will note deflections (spikes) on the base line. Each spike represents an echo-producing surface within the body from which sound has been reflected. The distance of each spike from the left side of the base line is proportional to the distance of the echo-producing surface from the skin of the patient. This type of sonography is employed in echoencephalography, examples of which will be shown below in the discussion of intracranial abnormalities. This type of echogram is made by holding an ultrasonic transducer more or less stationary against the patient's skin over the part being examined.

In the production of Grey scale sector scans, a transducer is moved over the part of interest and a cross-sectional image of body structures deep to the transducer is produced. This type of sonography has application in the neck (thyroid), abdomen (adrenal), and testes.

Real time scanning is similar to the type of cross-sectional scanning just described except that by means of mechanical or electronic manipulation, a moving image is produced. This technique is analogous to fluoroscopy in diagnostic radiology. For our purposes, real time scanning would be used for quick localization and study of intra-abdominal structures, although there are now real time devices (still in the developmental stage) which can produce exquisitely fine detail of such superficial structures as the thyroid and testes.

Diagnostic ultrasound has some inherent limitations of which the reader should be aware. High frequency sound waves cannot pass through air and are almost completely reflected at transducer-air or soft-tissue-air interfaces. As a result, a coupling agent such as oil or a gel must be introduced between the transducer surface and the skin. In addition, the sound waves cannot pass through hollow air-containing viscera such as stomach or intestines. As a result, such intra-abdominal organs as the pancreas and adrenals may be hidden from ultrasonic study. In such a case, a patient may have to be re-examined at a time when the stomach and/or intestines are free of gas. In some instances, it may not be possible at all to visualize adequately the retroperitoneal area. Another limiting factor is obesity. In diagnostic ultrasound, the quality of the diagnostic image often varies inversely as the size of the patient. In moderately obese patients, therefore, we may not be able to visualize the adrenals or other deep abdominal structures. It is of interest that in these patients computerized tomography

may be helpful in diagnosis because with this modality fat acts as a contrasting medium outlining intra-abdominal organs.

Bone may also cause difficulty in ultrasonography. Because of the great difference in acoustic properties between bone and soft tissues, sound waves are for the most part reflected rather than transmitted across bone-soft-tissue interfaces. It is difficult, therefore, to see such organs as the adrenals through a patient's rib cage. In the head, we cannot in the adult perform cross-sectional scans because of the 'impermeability' of the bone. In the young child, however, whose skull vault is thinner than the adult, this may be possible. Sufficient sound with which to obtain diagnostic information can be introduced into the head using the A-mode type of scanning.

Diagnostic ultrasound is a completely painless and harmless technique which may be repeated as many times as necessary. Diagnostic information obtained at ultrasonographic study may be recorded on Polaroid, X ray or 70 mm film.

2. ULTRASONIC INVESTIGATION OF THE ENDOCRINE SYSTEM

The remainder of this chapter will deal with the ultrasonic appearance of the various endocrine organs in which dysfunction may result in disorders of androgenization and fertility.

2.1. Intracranial structures

As mentioned above, intracranial structures must, for the most part, be examined with the A-mode technique of diagnostic ultrasound. There is a vast literature on echoencephalography which is available to the interested reader (Tenner and Wodraska, 1975, Uematsu and Walker, 1971). Since the advent of computerized tomography of the head, the popularity of echoencephalography has waned somewhat. However, echoencephalography is still, and will remain a useful technique. It is a relatively cheap (compared to computerized tomography), rapid, readily reproducible, non-ionizing diagnostic technique. Besides localization of midline structures and measurement of ventricular size, it can be used as the primary method for detecting the presence of

intracranial space occupying lesions. One very important feature of ultrasonography is that frequent studies can be performed to follow changes in ventricular size and the position of midline structures in patients who have sustained head trauma or who are recovering from intracranial surgery. These studies may be done at will without concern for radiation and overwhelming expense (Fig. 1).

Intracranial abnormalities may cause hypogonadism or precocious puberty in children or hypogonadism in the adult. Precocious puberty may be associated with brain tumors (gliomas, astro-

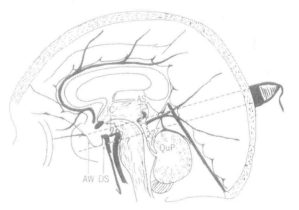
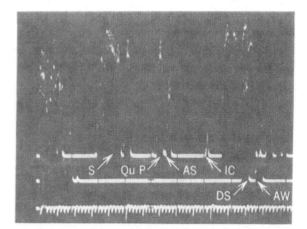

Figure 1. (a) An echoencephalogram of the upper brain stem made by placing a transducer midway between the external occipital protuberance and the vertex of the skull and aiming at the sella turcica (see b). The lower line seen in the illustration was made at a lower sensitivity setting of the equipment. The base line was then moved up the oscilloscope screen and the sensitivity raised. Each deflection from the line represents an echo produced from a structure through which the sound passed. (S = splenium; QuP = quadrigenimal plate; AS = aqueduct of Sylvius; IC = interpeduncular cistern; DS = dorsum sellae; AW = anterior wall of sella turcica.) (b) Cross-section of the brain showing the path through which the sound beam passed to produce the sonogram illustrated in (a).

cytomas) in the region of the third ventricle, brain stem, optic nerve or temporal lobe. Craniopharyngiomas and pinealomas may also induce precocious puberty, as may internal hydrocephalus from any cause. Craniopharyngioma, and hypothalamic and pituitary tumors per se may cause prepubertal hypogonadism. After puberty, hypogonadism may be secondary to pituitary neoplasm (e.g. chromophobe adenoma), craniopharyngioma or glioma (Daughaday, 1974). All of these neoplastic masses are amenable to detection by ultrasound. An example of a craniopharyngioma is illustrated in Fig. 2.

2.2. Thyroid

Ultrasonography of the thyroid is now a well established diagnostic technique (Miskin et al., 1975, 1976; Walfish et al., 1977). Both A-mode and cross-sectional studies are employed in the study of thyroid enlargements. With the increasingly sophisticated Grey scale equipment now available, it is possible to obtain very detailed images of the thyroid gland. Formerly, A-mode played a prominent role in establishing the consistency (solid or cystic) of thyroid masses, but nowadays this information is quickly ascertained from cross-sectional images alone.

Thyroid dysfunction is rarely the cause of infertility in the male. In a study of 1294 infertile men, Dubin and Amelar found that thyroid disease was a causative factor in only 0.6% (Amelar et al., 1977). Figure 3 illustrates sonograms of a normal neck at the level of the thyroid gland and a goitrous thyroid associated with hypothyroidism is illustrated in Fig. 4.

2.3. Adrenal gland

Excessive production of adrenal androgens may result from adrenocortico-hyperplasia, adenoma or carcinoma. In the prepubertal male, precocious puberty will result. In the postpubertal male however, there will be little of any outward physical signs of increased virilization.

It is possible to visualize the adrenal glands ultrasonically in a high percentage of patients (85%, Sample, 1977) in whom the examination is attempted. Scanning may be performed via the anterior

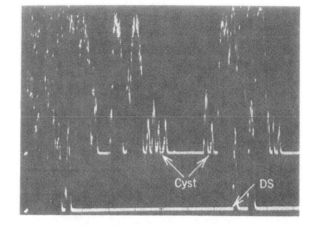

Figure 2. Craniopharyngioma. An echoencephalogram performed in the manner of that illustrated in Fig. 1(a) shows a cluster of echoes from the 'near' and 'far' walls of a craniopharyngioma which has undergone cystic degeneration. (Figures 1 and 2 are reproduced by permission from Tenner and Wodraska, 1975.)

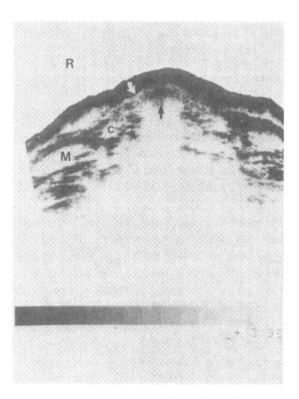

Figure 3. Normal neck. A transverse sonogram at the level of the thyroid gland is shown. (R = right side of patient; M = sternomastoid muscle; C = carotid sheath; black arrow points to the trachea; curved white arrow points to the right lobe of the thyroid gland.) Note the echo-free area deep to the trachea – sound does not pass through the air in this structure. The normal thyroid lobes are seen as a small cluster of echoes on either side of the trachea.

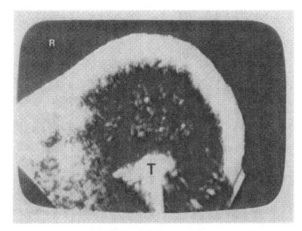

Figure 4. Goitre. Note the much enlarged thyroid gland surrounding the trachea (T). There are echoes in the gland because the enlargement is solid in nature.

or posterior abdominal walls, or from the patient's side while he is turned into the left or right decubitus position. Sample (1977) has described a modification of the decubitus scanning position with which the adrenals can be seen in the vast majority of cases. Figure 5 shows an example of a left adrenal adenoma visualized from the anterior abdominal wall.

2.4. Testes

Ultrasonic examination of the testes may be accomplished in one of two ways. A transducer may be moved over the testis held in the examiner's hand after coating the scrotum with an ultrasonic couplant, or they may be scanned through a water bath. The former technique yields better results especially when one of the newer, smaller high frequency transducers now available is used. With this technique it is possible to measure the thickness of the testis, assess its internal consistency, assess the nature of an intrascrotal swelling (solid or cystic) and follow the clinical course of an intrascrotal swelling. Testicular width can be assessed very accurately with ultrasonography. This is an important measurement as there is a direct correlation between width and sperm count (Miskin and Bain, 1978). (Fig. 6).

Not all testicular causes of infertility can be assessed ultrasonically, but such abnormalities as orchitis, varicocele and epididymitis can be visualized. The nature of such intrascrotal swellings as spermatocele, hydrocele, and hematoma can also

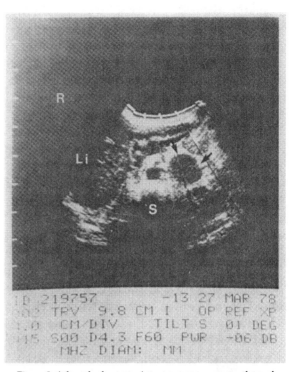

Figure 5. Adrenal adenoma. A transverse sonogram through the upper part of the abdomen shows a left adrenal adenoma (black arrows). The tumor is seen just antero-lateral to the lumbar spine (S). The round clear zone anterior to the spine is the abdominal aorta (Li = liver, R = right side of the patient). (Courtesy of Dr. Stephanie Wilson, Sunnybrook Hospital, Toronto.)

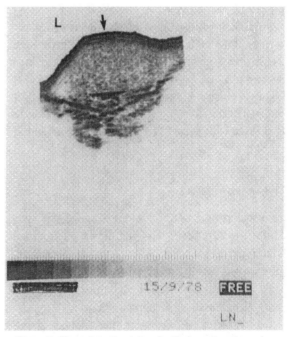

Figure 6. Normal testis. A longitudinal section through a normal testis is illustrated. The arrow points to the skin of the scrotum. Note the homogeneous internal echo pattern in this testis. The testis measures 2 cm in thickness.

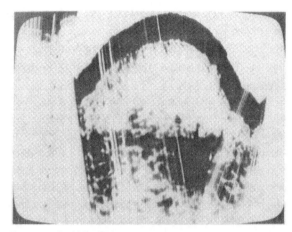

Figure 7. Orchitis. This swollen testis is 3.2 cm thick. The decreased number of echoes in it (compare with Figs. 6 and 7) is due to edema. (With an increase in fluid there are fewer interfaces from which sound can be reflected.)

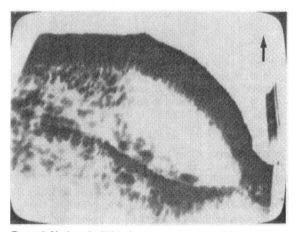

Figure 8. Varicocele. With the patient sitting (vertical arrow) and performing a Valsalva's maneuver, the dilated intrascrotal veins become distended and are seen as serpiginous structures at the deep surface of the testis. The testis in this case shows fewer than usual echoes because the sensitivity was turned down to illustrate better the varicocele deep to the testis.

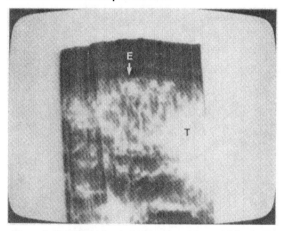

Figure 9. Epididymitis. A thickened nodular epididymis (E with an arrow pointing down) was visualized at the cranial end of the testis (T) in this patient with epididymitis.

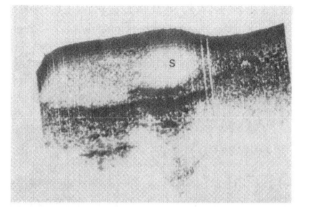

Figure 10. Spermatocele. A spermatocele (S) is visualized as an oval cystic area at the caudal pole of the testis.

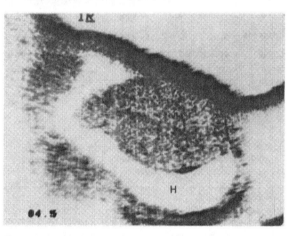

Figure 11. Hydrocele. Note how the hydrocele (H) surrounds the testis.

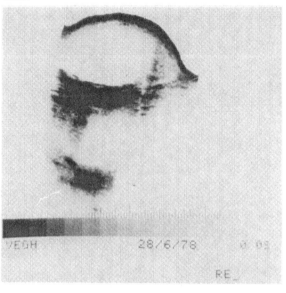

Figure 12. Hematoma. This patient was struck in the scrotum many years earlier. The resultant hematoma became encapsulated and is shown as a large oval sonolucent area. Only a small remnant of testicular tissue is seen at the caudal end of the hematoma (right side of sonogram).

be elucidated (Figs 7-12). It should be noted that if a varicocele is suspected clinically, the patient should be examined in a sitting position while performing Valsalva's maneuver in order that the varices of the varicocele will fill and therefore become visible ultrasonically.

3. CONCLUSIONS

Diagnostic ultrasound has limited but definite usefulness in andrology. In the head it can be used as a quick and efficient screening process for the assessment of a midline shift and the presence of a mass in the region of the sella turcica. In the event that a mass is found, however, more definitive studies such as computerized tomography, pneumoen-cephalography, and/or angiography would have to be done prior to surgery. Ultrasonography has little application in the study of thyroid gland diseases as they relate to andrology. Echography of the adrenal gland, however, may be very useful.

The most significant application of diagnostic ultrasound in andrology is in the examination of the testes. This technique allows for the assessment of the nature of a mass in the scrotum – one which may have bearing on fertility and/or androgenicity. We must appreciate however, that in a patient with normal size testes and oligospermia, the internal echo pattern of the testes looks no different than in a patient with normal sperm count. Undescended testes which are above the inguinal canal cannot be visualized ultrasonically.

REFERENCES

Amelar ID, Dubin L, Walsh P (1977) Male infertility, p 50. London: W.B. Saunders.

Daughaday WH (1974) The adenohypophysis. In: Williams RH, ed. The textbook of endocrinology, 5th ed, p 68. London: W.B. Saunders.

Miskin M, Bain J (1978) Use of diagnostic ultrasound in the evaluation of testicular disorders. In: Bain J, Hafez ESE, Barwin BN, eds. Progress in reproductive biology, Vol 3: Andrology – Basic and Clinical Aspects of Male Reproduction and Infertility, p 117-130. Basel: S. Karger.

Miskin M, Rosen IB, Walfish PW (1975) Ultrasonography of the thyroid gland. Radiol Clin North Am 13: 479.

Miskin M, Rosen IB, Walfish PW (1976) Using ultrasonics to visualize the thyroid. Med Opinion 5: 29.

Sample WF (1977) A new technique for the evaluation of the adrenal gland with grey scale ultrasonography. Radiology 124: 463.

Tenner MS, Wodraska GM (1975) Diagnostic ultrasound in neurology – methods and techniques. New York: John Wiley.

Uematsu S, Walker AE (1971) A manual of echoencephalography. Baltimore: Williams & Wilkins.

Walfish PG, Hazani E, Strawbridge HTG, Miskin M, Rosen IB (1977) Combined ultrasound and needle aspiration cytology in the assessment and management of the hypofunctioning thyroid nodule. Ann Intern Med 87: 270.

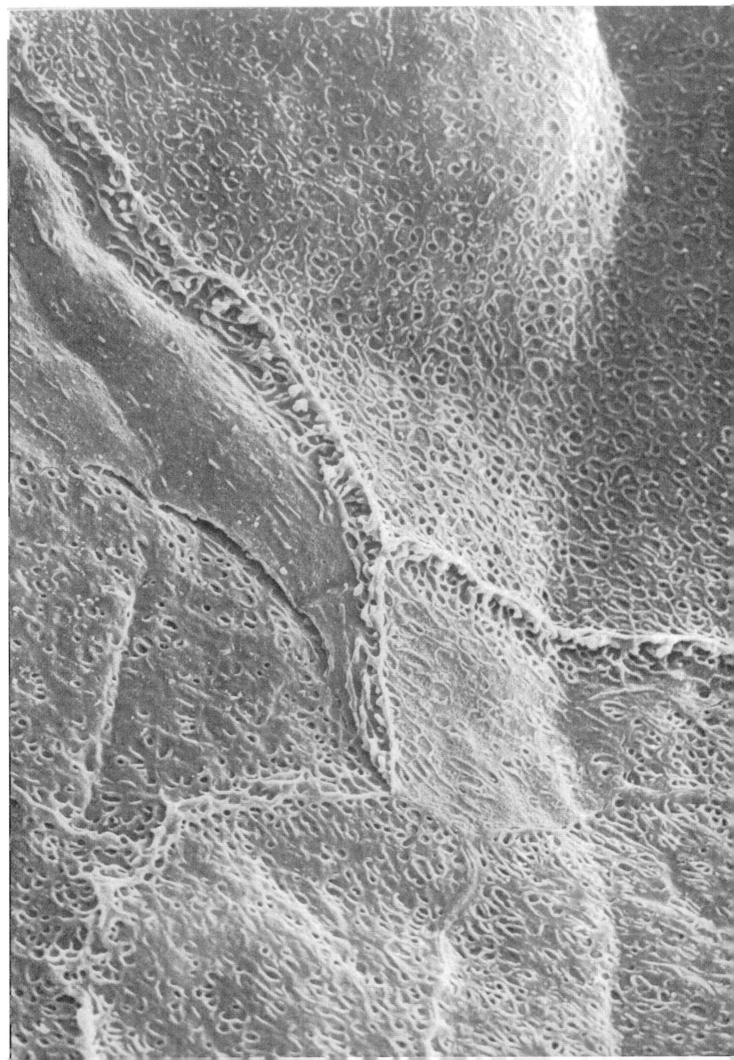

IV. SYSTEMIC DISORDERS

15. NEUROLOGICAL DISORDERS IN ANDROLOGY

P.O. LUNDBERG

INTRODUCTION

Neurological disorders may result in andrological problems through two different types of mechanisms, endocrine and neural. The central nervous system regulates the peripheral endocrine organs through the hypothalamus and pituitary gland. A neurological disorder occurring before puberty may cause endocrine dysfunction resulting in premature, retarded or absence of sexual development. In post-pubertal males a neurological disorder may affect the hypothalamo-pituitary endocrine regulation, resulting in atrophy of the testis and some of the accessory genital organs, infertility and reduction or loss of libido. Hypogonadism in patients with neurological disorders is usually associated with normal or decreased gonadotropin secretion but may occasionally be hypergonadotropic. Neural mechanisms are involved in the regulation of sexual libido, sexual behavior, sexual arousal and orgasm as well as in the transportation of the spermatozoa and the seminal fluid from the organs of production.

1. TERMINOLOGY

1.1. Libido and sexual behavior

The parts of the brain that are of most importance with respect to the central regulation of libido and sexual behavior are the limbic cortex and the hypothalamus. A minor lesion of the hypothalamus may result in a decrease or total loss of libido. Lesions of the limbic cortex may also result in aberrant sexual behavior. However, the mechanisms governing sexual libido and sexual behavior in man are not well understood and many other parts of the brain are also involved.

1.2. Erection

Sexual arousal is usually provoked by intracerebral mechanisms such as thoughts, or by external stimuli, e.g. visual, auditory, olfactory or tactile perceptions which through the spinal cord and peripheral nerves give rise to erection. This type of erection is called cerebral or psychic erection, and for this to occur the sense organs as well as the central nervous system, including the spinal cord, the reflex center in the spinal cord, and the peripheral nerves must be intact. However, there is also another type of erection, called reflex erection, which is provoked by tactile stimulation mainly of the genital region. Reflex erection depends solely on the peripheral nerves and the reflex center in the sacral spinal cord, and may thus occur even in the presence of lesions of the spinal cord above the reflex center.

Erection is mediated by parasympathetic fibers passing from sacral spinal cord segments 2-4 via the pelvic nerves (nervi erigentes). This neural mechanism is essential for reflex erection and is also involved in cerebral erection. Cerebral erection may also be brought about by impulses transmitted through the sympathetic nervous system leaving the spinal cord at the thoracolumbar junction via the hypogastric plexus. Both types of nerve fibers are cholinergic.

1.3. Emission

Seminal emission is the expulsion of secreted fluids from the prostate and seminal vesicles as well as the fluid from the testicles through the vasa deferentia into the proximal part of the urethra. Immediately before seminal emission takes place the proximal end of the urethra closes by contraction of the

internal bladder sphincter. Seminal emission and closure contraction of this sphincter are mediated by the sympathetic nervous system through nerve fibers arising from segments T11-L2 of the spinal cord and passing through the hypogastric plexus. Adrenalin secreted from the adrenal medulla may also play a part in this mechanism.

1.4. Ejaculation

Ejaculation is achieved by a series of contractions of the striated muscles in the pelvic floor, mainly the bulbocavernosus and ischiocavernosus muscles, which are innervated by somatic, spinal nerves from sacral spinal cord segments 2-4 through the pudendal nerve.

1.5. Orgasm

It should be noted that orgasm is not identical to ejaculation. Orgasm is difficult to define but could be described as the sum of a series of physiological reactions and sensations in the human body at sexual climax.

1.6. Innervation of the testes

The sympathetic nervous system innervates the testis through nerve fibers leaving the spinal cord at the thoracolumbar junction. The importance of these nerve fibers in man is unknown but complete spinal cord lesion involving this system may result in some testicular atrophy.

2. DIAGNOSIS OF SEXUAL AND GONADAL DYSFUNCTION IN PATIENTS WITH NEUROLOGICAL DISORDERS

2.1. History

2.1.1. Pubertal development. It is important to determine occurrence and timing of various growth and development parameters such as height and secondary sex characteristics. The onset of puberty varies considerably but precocious puberty can be said to exist if there are signs of sexual maturation before age 10. Puberty is considered retarded if sexual development has not been initiated by age 17.

2.1.2. Libido. The occurrence and frequency of sexual outlets such as masturbation or intercourse give a very rough estimation of degree of libido. Changes in libido are important and the libidinous state before the disorder became manifest should be determined. There may be a total lack of libido in a small number of patients with a hypothalamic lesion or complete destruction of the pituitary gland. Frank hypersexuality is very uncommon.

2.1.3. Potency. Erectile impotence is a reduction or lack of ability to achieve an erection. Impotence may be primary, if it has always been present, or secondary, if sexual function has previously been normal. Total impotence means a total loss of the erectile capacity. Partial impotence is an inability to maintain a full erection for a sufficient length of time or to attain a full erection of the entire penis. It may be absolute, which means impotence in all situations with all partners and also at masturbation, or may be relative, i.e. present only under certain circumstances or with a certain partner.

Priapism or persistent abnormal erection, is usually not caused by actual sexual stimulation, is not pleasurable and is often very painful. Commonly priapism is sustained for a long period but in certain neurological disorders it may fluctuate. In such patients it is often difficult to decide whether the priapism is spontaneous or results from lack of sexual inhibition, since these patients often have severe brain damage.

2.1.4. Ejaculation. Ejaculation may be premature, retarded or totally absent. Premature ejaculation occurs involuntarily before or immediately after vaginal intromission. Retarded ejaculation usually means difficulty in ejaculation even during strong sexual stimulation. Absent ejaculation or anejaculation exist when no ejaculatory contractions occur under any circumstances. Ejaculatory problems may be primary or secondary, absolute or relative, circumstances analogous to impotence. Partial ejaculatory failure, called dribbling, is sometimes seen in certain disorders of the spinal cord. Instead of a series of strong ejaculatory contractions with heavy expulsion of the semen, only a few weak contractions take place and semen dribbles from the tip of the penis.

Retrograde ejaculation refers to ejaculation of

the semen backward into the bladder. The reason for this dysfunction is usually non-closure of the internal bladder sphincter because of a neurological disorder. Retrograde ejaculation has to be differentiated from aspermia in which there is no production of semen at all. Most cases of aspermia are caused by lack of androgen stimulation secondary to a hypothalamo-pituitary disorder (Kjessler and Lundberg, 1974). In such cases the prostate gland and seminal vesicles are atrophied or underdeveloped.

2.1.5. Orgasm. Absence of the orgasmic experience is called anorgasm, which may also be primary or secondary, absolute or relative. In neurological disorders there may be a dissociation between ejaculation and orgasm. Some patients may have an ejaculation without orgasm, while others may have an orgasm without ejaculation. Ejaculation may be painful and there may be other quantitative or qualitative changes in the orgasmic experience.

2.2. Neurological examination and special tests
Two regions of the nervous system are of the utmost importance for normal gonadal and sexual function, namely the hypothalamo-pituitary region, including the optic and olfactory parts of the brain, and the lower part of the spinal cord, including somatic and autonomic nerves from this region. Following a general neurological examination, these two parts of the nervous system should be studied further by a number of clinical and laboratory test methods.

2.2.1. The visual system. A thorough ophthalmological examination is often necessary, especially when impingement upon the optic chiasm is suspected. The visual acuity and visual fields are of the greatest importance. The visual fields should be examined with a Goldman perimeter, where a number of objects differing in size, contrast and color can be used. In early cases, chiasmatic compression by a suprasellar tumor gives rise to a visual defect for small objects of low intensity that may only be detectable at a very careful examination.

2.2.2. The olfactory system. This can easily be tested by means of a series of test tubes containing substances such as coffee, oil of cloves, peppermint,

wintergreen oil, and so on. At least three different test substances should be used on each side.

2.2.3. Roentgenological examinations of the sellar region. A plain skull X ray in two projections, frontal and lateral, should be combined with polytomography of the sellar region if there is any suspicion of roentgenological changes. Its size, determined according to the di Chiro formula (di Chiro and Nelson, 1962) usually gives information not only about pituitary tumor expansion but also about underdevelopment of the pituitary due to lack of hypothalamic stimulation. If any neurological, ophthalmological or radiological findings give reason to suspect a brain disorder the next step in the roentgenological examination is computed tomography (Fig. 1). In a few cases where pituitary surgery is to be undertaken pneumoencephalography and arteriography will be necessary to determine the extent of a pituitary tumor and its vascular relationships.

2.2.4. Electroencephalography. Electroencephalography is of limited value in neurological assessment of andrological disorders. It may be essential, however, in the diagnosis of epilepsy and may also be of importance in some metabolic, infective and degenerative disorders.

2.2.5. Clinical examination of the lower segments of the spinal cord. The neurological examination should include an evaluation of sensory and motor function as well as of reflexes. In the genital region, especially on the glans penis, there are mucocutaneous end-organs which are very sensitive to vibration. A quantitative examination of the vibration sense with the aid of a biothesiometer is often the best method of investigating the sensory function in the genital region. However, the sensory examination should also include investigation of the sense of pain, by the pin-prick test, and of temperature, with a test tube containing cold water.

The bulbocavernosus and ischiocavernosus muscles can be voluntarily contracted and this contraction can be seen on inspection. The tone of the anal sphincter and contractions of the levator ani muscle on each side can easily be evaluated by palpation per rectum.

A number of reflexes are useful in the evaluation

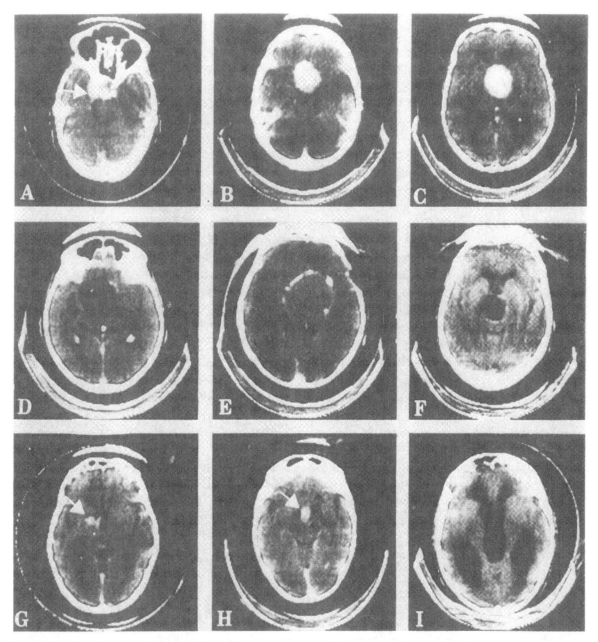

Figure 1. Examples of computed tomograms illustrating the importance of this method in the evaluation of patients with disorders of the suprasellar, parasellar and hypothalamic regions. All patients represented had hypogonadism as a major or presenting symptom. *Case A:* A 52-year-old man with an invasive pituitary adenoma. Serum prolactin concentration 2800 μg/l. Note the destruction of the sella turcica and the high attenuation after contrast enhancement into the temporal fossa to the left (arrow), indicating tumor invasion. This led to temporal lobe epilepsy. *Case B:* This 50-year-old patient had hypogonadism, hypothyroidism and progressive visual failure. A large suprasellar meningioma is seen. *Case C:* This male patient, now 21 years old, has a pituitary adenoma growing up into the hypothalamus. He has had visual defects since childhood. He is 195 cm tall but otherwise has pronounced hypopituitarism. Note the high attenuation of the tumor mass after contrast enhancement. *Case D:* A 61-year-old man with a cholesteatoma. Note the extremely low attenuation of the cholesterol-containing content. *Case E:* This man, now 59 years old, had an aspergilloma removed 5 years ago. Surgery was not radical, however, and now aspergillus is growing as a huge tumor mass. Note that the mass itself has the same attenuation as the brain tissue, but there are some calcifications around it. This patient had very few clinical symptoms besides pituitary insufficiency. *Case F:* A 67-year-old patient with a craniopharyngioma. This patient had a large cystic tumor at the midline. Note the low attenuation in the cyst and the higher attenuation in the capsule. *Case G:* Diabetes insipidus was the presenting symptom in this 53-year-old man. Later progressive hypothalamic symptoms as well as diplopia, ataxia and a defect of conjugate ocular deviation developed. Computed tomography showed a left-sided hypothalamic tumor (arrow) which at autopsy was found to be a reticulum cell sarcoma. *Case H:* A 48-year-old patient with sarcoidosis in the brain. The patient had several lesions but one was located at the midline in the hypothalamus (arrow). Note the high attenuation after contrast enhancement. *Case I:* This is a 31-year-old patient with hypogonadism caused by hydrocephalus secondary to stenosis of the aqueduct. Note the huge third ventricle.

of patients with suspected lesions in this region of the nervous system:

(i) *The scrotal reflex* is a local, axonal reflex. By application of a cold object to the scrotum a slow vermicellar contraction of the tunica dartos muscle is elicited. This reaction is often observed spontaneously immediately after the patient has undressed and it may sometimes also be provoked from a more widespread area including the perineum or the inner parts of the thigh. During full erection the dartos muscle is contracted.

(ii) *The cremasteric reflex* is a superficial, somatic, ipsilateral reflex. The afferent loop arises from the genito-femoral and ilioinguinal nerves; the reflex center lies in lumbar segments 1-2 and the response consists of a contraction of the ipsilateral cremasteric muscle. This leads to an elevation of the ipsilateral testicle. The cremasteric muscle is contracted during full erection. The reflex is best elicited by stroking the skin of the upper inner part of the thigh with a blunt point. It is absent both in lesions of the central motor neuron and in lesions interrupting the peripheral relfex arc.

(iii) *The bulbocavernosus reflex* is a spinal, somatic and bilateral reflex. The afferent and efferent loops are mediated through the pudendal nerve, the reflex center lies in sacral cord segments 2-3 and the response consists of a contraction of the bulbo-cavernosus muscle and some other striated muscles of the pelvic floor. The reflex is best elicited by pinching the dorsum of the glans penis. Lesions interrupting the reflex are result in absence of this reflex. Damage to the central motor neuron may lead to an exaggerated reflex response. In certain cases pinching of the glans penis may result in a contraction of several muscles in the legs on both sides.

(iv) *The superficial anal reflex* is somatic, ipsilateral and is mediated through branches of the pudendal nerve; the reflex center is located in sacral cord segments 2-4 and the response leads to a contraction of the external anal sphincter muscle or sometimes even the ischiocavernosus and bulbocavernosus muscles. The reflex is best elicited by stroking the skin in the perineal region on each side with a blunt point. Lesions interrupting the reflex arc result in loss of the reflex response. Central motor neuron lesions may cause exaggeration of this reflex.

(v) *The internal anal reflex* is supplied by sympathetic post-ganglionic nerve fibers going through the hypogastric nerves and presacral plexus. The reflex center is probably located in lumbar cord segments 1-2. The reflex is best elicited by dilation of the anal sphincter with a gloved finger. This leads to a contraction of the anal sphincter. Damage to the hypogastric nerves, presacral plexus or lumbar spinal cord results in absence of the reflex.

2.2.6. Roentgenological examinations of the spinal cord. A plain X-ray of the spine, especially of the lumbosacral region, including the sacrum, should be performed in appropriate cases. If there is any suspicion of spinal cord compression or rhizopathy, meyolography with air or water-soluble positive contrast medium should be the next step.

2.2.7. Urodynamic investigations. Mictometry and carbon dioxide cystometry are often of interest in these cases, as many of the patients also have urinary dysfunction. Cystoscopy, including testing of the bladder sensitivity, is also helpful.

2.2.8. Electromyography. The muscles of the pelvic floor can be examined by electromyography. In certain cases it may be of value to make recordings from the striated urethral sphincter, the anal sphincter and the levator ani muscles during voluntary contraction, cystometry or sometimes even during ejaculation induced by masturbation.

3. CENTRAL NERVOUS SYSTEM DISORDERS WITH HYPOGONADISM OR PRECOCIOUS PUBERTY

3.1. Malformations of the brain and pituitary gland

The development of a normal adenohypophysis is highly dependent on the development of the neurohypophysial anlage. The optic system and the olfactory (rhinencephalic) system are very closely connected with the hypothalamus from an ontogenetic, a functional and morphological point of view. Malformations of these parts of the brain often result in a lack of sexual development. A number of malformation syndromes thus exist in which hypogonadism is one facet of what is often

very complex symptomatology.

The simplest of these malformations is non-fusion of the two pituitary anlagen. In these cases the neurohypophysis is seen as a small nodule at the bottom of the hypothalamus. This is called dystopia of the neurohypophysis. Since there is no normal development of the anterior pituitary there is no real sella turcica and only a shallow depression is seen on the skull X ray. This phenomenon has been called dysplasia of the sella turcica (Lundberg and Gemzell, 1966) Symptoms of partial hypopituitarism may exist. Anophthalmia, which may be hereditary, and hypoplasia of the optic nerves and tracts is a much more severe anomaly associated with panhypopituitarism and sometimes diabetes insipidus and other hypothalamic symptoms. Other serious defects in the face, the head or the rest of the body are often present and in some cases chromosomal aberrations have been found. In diencephaloschisis the floor of the third ventricle is absent.

In anencephaly a hypophyseal primordium is always present, but there is no fully developed pituitary gland. Microcephaly also gives rise to a hypothalamo-pituitary anomaly. Patients with more severe malformations usually die at a young age. However, an increasing number of microcephalic patients are reaching adulthood.

Olfactogenital dysplasia (Hypogonadotropic hypogonadism with anosmia, Kallmann's syndrome, de Morsiers' syndrome): In studying the genetic aspects of primary eunuchoidism, Kallmann et al. (1944) found a number of familial cases of eunuchoidism associated with color blindness, anosmia and synkinesia. In a review of cranioencephalic malformations, based on personal and previously published cases, de Morsier (1954) stated that malformations of the olfactory parts of the brain usually were combined with hypogonadism. He thus outlined the nosological entity olfactogenital dysplasia.

It is now apparent that olfactogenital dysplasia represents different neuroendocrine syndromes in which a more or less pronounced congenital cerebral malformation including an anomaly of the olfactory region of the brain, is combined with a hypothalamo-pituitary defect resulting in hypogonadism. The clinical symptomatology may therefore vary. The central nervous defect is not usually very apparent and some patients are not even aware of their olfactory malfunction. This is the reason why a test of olfactory function should always be included in the examination in a case of hypogonadism or infertility of unknown origin. In some cases only hyposmia will be found, but most patients with this syndrome are totally anosmic.

Most of the cases with simple symptomatology (hypogonadism with anosmia or hyposmia) are hereditary. Sporadic cases occur in which hypogonadism and anosmia are combined with different degrees of mental retardation, epilepsy and/or visible abnormalities of the face, skull, eyes or other parts of the body.

Most hereditary cases are males. From statistical genetic analysis as well as from the occurrence of father-to-son transmissions, an autosomal dominant inheritance seems probable. The karyotype in males is usually 46 XY but isolated cases of XXY/XY mosaicism have been found. D-trisomy may be combined with an absence of olfactory bulbs. The frequency of the syndrome has been estimated to be 0.2% of all newborn males.

A delay of puberty is usually the presenting symptom if mental retardation or visible malformations are not apparent. At adult ages more or less marked hypogonadism is present with small to medium-sized testes, often cryptorchidism, a small penis, sometimes gynecomastia, and underdevelopment of sexual hair. The patients have aspermia or a reduced volume of semen with azoospermia. The body proportions are usually eunuchoid and some of the patients have above average height. Testicular biopsy shows arrested spermatogenesis, often at the primary spermatocyte stage, with normal spermatogonia and Sertoli cells. The Leydig cells are sparse or hypotrophic. The serum and urinary concentrations of FSH and LH are low, serum testosterone concentration is decreased and sex hormone binding globulin (SHBG) is normal. In most cases the serum gonadotropins respond well to LH-RH but not to clomiphene. The testes usually respond to treatment with chorionic gonadotropin. Untreated men are usually sterile, but a number of patients have become fathers after treatment and some untreated fathers with the syndrome do also exist.

3.2. Hypothalamic disorders

The unique position of the hypothalamus in the center of the brain and the fact that so many centers of vital body regulation are located in the hypothalamus make symptomatology in hypothalamic disorders very complex (Bauer, 1959). A number of symptoms and symptom complexes which can be divided into different groups and which occur in purely hypothalamic disorders are listed in Table 1. One major group of symptomatology is that of endocrine dysregulation, which occurs mainly by hypothalamic influence on the pituitary. Another group comprises symptoms of autonomic dysregulation, mediated by the sympathetic and parasympathetic nervous systems. Other symptoms are more complex such as dysfunction of the regulation of food and water intake and of thermoregulation.

Progressive hypothalamic lesions or tumors growing into the hypothalamus will eventually give rise to symptoms from other structures of the brain. The most important of these are symptoms of compression of the optic nerves, the chiasm or the optic tracts. Visual field examination is therefore essential in the assessment of patients with hypothalamic disorders. Tumors invading the frontal lobes will sooner or later give rise to mental symptoms, the so called frontal lobe syndrome. Tumors growing into the mesencephalon will cause symptoms from that part of the brain such as oculomotor dysfunction and pyramidal signs. Compression of the aqueduct of Sylvius will give rise to increased pressure in the ventricular system, with hydrocephalus and dilation of the lateral ventricles and the third ventricle. If there is compression of the foramen of Monro the pressure in one or both lateral ventricles will be increased. Expansion of a tumor or compression of the cerebrospinal circulatory system will result in increased intracranial pressure, causing headache, vomiting, somnolence or even death.

Precocious puberty or hypogonadism may very well be early or even presenting symptoms of hypothalamic disorders. When it is suspected that hypogonadism is of hypothalamic (or pituitary) origin, three investigations in addition to the clinical examination are essential. These are examination of the visual fields, plain X ray of the skull and computed tomography. Computed tomography has

proved to be extremely valuable in these cases, since it may not only reveal a hypothalamic lesion but also give a clue as to the lesion's etiology. Computed tomography is also of value for the detection of

Table 1. Clinical symptoms of hypothalamic disorders.

1) Gonadal dysfunction
   a) precocious puberty
   b) retarded puberty
   c) gonadal atrophy with secondary hypogonadism
   d) decrease or loss of libido

2) Thyroid dysfunction; hypothyroidism

3) Adrenal gland dysfunction
   a) adrenal gland insufficiency
   b) Cushing's disease

4) Growth disorders
   a) hypothalamic dwarfism
   b) gigantism
   c) acromegaly

5) Hyperprolactinemia

6) Hyperpigmentation

7) Increase in body hair

8) Disorders of salt and water metabolism
   a) diabetes insipidus of central origin
   b) primary polydipsia (compulsive water drinking)
   c) adipsia; inappropriate secretion of antidiuretic hormone ('antidiabetes insipidus')
   d) adipsia, hypernatremia and persistent hyperosmolarity (neurogenic hypernatremia)

9) Disorders of regulation of food intake
   a) hyperphagia
   b) obesity with or without hyperphagia (combined with hypogonadism called Fröhlich syndrome or dystrophia adiposogenitalis)
   c) diencyphalic syndrome of early childhood (emaciation)
   d) secondary anorexia nervosa

10) Disorders of thermoregulation
   a) hyperthermic crises
   b) hypothermia and poikilothermia

11) Disorders of autonomic dysregulation
   a) dyshidrosis
   b) persistent pilo-erection
   c) disturbances of sphincter control
   d) impotence

12) Sleep disorders
   a) somnolence
   b) disorders of sleep rhythm
   c) constant alertness
   d) periodic hypersomnia and hyperphagia (Kleine-Levin syndrome)

13) Hypothalamic crises and episodes of rage

14) Psychic disturbances

many other cases such as hydrocephalus, infections and some vascular lesions. In Fig. 1 a number of typical examples of its use are given.

3.3. Tumors of the hypothalamus (Table 2)

Pituitary tumors will not be discussed in this chapter; however, an undiagnosed tumor of the pituitary may expand into the hypothalamus and give rise to a number of hypothalamic symptoms by compression of hypothalamic tissue (Fig. 1C). Since those parts of the hypothalamus that contain the centers of regulation of the pituitary function are located in the hypothalamic region closest to the pituitary in the tuber cinereum and the basal anterior hypothalamus, it is often difficult to decide whether, for example, hypogonadism or hypothyroidism in such a case is caused by the hypothalamic or the pituitary portion of the tumor (Korsgaard et al., 1976; Lundberg and Wide, 1974). Diabetes insipidus is a hypothalamic and not a pituitary symptom. Diabetes insipidus in a case of pituitary tumor indicates hypothalamic involvement, or at least destruction of the upper part of the pituitary stalk. If a pituitary tumor grows into the hypothalamus a compression of the chiasm almost always occurs, giving rise to visual field defects. Pituitary adenomas may be ectopic, i.e. located primarily outside the sella turcica. Such a tumor may invade the hypothalamus without causing any

Table 2. Tumors of the hypothalamus.

1) Pituitary adenomas expanding into the hypothalamus
2) Ectopic pituitary adenomas
3) Craniopharyngiomas
4) Pinealomas
5) Hypothalamic hamartomas
6) Infundibulomas
7) Atypical teratomas
8) Malignant teratomas
9) Hypothalamic gliomas
10) Optic nerve gliomas
11) Ependymomas
12) Ganglioneurinomas
13) Suprasellar meningiomas
14) Malignant hemangiotheliomas
15) Cerebral reticulum cell sarcoma
16) Colloid cysts
17) Metastatic tumors
    a) bronchogenic carcinomas
    b) choriocarcinomas
    c) leukemic infiltrates
    d) plasmocytomas

changes of the sella turcica. Pituitary adenomas may also grow in an invasive way destroying adjacent bone structures and infiltrating the brain, the hypothalamus as well as the temporal lobes. Such tumors hypersecrete prolactin (Lundberg et al., 1977a) (Fig. 1A).

Craniopharyngiomas are congenital tumors that are usually manifested clinically in late childhood or early adolescence. Retarded puberty may therefore be the first sign. Craniopharyngiomas are believed to arise out of residual tissue from Rathke's pouch. Part of the tumor may be solid, but more often it consists of cysts with an amorphous non-vital content. These cysts may expand rapidly and may become very large (Fig. 1F). Alarming symptoms with very severe visual loss, somnolence and signs of raised intracranial pressure will eventually appear. In such a case the presence of hypogonadism indicates that the lesion is primarily a craniopharyngioma or another type of tumor in the hypothalamic region. Sometimes the tumor cysts start to expand in adulthood, in which case the symptomatology may progress more slowly, the clinical picture then being very similar to that of a pituitary adenoma.

Suprasellar meningiomas may give endocrine symptoms both by compressing the hypothalamic floor and by extension into the sella turcica (Fig. 1B).

Pinealomas also occur mainly in children. Instead of hypogonadism, precocious puberty is the main endocrine symptom in this group of patients. Because of its location the tumor seldom causes chiasmatic compression but may give rise to oculomotor symptoms by compressing the mesencephalon.

Teratomas and so-called germinomas (Camins and Mount, 1974; Simson et al., 1968) are not uncommon in the hypothalamic region and usually lead to clinical symptoms in childhood occasionally with a malignant course.

A very special type of malformation tumor is the hamartoma of tuber cinereum (Lin et al., 1978). Precocious puberty is usually the presenting symptom in this group of patients.

Hypothalamic gliomas occur especially in early childhood, causing the so-called early childhood diencephalic syndrome, in which emaciation is the most obvious symptom (Menezes et al., 1977).

Hypothalamic gliomas occurring at an adult age give rise to a very varied clinical picture. In some cases an optic nerve glioma will grow into the hypothalamus, giving endocrine symptoms. Optic gliomas are especially common among patients with Recklinghausen's syndrome. A visual defect is the first symptom.

A number of other types of tumors occur in the hypothalamus, as shown in Table 2. Among the metastases, bronchogenic carcinomas are the most common. Leukemic infiltrates of the hypothalamus also occur, especially in childhood leukemia (Greydanus et al., 1978).

3.4. Non-tumorous disorders of the hypothalamus (Table 3)

3.4.1. Post-traumatic hypothalamic bleeding.

Traumatic lesions of the hypothalamus and pituitary are fairly common in cerebral concussion (Ceballos, 1966). The pituitary stalk may rupture, with severe haemorrhage into the pituitary. Haemorrhage in the hypothalamus alone is less common. Extensive hypothalamic bleeding will lead to a rapid death, but sometimes less severe bleeding may result in scar formation and atrophy of the hypothalamus, with hypogonadism, obesity and vegetative dysfunction as symptoms.

3.4.2. Suprasellar aneurysms.

Arterial aneurysms or arteriovenous malformations of the suprasellar and hypothalamic region may give rise to symptoms similar to those of a suprasellar pituitary tumor. Usually no bleeding will have occurred but the aneurysm itself may be large.

3.4.3. Ruptured aneurysms of the anterior communicating artery.

Subarachnoid haemorrhage from a ruptured arterial aneurysm may lead to hypothalamic damage resulting in hypothalamo-pituitary insufficiency. This is especially common in the case of a ruptured aneurysm of the anterior communicating artery.

3.6.4. Acute asphyxia and increased intracranial pressure

may lead to minute hemorrhages and necrosis in the hypothalamus, giving rise to hypothalamic dysfunction, the main symptoms being hypogonadism and obesity.

Table 3. Non-tumorous disorders of the hypothalamus.

1) Post-traumatic hypothalamic bleeding
2) Suprasellar aneurysms
3) Ruptured aneurysms of the anterior communicating artery
4) Acute asphyxia
5) Increased intracranial pressure
6) Spontaneously arrested infantile hydrocephalus (pituitary pseudotumor)
7) Delayed radiation necrosis of the hypothalamus
8) Meningoencephalitis (mainly tuberculosis)
9) Mycotic infections (mainly aspergillomas)
10) Sarcoidosis
11) Histiocytosis-X

3.4.5. Spontaneously arrested infantile hydrocephalus.

Non-tumorous obstruction of the aqueduct of Sylvius in early childhood caused by encephalitis or a trauma at birth, may give rise to hydrocephalus which becomes arrested (Hagberg, 1962). The consequence of such a lesion from the pathological point of view is a moderate or pronounced hydrocephalus with dilation of the lateral ventricles and the third ventricle. Bulging of the floor of the third ventricle into the sella turcica also often occurs, leading to a roentgenological change of the latter structure which may be erroneously interpreted as a pituitary tumor. The term pituitary pseudotumor has therefore been recommended for such cases (Avman et al., 1978). As long as the cranial sutures are still open, the head is growing. If the pressure in the ventricular system becomes normal again the growth of the head is arrested. In adults one may see roentgenological signs of the pressure on the skull in the form of enhanced digitate impressions and diasthesis of some cranial sutures. Hypogonadism is more common than precocious puberty in these cases (Fig. 11).

3.4.6. Delayed radiation necrosis of the hypothalamus.

After irradiation of the brain, especially when this has been directed to the hypothalamic area, but also after irradiation of tumors of the eye or middle ear, or brain tumors in the posterior fossa, delayed radiation damage to the hypothalamus may occur (Samaan et al., 1975). The question may arise whether progressive hypothalamic insufficiency is caused by radiation necrosis or by expansion of the tumor.

3.4.7. Meningoencephalitis.

A number of meningitic and meningoencephalitic lesions that are located at

the basal cisterns may give rise to hypothalamic dysfunction in the late course of the disease. This is especially common in tuberculosis meningitis, where calcifications in the basal cisterns may be found (Shizume et al., 1977). It may also occur following a number of other infectious diseases such as luetic, pneumococcal and β-hemolytic streptococcal infections. Encephalitis from poliomyelitis virus and Coxsackie B5-virus may also cause a hypothalamic lesion. For unknown reasons, in addition to obesity, hypogonadism, autonomic dysfunction and sleep disorders, an increase in body hair is often seen in these cases.

3.4.8. Mycotic infections. Mycotic infections of the hypothalamus are rare. Aspergillus may grow in tumor formation as an aspergilloma (Fig. 1E).

3.4.9. Sarcoidosis. Sarcoidosis of the brain is not uncommon. The lesions may be situated almost anywhere in the brain and also in the hypothalamic region (Fig. 1H). They often occur in the walls of the third ventricle (Stuart et al., 1978).

3.4.10. Histiocytosis-X. This is a granulomatous lesion. The granulomas contain collections of phagocytes, mononuclear inflammatory cells and glial elements. Cholesterol is deposited into some of the cells. Histiocytosis-X is very often found in the hypothalamus, partly as scattered lesions in the walls of the third ventricle, but also as a small nodule located at the infundibulum. This may result in a very interesting clinical picture of retarded pituitary development. There may be a morphologically completely normal but undersized adenohypophysis that does not produce sufficient amounts of pituitary hormones because of interruption of the portal vessels resulting in inability of the releasing hormones to reach the anterior pituitary. Histiocytosis-X usually has its onset before puberty. The lesion is often localized to the pituitary stalk. In these cases the pituitary fossa will not develop normally, and in adults this underdevelopment of the pituitary is manifested as an abnormally small pituitary fossa. This sign is of great importance for differential diagnosis (Lundberg et al., 1977b).

3.5. Pubertas praecox

True precocious puberty is defined as abnormally early pubertal development which does not differ, apart from its early onset, from normal isosexual pubertal development. It may be idiopathic or caused by an apparent central nervous disorder. Only the latter group will be considered in this chapter.

The process of precocious sexual development may start as early as 6 months of age. In most cases, however, the first symptoms appear after the age of 3 years and by definition in boys before 10 years of age. In boys the most common underlying pathology is a tumor of the hypothalamus or pineal region (Thamdrup, 1961 and Table 4). In the tuber cinereum, which is a part of the basal hypothalamus, a certain type of congenital malformation tumor – a hamartoma – may be found. Immunofluorescence studies with use of specific antibodies to LH-RH have shown the presence of this hormone in such tumors (Judge et al., 1977). However, most cases of precocious puberty of central origin are not caused by this specific tumor. Localization of any tumor to the basal and posterior parts of the hypothalamus or the pineal region seems to be a critical causal factor. Tumors located in the anterior, upper or lateral parts of the hypothalamus do not usually give rise to precocious puberty.

The pathophysiological background probably is not a pathological production of releasing hormones by tumor cells but a blockade of inhibitory mechanisms normally operative at prepubertal ages. This can also explain why hydrocephalus, arachnoid cysts and post-traumatic lesions in the hypothalamus may be the only pathological finding.

Although sexual development may be complete, resulting in the formation of mature spermatozoa in the testis, in most cases it is partial. Body weight is usually increased and blood and urinary hormone values generally correspond to the different stages of sexual development. The results of hypothalamo-pituitary stimulation tests vary in relation to the underlying disorder (Chaussain et al., 1978).

Epileptic seizures are fairly common even in early cases. Of specific interest is the occurrence of fits of laughter (Hann, 1978). Some of the patients are mentally retarded. In the tumor cases further symp-

Table 4. True precocious puberty of central nervous origin in 55 boys (own cases and cases from the literature 1952-77).

Pathology	Number	Age at first sign of puberty (range and mean in years)	
Hamartoma of tuber cinereum	13	½-7	(3.3)
Hypothalamic teratoma	2	8-10	
Hypothalamic astrocytoma	1	9	
Hypothalamic spongioblastoma	1	7	
Hypothalamic ependymoma	1	9	
Hypothalamic choriocarcinoma	2	7-9	
Hypothalamic tumor, not verified	5	2/12-2	(10/12)
Optic glioma	2	½-9	
Pinealoma	7	3-10	(7.7)
Teratoma of pineal gland	1	7	
Tumor of the pineal gland, not verified	2	6½-7½	
Tuberosis sclerosis	2	2½-8	
Neurofibromatosis	2	7½-9	
McCune-Albright syndrome	3	2½-5½	(4.3)
Hydrocephalus	4	½-8	(4.4)
Post-traumatic hypothalamic lesion	2	5-10	
Arachnoiditis of the chiasm	2	2½-5	
Suprasellar cyst	3	3-9	(6.8)

toms of tumor growth develop, such as signs of compression of the optic chiasm or optic tracts, evidence of a mid-brain lesion (e.g. paralysis of conjugate upward gaze and pupillary disturbances) and increased intracranial pressure (e.g. headache, vomiting and somnolence). The prognosis is dependent upon the underlying disorder. Sometimes the tumor is curable, but in most cases it leads to death within a few years.

A peculiar form of precocious puberty of central origin is the so-called McCune-Albright syndrome. This syndrome, which is much more common in girls than boys, also includes polyostotic fibrous dysplasia and brown, non-elevated areas of skin pigmentation. These two conditions are often unilateral and found on the same side of the body. The bone lesions lead to pathological fractures. In the McCune-Albright syndrome an excess production of ACTH or growth hormone (GH) may occur, resulting in Cushing's disease or gigantism/acromegaly.

small stature with acromicria (i.e. small hands and feet), hypogonadism, congenital muscular hypotonia and mental retardation (Prader et al., 1956). The mental retardation is moderate with an IQ of 30-70 (S-D or WISC). Bone development is usually retarded, resulting both in stature below the mean for the age and acromicria. A high-arched palate and dental malformations are common, as well as strabismus and a number of other minor 'stigmata'. A small penis, hypoplasia of the scrotum and bilateral cryptorchidism are present in most male cases. Testicular biopsies at prepubertal ages display normal conditions for the age. Most cases described have been children. In adulthood severe sexual underdevelopment is present and the patients remain sterile. The serum FSH, LH and testosterone concentrations are low normal to subnormal. The responses to LH-RH and clomiphene may vary (Tolis et al., 1974). In most cases the karyotype is normal. Neuropathological studies are still lacking.

4. HEREDITARY NEUROLOGICAL SYNDROMES WITH HYPOGONADISM

4.1. Prader-(Labhart)-Willi syndrome (hypotonia-oligophrenia-hypogonadism-obesity)

This syndrome consists of oligophrenia, obesity,

4.2. Laurence-Moon-Bardet-Biedl syndrome

The cardinal symptoms in this syndrome are retinitis pigmentosa, polydactyly, mental retardation, obesity and hypogonadism. The syndrome is hereditary, with an autosomal recessive mode of transmission. The pigmentary retinopathy is generally discovered at school age because of a decrease in

visual acuity, which is often preceded by night-blindness. The visual acuity deteriorates to blindness towards the age of 30 years. Most of the adult males display testicular hypoplasia, a female distribution of body hair and more or less complete absence of libido and erectile potency. Sometimes gynecomastia is present and the body proportions may be eunuchoid. Data concerning hormone levels in this syndrome, though incomplete, suggest hypogonadotropic hypogonadism. Diabetes mellitus and hypothyroidism may be found. The syndrome seems to occur in Central Europe more often than elsewhere. In Switzerland the incidence is estimated at 1:160,000 (Klein and Amman, 1969).

In Sweden a somewhat different syndrome has been described by Alström et al. (1959). Instead of polydyctaly and mental retardation, neural deafness is a feature of the syndrome. The hypogonadism is of the hypergonadotropic type and testicular biopsy shows germinal cell aplasia.

4.3. Börjeson-Forssman-Lehmann syndrome

This is probably an X-linked, recessively inherited syndrome characterized by grave mental retardation (idiocy), hypogonadism, dwarfism, epilepsy, a grotesque physical appearance with enormous ears and a number of other abnormalities. The panniculus adiposus is abnormally increased and the skin and subcutaneous tissue in the face swollen. The testes are small and autopsy has revealed advanced tubular fibrosis, interstitial fibrosis and Leydig-cell hyperplasia (Brun et al., 1974).

4.4. Cerebellar ataxia and hypogonadism

The coexistence of hypogonadism and different types of heredoataxias has been described in a number of patients (Neuhäuser and Opitz, 1975; Sylvester, 1972). In most cases the neurological syndrome has been Friedreich's ataxia, but other heredoataxias have been the main disorder in some patients. Puberty usually is absent or retarded, with small testes and lack of pubic hair. The serum testosterone and gonadotropin concentrations are low and testicular biopsy shows spermatogenic arrest. Aspermia and lack of libido and potency are characteristic features in these cases. Hypogonadotropic hypogonadism has also been described in

hereditary polyneuropathy of the Charcot-Marie-Tooth type, in the Moebius syndrome (congenital bilateral paralysis of the facial and abducens nerves (Olson et al., 1970)) and in a number of other hereditary neurological disorders.

4.5. Hypergonadotropic hypogonadism in hereditary neurological disorders

A number of hereditary neurological syndromes exist usually combined with more or less pronounced mental retardation or progressive dementia, with hypergonadotropic hypogonadism as a salient feature. The most well-known of these syndromes is myotonic dystrophy (see below), which is not uncommon. However, most of the other syndromes are rare and some are only confined to an occasional family. A number of these syndromes have recently been studied and the type of hypogonadism compared (Lundberg, 1973; Lundberg et al., 1978). Thus, the clinical picture of hypogonadism was similar in one sibship in which the main neurological defect was respectively a myopathy, a polyneuropathy and a spastic tetraparesis. The hypogonadism was sometimes congenital, with absence of pubertal development, but in most cases it was acquired, with normal pubertal development, but subsequent atrophy of the gonads. Females presented a picture of premature menopause. Serum FSH and LH concentrations were high and the response to LH-RH was exaggerated, similar to the findings in Klinefelter's syndrome. The serum testosterone concentrations were lower than normal, but not as low as is usually seen in hypogonadotropic hypogonadism. The patients usually had developed sexual interest.

Hypergonadotropic hypogonadism may also be seen in the Marinesco-Sjögren syndrome (cerebellar ataxia, congenital cataract and mental retardation (Skre and Berg, 1977) and ocular myopathy (Lundberg, 1966).

4.6. Myotonic dystrophy (dystrophia myotonica, myotonia atrophica, Steinert's disease)

This disorder is characterized by progressive muscular atrophy, myotonia, mental defects, cataracts and hypogonadism. It is a hereditary disorder with an autosomal dominant trait. The incidence has been

estimated to be between 1 and 5 per 100,000.

The muscular disorder may be manifested in early infancy, with difficulty in nursing, attributable to bilateral facial weakness. Half of the cases have distinct muscular weakness at puberty. Facial signs (the so-called facies myotonica), are typical. The face is expressionless and the forehead smooth, the eyelids droop, the cheeks are sunken, the mouth is open and the neckline is indistinct, the latter because of atrophy of the sternocleidomastoid muscle. The progressive muscular wasting and weakness also involve many arm and leg muscles. Myotonia is present and is manifested as a prolonged after-contraction persisting in the muscle after voluntary contraction, especially after clenching of the fists. It may also be seen as a persistent, localized muscular contraction on percussion of the affected muscle, e.g. the thenar muscles. The electromyographic pattern is pathognomonic.

A star-shaped cataract of the lens appears sooner or later in most cases. This may not lead to visual impairment until later in life and often the cataract is therefore only discovered on examination. Many of the patients have more or less pronounced progressive mental deficiency. This may be mild and may affect only certain aspects of the mind, such as judgement.

Puberty is usually normal in myotonic dystrophy. Frontal baldness subsequently develops later and is an almost obligatory finding in the adult male. However, a decrease of body hair, gynecomastia and eunuchoid body proportions are uncommon. All males are probably fertile from the beginning and about 70% actually become fathers. Sexual activity is normal or may even be excessive. The sexual life of the patients may be complicated by a progressive loss of judgement. Later there may be a decrease in libido and erectile potency.

The testes may be normal on palpation just after puberty. Clinically noticeable atrophy then occurs and they become small and soft. Histopathological examination of the testes at different ages postpuberty shows disorganization of spermatogenesis followed by a progressive decrease in spermatogenic activity, degeneration of germ cells and Sertoli cells and finally complete tubular sclerosis.

The serum testosterone concentration is low or normal, as is the urinary excretion of 17-ketosteroids. The serum FSH level is regularly elevated in the adult male. Serum LH may be normal but is often increased, and the response to LH-RH is supranormal. The testicular pathology is not normalized by treatment with human chorionic gonadotropin (HCG).

5. DISORDERS OF THE NERVOUS SYSTEM WITH SEXUAL DYSFUNCTION AS THE PREDOMINANT ANDROLOGICAL SYMPTOM

5.1. Sexual dysfunction in patients with cerebral lesions outside the hypothalamic area

Sexual dysfunction often occurs in patients as a result of focal or diffuse cerebral lesions, both cortical and subcortical. Thus a decrease in libido and potency has been reported after vascular lesions and tumors, following a single brain injury (de Morsier and Gronek, 1972) or in patients with repeated brain injuries such as boxers with traumatic encephalopathy, and in patients with degenerative disorders such as Parkinson's and Alzheimer's disease. It is often difficult to evaluate these cases, however, since the brain lesion may be hard to delineate and is often widespread, and since the patients often present with a number of severe psychiatric symptoms and may be severely physically disabled.

In most cases it appears that the temporal lobes or the limbic cortex are involved in sexual function. Impotence has never been proved in pure frontal lobe lesions. On the contrary, in such cases, as after frontal leukotomy, increased sexual activity has been reported. On the other hand, impotence has often occurred after temporal lobe surgery and in patients with temporal lobe tumors impotence may precede other symptoms. Impotence often occurs after surgical interruption of the ansa lenticularis for parkinsonism and is especially frequent after bilateral operations. It is probable that the localization of the lesion is more important than its pathological features. It is also quite clear that the premorbid personality plays a very important role.

Besides changes in libido and potency, alterations of sexual behavior, as well as delusions, confabulations and hallucinations with a sexual content have been reported in patients with brain lesions, especially when the lesion has involved the temporal lobes.

5.2. Epilepsy

Patients with epilepsy present special problems with respect to sexual dysfunction (Saunders and Rawson, 1970). Genital sensations as well as motor activity in the genital region and a feeling of orgasm can occur as a focal epileptic manifestation. Orgasm can provoke an epileptic fit. An increase in sexual arousability and in sexual activity may be present in the post-paroxysmal phase after an epileptic fit. It has been found that sexual problems occur mainly in patients with temporal lobe epilepsy and in those having psychomotor epileptic fits. In such cases there may be a decrease in libido and potency without any signs of a major brain lesion. However, if there is gross damage to the temporal lobes, especially if bilateral, the sexual problems may be more pronounced.

Sexual problems in these patients have been eliminated after temporal lobe surgery; however, anticonvulsive drugs usually do not improve sexual performance. Some antiepileptic drugs have a definite negative influence on libido. A decrease in androgen metabolites in the urine has been reported in males with epilepsy on phenobarbital or phenytoin. This has been explained by an increase in steroid hormone metabolism due to induction of liver enzymes caused by the anticonvulsants. Phenytoin increases the sex hormone binding globulin, resulting in a reduction of active sex steroids circulating in the blood (Victor et al., 1977). Other anticonvulsants do not seem to have such important negative effects on steroid binding and metabolism. It is therefore suggested that if an epileptic patient on phenobarbital or phenytoin complains of a decrease in libido or impotence, his medication should be changed to carbamazepine or a benzodiazepine. On rare occasions a patient with epilepsy may experience the epileptic attack as pleasurable, especially if there is a focal genital component in the epileptic fit. Other patients may experience the unconsciousness occurring during the fit as a form of sexual gratification and sometimes, therefore epileptic fits may be self- induced. A patient may provoke an attack by masturbation or even by imaginative thoughts. Self-induced photostimulation of an epileptic attack, for example at a discotheque, is not uncommon.

Both sexual dysfunction and sexual deviations may appear interictally, especially in the post-paroxysmal phase. Sexual problems are usually overlooked in patients with epilepsy. However, the frequency of some kind of sexual problem is high. In temporal lobe epilepsy it is estimated at about 50%, and this is the most common form of focal epilepsy. Since epilepsy is a very common neurological manifestation, sexual dysfunction and disorders of sexual behavior in epilepsy comprise one of the most important fields of sexology for the neurologist.

5.3. Multiple sclerosis

Multiple sclerosis is characterized by a widespread occurrence of lesions in the central nervous system giving rise to disseminated neurological symptoms. These neurological symptoms occur mainly in episodes. Usually some improvement takes place after each episode. The prognosis is extremely variable. In one case there may be just one single episode with no apparent residual symptoms, and in another case rapid deterioration may lead to total physical disability. the most prominent features are weakness and loss of control of the limbs, sensory symptoms, incoordination and visual defects. Symptoms from the autonomic nervous system may be pronounced, however, and may also appear early in the course of the disease. Most of the patients sooner or later develop transitory or persistent urinary troubles such as urgency, incontinence or urinary retention. Constipation is also common and bowel incontinence may occur.

Sexual activity changes in almost all male patients with advanced multiple sclerosis (Lilius et al., 1976). The interest in sexual intercourse, its frequency and the satisfaction of coitus are reduced in more than half of the cases. A common symptom is loss or weakness of erection (Vas, 1969). This is a residual symptom between episodes in at least half of the male patients with advanced multiple sclerosis and may occur transiently even in early and mild cases. Retarded or absent ejaculation and orgasmic difficulties are also reported in one third to one-half of advanced multiple sclerosis patients. However, changes of sensory perception may also constitute a severe problem for the patients (Lundberg, 1978). During certain episodes the patient may have intense paresthesiae and dysesthesiae in

certain areas of his body surface. If the external genitalia are involved, or other parts of the body that come in contact with the partner during sexual activity, the tactile stimuli may be very disagreeable. Fortunately, these sensory symptoms are usually transitory. Treatment with local anesthetics or certain drugs such as carbamazepine may be used during the acute phase.

When loss of libido is the main problem there is probably a lesion in the brain. Thus, lesions of the nerve tracts conveying impulses to and from the genital organs, and lesions in those parts of the brain regulating sexual libido and orgasm may very well explain why patients with multiple sclerosis often have severe sexual problems. However, multiple sclerosis may also affect the sex-life of a patient in other ways. In advanced cases the occurrence of limb paresis, spasticity, ataxia and decreased visual function may result in severe sexual incapacity by making ordinary sexual activity difficult or even impossible. Psychological problems connected with the disability and social changes in these patients may also affect sexual relationships.

5.4. Paraplegia and tetraplegia

Tetraplegia is caused by a lesion in the cervical part of the spinal cord and paraplegia by a lesion in the thoracic or lumbar area of the cord. In many cases the lesion is traumatic and involves only a restricted part of the spinal cord, but often a more widespread myelopathy may be present. If the lesion is complete, there is no longer any connection between the brain, the upper part of the medulla and the underlying segments of the body. In complete lesions some nerve paths may still be functioning. Besides an interruption of the long ascending and descending nerve tracts, the nerve centers at the site of the lesion are usually also destroyed.

The effect of a spinal cord lesion on the sexual function of a patient is very much dependent upon the level at which the lesion is located. If there is destruction of the genital reflex centers in the lower part of the medulla – a so-called lower motor neuron lesion – no or very little sexual function can remain. In lesions of the upper part of the medulla, reflex erection and ejaculation may still be possible, despite the fact that the patient might no longer have any sensory perception in his genital organs. As stated above, erection may be brought about by two different mechanisms, the cerebral and the reflex erection operating at different levels. In some cases, therefore, erection provoked by psychic influences and visual stimulation may still be possible despite a loss of reflex erection. In some patients with a complete lesion in the lower part of the medulla, with paresis of the striated ejaculatory muscles in the genital region, semen may still be produced and on sexual stimulation dribbling of semen from the tip of the penis may be seen.

From most clinical case material it is reported that about 80% of the patients with all types of spinal cord lesions retain at least some erectile capacity, but only 10% experience ejaculation. Spontaneous activity after a traumatic spinal cord lesion is usually low. However, it has been proven that rehabilitation may be very helpful for such patients and that many paraplegics and even tetraplegics may have a quite satisfactory sexual life. Rehabilitation is especially liable to be successful in patients with partial or high cord lesions.

Technical devices may be of help. Erection and sometimes ejaculation can be attained with the aid of vibrators. Electroejaculation, that is electrical stimulation of the nerves near the prostate gland and seminal vesicles through a probe inserted in the rectum, has also been induced. Even if it is impossible for a patient to impregnate his partner and ejaculate intravaginally, conception may be brought about by artificial insemination from a paraplegic patient through electroejaculation.

Testicular function has been studied in a number of men with spinal cord injuries. Germinal cell hypoplasia with spermatogenic arrest has been documented in a large proportion of these patients (Kikuchi et al., 1976). Low spinal cord lesions, i.e. lesions below the point of sympathetic outflow from the spinal cord, are less likely to result in testicular disorders. Serum FSH, LH and testosterone concentrations and the response to HCG stimulation are usually quite normal in patients with spinal cord injuries. Testicular disorders in these cases are therefore considered to be secondary to a disturbance of sympathetic nervous activity.

5.5. Malformations of the spinal cord

Spina bifida is a congenital malformation with

incomplete closure of the bony spine, most commonly in the lumbosacral area. It is often associated with developmental defects of the meninges and the spinal cord. There may be a meningocele, i.e. a sac-like mass covered by the skin and containing the meninges protruding at the side of the spina bifida. The mass is called a myelomeningocele if it includes a malformation of the spinal cord and nerve roots, and a myelocele if the spinal cord itself is exposed, uncovered by skin.

Impotence and ejaculatory failure are usually present in spina bifida and there is often pronounced sensory loss in the genital region. Only about one third of boys with spina bifida are reported to masturbate (Dorner, 1977). Interest in the opposite sex has been stated to be lower in this group of patients than in adolescents with, for example, cerebral palsy. Less severely handicapped males seem to have a satisfactory sexual life and some of these men have fathered children (Laurence and Beresford, 1975).

Spinal cord malformations may also occur in the upper part of the spine, the most frequent of these being basilar impression and the so-called Arnold-Chiari syndrome (de Barros et al., 1975). In this group of patients absolute or relative impotence is very common. This is probably caused by damage to the long descending spinal path regulating cerebral erection. Gonadal function is often normal in these cases and many have become fathers.

Another type of spinal malformation is syringomyelia. This condition is marked by abnormal cavities in the spinal cord usually in the central part of the medulla. These cavities are rarely present in the lower part of the medulla, where the genital reflex centers are located, but in certain instances the long descending nerve tracts may be involved, resulting in a defect of cerebral erection as well as difficulties in micturition, mainly urinary retention.

5.6. Myelopathies

Besides the spinal cord malformation syndromes, the more or less complete spinal cord compression syndromes giving rise to paraplegia or tetraplegia, and mulitple sclerosis, there are several types of myelopathies of different origin. Sexual dysfunction may be present in many patients with cervical spinal cord injuries without paralysis (Perese et al., 1976),

in patients with subacute combined myelopathy due to lack of vitamin B_{12}, in tabes dorsalis and in myelopathies due to infections and vascular disorders (Schneider, 1974). Impotence is also common in the Shy-Drager syndrome.

5.7. Polyneuropathies

Polyneuropathies, i.e. systemic disorders of the peripheral nerves, both spinal and cranial nerves, may have very variable etiologies. The immediate cause may be infectious, toxic or metabolic, or malnutrition. Polyneuropathy is often a part of a heredodegenerative syndrome where the pathophysiology probably is an inborn error of metabolism. Symptoms may be motor as well as sensory. Somatic nerves are usually involved, but certain metabolic disorders preferably affect the peripheral autonomic nerves. Diabetic polyneuropathy and alcoholic polyneuropathy are the most common forms of polyneuropathies. In the diabetic type autonomic nerves are usually involved to a much greater extent than in alcoholic polyneuropathy. To differentiate sexual dysfunction in such cases a study of the genital reflexes may be helpful. The bulbocavernosus reflex, which is a somatic reflex, is usually normal in diabetic polyneuropathy but may be pathological in the alcoholic type.

The relationship of diabetes mellitus to andrological disorders is discussed in Chapter 5.

5.7.1. Alcoholic polyneuropathy

Sexual problems in alcoholism are very common, but in most cases the psychosocial situation of the alcoholic and the acute alcoholic intoxication rather than neuropathic lesions give rise to sexual difficulties. In chronic alcoholism 10% of the patients are reported to have alcoholic polyneuropathy. This polyneuropathy mainly involves the somatic peripheral nerves. Therefore, apart from impotence, ejaculatory difficulties in the form of retarded or absent ejaculatory contractions are a common complaint in these patients. Reflexes of the genital region, such as the bulbocavernosus reflex, are often affected. If the alcoholism itself can be treated, the prognosis in alcoholic polyneuropathy is much better than that in diabetic polyneuropathy. A vitamin deficiency, especially of

vitamin B_1, plays a considerable part in the pathophysiology. Vitamin injection should therefore always be given if alcoholic polyneuropathy is suspected.

5.7.2. Heredodegenerative neurological disorders with polyneuropathy

Sexual function has been investigated very little in these types of disorders. Primary amyloidosis with polyneuropathy is a syndrome in which the autonomic peripheral nerves are involved in a considerable number of the patients, and therefore genito-urinary troubles may be prominent symptoms. Total impotence is reported to occur in two-thirds of male patients, a symptom which may appear early in the disease. Histological examination of the testes has shown spermatogenic arrest and deposits of amyloid in the small vessels (Andersson and Hofer, 1974).

5.8. Sacral rhizopathies

Disorders involving the peripheral nerves, connecting the centers of erection and ejaculation in the spinal cord with the sex organs, usually only partially interrupt efferent and afferent nerve fibers. These so-called rhizopathies generally involve only one or a few lumbosacral nerves on one side. The unilateral rhizopathy of sacral nerves 2 and 3 gives an ipsilateral sensory defect of all qualities in parts of the penis and scrotum (Bohm et al., 1956). Only in patients in whom these nerves have been bilaterally affected may the ability to produce or to maintain an erection be seriously affected and ejaculation become impossible. However, another type of problem may exist in these patients. They may have severe pain radiating into the genital organs. This pain may be intensified at the moment of orgasm and thus greatly influence the sexual life of the patient. Radiating pain from the spine during movements may also complicate sexual activity.

The sacral nerve roots are sometimes involved in inflammatory reactions of the meninges, which may be of varying origin. Such reactions have been observed as a complication of contrast myelography. Unfortunately, the symptoms in these cases are usually bilateral, leading to both a sensory defect and a loss of sexual function.

Another cause of sacral rhizopathy may be herpes zoster infection. Herpes zoster may occasionally involve the bladder, the anus and the genital region (Jellinek and Tulloch, 1976). In such cases persistent pain may result in severe sexual incapacity. There is usually both sensory loss, paresis of some of the muscles in the pelvic area and loss of some of the genital reflexes. The site of the underlying disorder can usually be located by a thorough neurological examination.

5.9. Priapism

Priapism is often caused by a blood disorder, intoxication or infection. Priapism due to these factors is as a rule very painful and may lead to permanent damage through thrombotic changes of the cavernous bodies. However, a number of acute and chronic neurological affections may result in a less pronounced, sometimes fluctuating priapism. In such cases it may be difficult to decide whether the priapism is spontaneous or results from a lack of sexual inhibition. In contrast to the other forms of priapism it may be combined with annoying demands for sexual gratification – a true hypersexuality.

Neurogenic priapism may be short-lasting and appear as a focal part of an epileptic fit, though this is very rare. It may be an early symptom of some acute neurological disorder such as encephalitis, medullary compression or lead poisoning. It may also suddenly occur in certain chronic diseases such as neurometabolic disorders, multiple sclerosis, tabes dorsalis or Behcet's syndrome.

6. CONCLUDING REMARKS

The most important andrological symptoms that point to a neurological disorder are precocious as well as delayed puberty, primary as well as secondary hypogonadism and decrease in libido as well as impotence or ejaculatory failure. Infertility may also be the presenting symptom. Therefore, a neurological examination, a neuroendocrine evaluation and a number of test procedures, including roentgenological examinations of certain parts of the brain and spinal cord, are important diagnostic tools in these cases.

The andrologist may diagnose a disease of the central or the peripheral nervous system as the cause of his patient's complaints. His patient may also have neurological symptoms as a part of a hereditary syndrome.

REFERENCES

Alström CH, Hallgren B, Nilsson LB, Åsander H (1959) Retinal degeneration combined with obesity, diabetes mellitus and neurogenesis deafness: a specific syndrome (not hitherto described) distinct from the Laurence-Moon-Bardet-Biedl syndrome: a clinical, endocrinological and genetic examination based on a large pedigree. Acta Psychiat Scand 34, Suppl 129: 1.

Andersson R, Hofer P-Å (1974) Genitourinary disturbances in familial and sporadic cases of primary amyloidosis with polyneuropathy. Acta Med Scand 195: 49.

Avman N, Erdogan G, Kanpolat Y (1978) Pituitary pseudo-tumor. Surg Neurol 9: 107.

de Barros MC, da Silva WF, de Azevedo Filho HC, Spinelli C (1975) Disturbances of sexual potency in patients with basilar impression and Arnold-Chiari malformation. J Neurol Neurosurg Psychiat 38: 598.

Bauer HG (1959) Endocrine and metabolic conditions related to pathology in the hypothalamus: a review. J Nerv Ment Dis 128: 323.

Bohm E, Franksson C, Petersén I (1956) Sacral rhizopathies and sacral root syndromes (SII-SV). Acta Chir Scand, Suppl 216: 1.

Brun A, Börjeson M, Forssman H (1974) An inherited syndrome with mental deficiency and endocrine disorders. A patho-anatomical study. J Ment Defic Res 18: 317.

Camins MB, Mount LA (1974) Primary suprasellar atypical teratoma. Brain 97: 447.

Ceballos R (1966) Pituitary changes in head trauma. Analysis of 102 consecutive cases of head injury. Alabama J Med Sci 3: 185.

Chaussain JL Savage MO, Nahoul K, Brijawi A, Canlorbe P, Job JC (1978) Hypothalamo-pituitary-gonadal function in male central precocious puberty. Clin Endocrinol 8: 437.

di Chiro G, Nelson KB (1962) The volume of the sella turcica. Am J Roentgenol Radiat Ther Nucl Med 87: 989.

Dorner S (1977) Sexual interest and activity in adolescents with spina bifida. J Child Psychol Psychiat 18: 229.

Greydanus DE, Burgert EO, Gilchrist GS (1978) Hypothalamic syndrome in children with acute lymphocytic leukemia. Mayo Clin Proc 53: 217.

Hagberg B (1962) The sequelae of spontaneously arrested infantile hydrocephalus. Dev Med Child Neurol 4: 583.

Hann J (1978) Präparoxysmale Lachanfälle bei hyperplastischer Missbildung des Hypothalamus. Arch Psychiat Nervenkr 225: 107.

Jellinek EH, Tulloch WS (1976) Herpes zoster with dysfunction of bladder and anus. Lancet ii: 1219.

Judge DM, Kulin HE, Page R, Santen R, Trapukdi S (1977) Hypothalamic hamartoma. A source of luteinizing-hormone-releasing factor in precocious puberty. New Engl J Med 296: 7.

Kallmann FJ, Schoenfeld WA, Barrera SE (1944) The genetic aspects of primary eunuchoidism. Am J Ment Defic 48: 203.

Kikuchi TA, Skowsky WR, El-Toraei I, Swerdloff R (1976) The pituitary-gonadal axis in spinal cord injury. Fertil Steril 27: 1142.

Kjessler B, Lundberg PO (1974) Dysfunction of the neuro-endocrine system in nine males with aspermia. Fertil Steril 25: 1007.

Klein D, Amman F (1969) The syndrome of Laurence-Moon-Biedl and allied diseases in Switzerland. Clinical, genetic and epidemiological studies. J Neurol Sci 9: 479.

Korsgaard O, Lindholm J, Rasmussen P (1976) Endocrine function in patients with suprasellar and hypothalamic tumours. Acta Endocrinol 83: 1.

Laurence KM, Beresford A (1975) Continence, friends, marriage and children in 51 adults with spina bifida. Dev Med Child Neurol 17, Suppl 35: 123.

Lilius HG, Valtonen EJ, Wikström J (1976) Sexual problems in patients suffering from multiple sclerosis. Scand J Soc Med 4: 41.

Lin SR, Bryson MM, Goblen RP, Fitz CR, Lee YY (1978) Radiologic findings of hamartomas of the tuber cinereum and hypothalamus. Radiology 127: 697.

Lundberg PO (1966) Observations on endocrine function in ocular myopathy. Acta Neurol Scand 42: 39.

Lundberg PO (1973) Hereditary myopathy, oligophrenia, cataract, skeletal abnormalities and hypergonadotropic hypogonadism. Eur Neurol 10: 261.

Lundberg PO (1978) Sexual dysfunction in patients of multiple sclerosis. Sex Disab 1: 218.

Lundberg PO, Drettner B, Hemmingsson A, Stenkvist B, Wide L (1977a) The invasive pituitary adenoma. Arch Neurol 34: 742.

Lundberg PO, Gemzell C (1966) Dysplasia of the sella turcica: clinical and laboratory investigations in three cases. Acta Endocrinol 52: 478.

Lundberg PO, Nilsson A-C, Wide L (1978) Hypergonadotropic hypogonadism in oligophrenia. Acta Med Scand 204: 115.

Lundberg PO, Olsson Y, Sundström C (1977b) Cerebral histio-cytosis-X with endocrine symptoms. Uppsala J Med Sci 82: 195.

Lundberg PO, Wide L (1974) The results of some neuro-endocrinological investigations in patients with anatomically verified hypothalamic disorders. Gin Pol 45: 953.

Menezes AH, Bell WE, Perret GE (1977) Hypothalamic tumors in children. Child's Brain 3: 265.

de Morsier G (1954) Etudes sur les dysraphies crânioencéphaliques. Schweiz Arch Neurol Psychol 73: 309.

de Morsier G, Gronek G (1972) Sur 92 cas de troubles sexuels post-traumatiques. Ann Médico-psychol 2: 653.

Neuhäuser G, Opitz JM (1975) Autosomal recessive syndrome of cerebellar ataxia and hypogonadotropic-hypogonadism. Clin Gen 7: 426.

Olson WH, Bardin CW, Walsh GO, Engel WK (1970) Moebius syndrome. Neurology 20: 1002.

Perese DM, Prezio JA, Perese EF (1976) Sexual dysfunction caused by injuries of the cervical spinal cord without paralysis. Spine 1: 149.

Prader A, Labhart A, Willi H (1956) Ein Syndrom von Adipositas, Kelinwuchs, Kryptorchismus und Oligophrenie nach myatonieartigem Zustand in Neugeborenenalter. Schweiz Med Wschr 86: 1260.

Samaan NA, Bakdash MM, Caderao JB, Cangir A, Jesse RH, Ballantyne AJ (1975) Hypopituitarism after external irradiation. Ann Intern Med 83: 771.

Saunders M, Rawson M (1970) Sexuality in male epileptics. J Neurol Sci 10: 577.

Schneider E (1974) Störungen der Sexualfunktion bei nicht-traumatischen Rückenmarkserkrankungen. Fortschr Neurol Psychiat 42: 562.

Shizume K, Harada Y, Ibayashi H, Kumahara Y, Shimizu N, Hibi I, Imura H, Miura K, Saito S, Yoshida S, Tomita A, Nakagawa K, Demura H (1977) Survey studies on pituitary disease in Japan. Endocrinol Jpn 24: 139.

Simson LR, Lampe I, Abell MR (1968) Suprasellar germinomas. Cancer 22: 533.

Skre H, Berg K (1977) Linkage studies on the Marinesco-Sjögren syndrome and hypergonadotropic hypogonadism. Clin Gen 11: 57.

Stuart CA, Neelon FA, Lebovitz HE (1978) Hypothalamic insufficiency: the cause of hypopituitarism in sarcoidosis. Ann Intern Med 88: 589.

Sylvester PE (1972) Spino-cerebellar degeneration, hormonal disorder, hypogonadism, deaf mutism and mental deficiency. J Ment Defic Res 16: 203.

Thamdrup E (1961) Precocious sexual development. A clinical study of 100 children. Copenhagen: Munksgaard.

Tolis G, Lewis W, Verdy M, Friesen HG, Solomon S, Pagalis G, Pavlatos F, Fessas PH, Rochefort JG (1974) Anterior pituitary function in the Prader-Labhart-Willi (PLW) syndrome. J Clin Endocrinol Metab 39: 1061.

Vas CJ (1969) Sexual impotence and some autonomic disturbances in men with multiple sclerosis. Acta Neurol Scand 45: 166.

Victor A, Lundberg PO, Johansson EDB (1977) Induction of sex hormone binding globulin by phenytoin. Br Med J 668: 934.

16. ANDROLOGICAL DISORDERS IN NEPHROLOGY

G. BUCCIANTE and A. BERNARDI

As our fundamental knowledge of the biochemical and physiological functions of the kidney increases, we are becoming more aware of the complex relations existing between the kidney and numerous endocrine glands. The effect of chronic renal failure on the parathyroid gland has been known for many years. Variations in aldosterone production in pathologic situations involving renal malfunctioning and the alteration of thyroid function in various renal diseases are other examples of this inter-relationship.

One aspect not yet completely understood is the effect of the kidney on testicular function. In some congenital nephropathies (Fanconi syndrome, renal tubular acidosis and nephrogenic diabetes insipidus) there is an associated retardation of growth and sexual development, most pronounced when there is some degree of renal insufficiency present. However, even in acquired renal disease, there is often profound alteration in testicular function.

1. TESTICULAR ALTERATIONS IN CHRONIC RENAL INSUFFICIENCY

The first signs of testicular insufficiency and disturbances of sexual function appear when renal insufficiency has reached an advanced stage, as defined by a reduction in the glomerular filtration rate (GFR) to below 7-8 ml/min, with clinical signs of uremia present, i.e. increased blood urea nitrogen (BUN), weakness, anemia, muscular atrophy, neuropathy and osteodystrophy. The categories of renal disease causing chronic renal failure are listed in Table 1.

Other symptoms attributable to alteration in gonadal function are: reduced libido, reduced frequence of sexual activity and difficulty in achieving and maintaining an erection, often resulting in complete impotence. This information may be difficult to obtain due to the prevalence of uremic symptoms.

In addition to a reduction in body weight, the physical examination in these patients reveals loss of muscular mass and marked testicular atrophy, defined as a reduction in testicular dimensions to less than 3.6×2.1 cm. If the patients with renal insufficiency are at the age of puberty there is an associated retardation of growth and development (Broyer et al., 1972; Mehls et al., 1978) (Fig. 1).

The institution of a treatment program of hemodialysis (HD) or peritoneal dialysis (PD) brings about an improvement in the biochemical parameters of uremia and its clinical aspects as well. Nausea and vomiting disappear, and there is the desire to start a normal diet. General well-being of the patient improves and there is a reduction in the anemic state. Nevertheless, only a few patients recover their libido and sexual potency to a level

Table 1. Categories of primary renal diseases causing chronic renal failure.

Glomerulonephritis
Pyelonephritis
Nephropathy caused by drugs of nephrotoxic agents
Cystic kidney disease
Cystinosis
Oxalosis
Congenital hypoplasia and dysplasia
Agenesis of abdominal muscles
Reno-vascular disease
Diabetes mellitus
Myelomatosis
Amyloidosis
Collagen-vascular disease
Cortical or tubular necrosis
Tuberculosis
Nephrocalcinosis
Tumor
Trauma

J. Bain and E.S.E. Hafez (eds.), Diagnosis in andrology, 215-223. All rights reserved.
Copyright © 1980 by Martinus Nijhoff Publishers bv, The Hague/Boston/London.

achieved prior to the onset of uremia. The majority of the patients who have undergone HD note a further reduction in libido with sexual activity becoming less frequent.

In extreme cases there is marked testicular atrophy and frequently gynecomastia, while hair distribution, rate of growth and voice remain normal.

Patients being treated with HD are classified into four groups based on the degree of altered libido (Rager et al., 1975):

Class I   – normal libido;
Class II   – slight reduction in libido;
Class III – severe reduction in libido;
Class IV   – impotence.

Patients treated with HD are distributed primar-ily among classes II, III and IV, while subjects who have undergone renal transplant are almost entirely in class I. Subjects who were previously part of class II, III or IV, after undergoing successful renal transplant have a gradual reversal of their symptoms as the renal function normalizes. Nothwithstanding steroid and immunosuppressive therapy, there is a restoration of libido and sexual function to levels preceding the onset of renal insufficiency as well as normal sperm production. Many patients become fertile again, often with pregnancy resulting. Therapeutic abortions have been performed in some of these cases because of the fear of chromosomal abnormalities due to the immunosuppressive

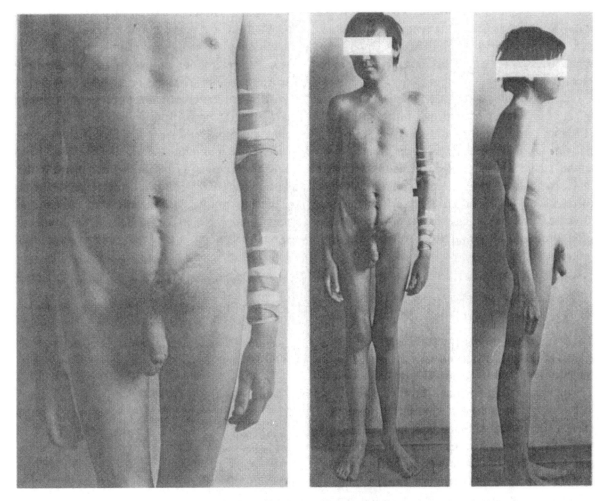

Figure 1. Twenty-year-old man treated with regular hemodialysis since 11 years of age because of pyelonephritis due to vesico-ureteric reflux and vesical extrophy. He received renal graft from living donor at 13 years of age; graft failure occurred 4 years later and then he returned to regular hemodialysis. Onset of pubescence was seen at 19 years of age. Virilization is incomplete: penis and right testicle are normal sized (left testicle was removed concurrently with kidney transplantation) but beard is absent; axillary hair is scanty; muscle development is poor; gynecomastia can be seen. Height 157.5 cm; weight 40 kg.

Table 2. Testicular function in various stages of renal disease.

Renal status	Signs and symptoms related to testicular function
Chronic renal failure	Reduced libido
	Impotence
	Decreased testicular size
	Retarded growth and development
Hemodialysis or peritoneal dialysis	Disappearance of uremic symptoms
	Persistence or accentuation of reduced libido and potency
	Testicular atrophy
	Gynecomastia
Renal transplantation with adequate function	Gradual restoration of libido and potency
	Normalization of objective data

2. LABORATORY DATA

The biochemical and hematological alterations of uremia are: increases in nitrogenous compounds (urea, creatinine, uric acid and methylguanidine), water retention, electrolyte alterations (hyperkalemia, hypocalcemia, hyperphosphatemia, hypomagnesemia), altered acid-base balance (reduced alkaline reserve and metabolic acidosis), and anemia.

The levels of gonadotropins (LH and FSH) and testosterone vary with the clinical condition and therapy employed. Similarly, patient responses to both stimulation tests with LH-RH, clomiphene and HCG, and inhibition tests with testosterone have been found to vary. Hemodialysis and renal transplantation markedly affect the baseline values found in the uremic patient. This is especially demonstrable with hemodialysis and renal transplantation, where the baseline values of patient responses are markedly affected.

In males with chronic renal insufficiency untreated with hemodialysis, the levels of testosterone are consistently low (average value equalling about 50% of normal minimum) (Guevara et al., 1969; Holdsworth et al., 1977) (Fig. 2a).

The average values for LH are elevated although levels vary significantly from case to case (Chen et al., 1970; Holdsworth et al., 1977), only infrequently are normal or low normal values found (Guevara et al., 1969; Phadke et al., 1970) (Fig. 2b). The titers of FSH are predominantly within normal limits or just above normal (Guevara et al., 1969), while urinary gonadotropins are low (approximately 3 U/24 hr

HMG), as a consequence of the direct reduction in GFR (Fig. 2c). Seminal fluid examination reveals marked oligospermia, and histological studies show a severe reduction of the germinal epithelial layer.

In patients treated with hemodialysis, LH remains elevated (Distiller et al., 1975; Sawin et al., 1973) or within the upper range of normal. FSH values also remain relatively unchanged from pretreatment levels (Holdsworth et al., 1977; Lim and Fang, 1975), with some patients having values slightly above normal (Sawin et al., 1973; Stewart-Bentley et al., 1974). Factors which influence these values are age and duration of renal insufficiency.

Testosterone and 5-α-DHT are also low in patients treated with HD, with values averaging about half that of normal subjects. Such levels undergo a continual reduction with progression of dialytic therapy (Lim and Fang, 1975). There does not seem to be any uniform change in testosterone before and after dialytic treatment (Distiller et al., 1975). The concentration of testosterone undergoes a transitory increase at the end of the dialysis session due to momentary increases in testosterone production (Stewart-Bentley et al., 1974). Lower values are seen in patients who undergo treatment three times weekly when compared to those who receive treatment twice weekly (Mies et al., 1975). Only in a few cases did normal testosterone values persist during the first year of HD therapy.

It seems that testosterone binding is increased while there is a reduction in testosterone production (hence free testosterone is reduced) (Vermeulen et al., 1969). Stimulation tests with HCG cause an increase in testosterone but below that of normal subjects (Fig. 3).

Administration of clomiphene has given very inconsistent results due to the variation of dosages used by different researchers. In general, an increase in serum levels on gonadotropins and testosterone has been noted.

After stimulation with LH-RH the values of LH increase sharply as observed in normal subjects but these levels remain elevated for a longer period with respect to controls (Mies et al., 1975). The response of FSH to LH-RH is, according to the majority of authors, significantly elevated and protracted in patients undergoing HD and PD compared to that of normal individuals (Mies et al., 1975) (Fig. 4).

In general, the response to LH-RH is modified by

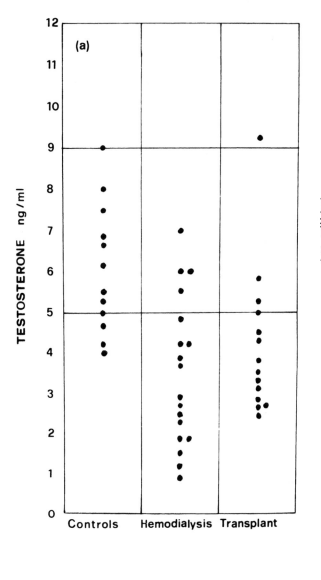
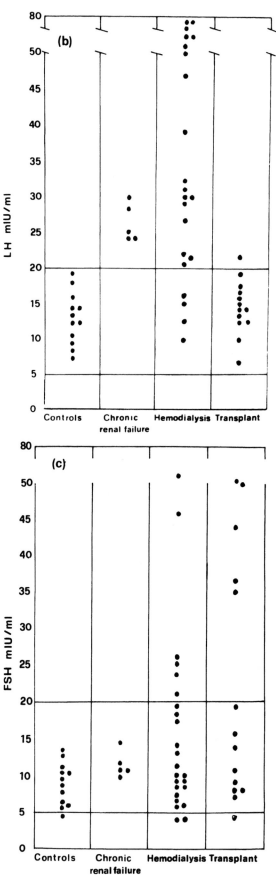

Figure 2. (a) Testosterone values in normal men, in uremic patients treated by hemodialysis, and in patients with renal transplantation. (b) LH values in normal men, in uremic patients, in patients treated by hemodialysis, and in patients with renal transplantation. (c) FSH values in normal men, in uremic patients, in patients treated by hemodialysis and in patients with renal transplantation. In transplanted men, blood samples were obtained 2 to 12 months after transplant.

a dialysis session. In evaluating the gonadotropins response to LH-RH, Distiller et al. (1975) have established the following criterion:

Index of abnormality = Sum of the percentage deviation of the average normal values of LH and FSH obtained after 0, 30, 60 and 120 min.

This index is directly correlated with the efficiency of dialytic therapy, based on the reduction of urea and creatinine obtained.

The metabolic clearance of testosterone (MCRT) is generally increased in HD patients. The MCR of LH is significantly reduced in patients with renal insufficiency (Holdsworth et al., 1977). The production of LH is significantly higher than normal.

Some patients treated with HD show a clear increase in prolactin levels that does not correlate with the presence of gynecomastia (Nagel et al., 1973; Sawin et al., 1973).

After transplantation with a functional kidney, LH decreasing and testosterone increasing become normal after several months, while FSH increases for approximately 8-10 months after transplant, and thereafter declines progressively with improvement in spermatogenesis reaching normal levels as the sperm count approaches normal.

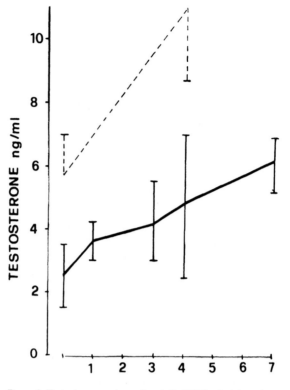

Figure 3. Testosterone values after daily HCG administration in dialyzed patients. The mean plasma testosterone levels were significantly lower than those seen in the normal men (dashed line).

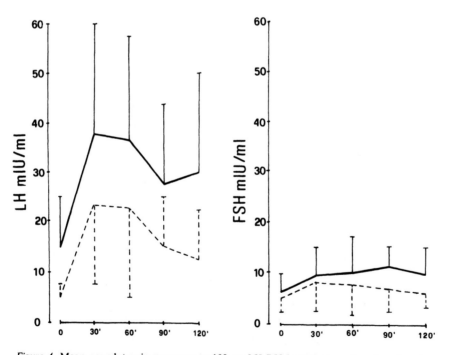

Figure 4. Mean gonadotropin responses to 100 μg LH-RH in patients undergoing chronic hemodialysis. Uremic patients (bold line) tend to have an exaggerated response when compared to normal men (dashed line). The horizontal axis indicates minutes after the LH-RH injection.

In stimulation tests with LH-RH, the response is within normal limits, while basal values may remain slightly elevated in the first few months after transplant, successively approaching that of normal subjects.

Seminal fluid examination on subjects undergoing HD shows a reduction in volume, rarely exceeding 0.8 ml (Lindsay et al., 1968), and occasional difficulty is encountered in obtaining a specimen. The sperm count in uremics, even when dialyzed, is usually about 3 million/ml, often barely reaching 1 million/ml. Sperm motility is also reduced and from 30 to 60% are anomalous forms (Phadke et al., 1970). After renal transplantation the volume of seminal liquid increases until it reaches normal values, the sperm count rises dramatically motility is excellent and few anomalous forms are found.

Testicular biopsy shows hypotrophy or atrophy in uremic men treated with hemodialysis, inter- and peritubular fibrosis and depressed spermatogenic activity with persistence of cells in every stage of maturation. The seminiferous tubules are small or atrophied, the interstitial tissue appears increased, the number of Leydig cells is reduced, and sometimes only Sertoli cells are present. The basal membrane is thickened and lipochrome depositions are found within the Leydig cells. Maturation does not proceed beyond the level of spermatocytes of the first order, numerous spermatogonia remaining in the tubules.

After a successful renal transplantation testicular biopsy reveals adequate cellularity, improved spermatogenesis and normal Leydig cells in both number and shape. Maturation is complete and the basal membrane is of normal thickness.

3. UREMIC INTOXICATION

Many of the clinical aspects of uremia are the result of the accumulation of various products of cellular catabolism such as urea, creatinine, urates and possibly other substances still unknown. In addition, there are alterations in the normal exchanges of water and electrolytes which further burdens the uremic patient. The effects of the uremic syndrome are manifested at the biochemical level, creating interference with enzymatic and cellular functions with subsequent alterations of tissues and organs (Teschan, 1970).

Gonadal failure in CRF is considered part of the phenomenon of general intoxication due to accumulation of the above mentioned substances. In particular, toxic products of low molecular weight have been strongly implicated as causing inhibition of many enzymatic reactions in various organ systems.

These effects probably also occur at the level of the testes with a consequent deterioration of testicular function, particularly reduced testosterone production. A rapid but transitory improvement in the production of this hormone immediately after dialysis has been observed, implicating some dialyzable factor or factors as responsible for testicular failure in uremia (Stewart-Bentley et al., 1974).

4. PROTEIN DEFICIENCY

Protein deficiency can casuse reduced libido and impotence consequent to a reduction in pituitary gonadotropins (Paulsen, 1974). In renal insufficiency, protein deficiency may result from: decreased dietary intake worsened by anorexia, nausea and vomiting, and proteinuria. Protein depletion can be prevented or ameliorated by a number of specially designed diets (Giordano, 1963; Giovannetti, 1964). The reduction in the amount of body protein serves indirectly to aid the uremic patient by reducing the overall protein requirement to a lower level. The need for dietetic restriction is particularly required in those patients with chronic renal insufficiency who are not undergoing dialysis. Once dialysis has been instituted the protein intake can be increased to almost normal levels. In most cases, a rise in serum gonadotropins occurs after initiation of dialysis. The state of protein malnutrition may be responsible for the depression of testicular function by lowering production of pituitary gonadotropins. After dialysis, with resumption of normal protein intake, this insufficiency may be overcome. In many uremics there are unequivocal signs of primitive testicular insufficiency as shown by the fact that nutrition itself cannot always correct the testicular insufficiency.

5. ZINC DEFICIENCY

Patients suffering from chronic uremia, including those undergoing dialysis on a regular or intermittent basis are deficient in zinc. Zinc deficiency can produce growth retardation and hypogonadism in laboratory animals. A similar syndrome has also been observed in young men in whom administration of zinc reestablished normal sexual development. Studies indicate that zinc may be essential for the full activity of pituitary gonadotropins on the testes, or that zinc deficiency alters the activity of the enzymes necessary for the conversion of testosterone to the active form, dihydrotestosterone (Antoniou et al., 1977). Patients who were dialyzed against solutions with added zinc showed a marked improvement in sexual potency, with elevation of plasma testosterone and reduction of plasma FSH and LH. Sexual function deteriorated within 4 weeks of suspension of zinc supplements (Antoniou et al., 1977). The cause of zinc deficiency in hemodialyzed patients may be related to reduction of dietary protein, inadequate gastrointestinal absorption of zinc or adherence to the dialysis membrane (Antoniou et al., 1977). Zinc deficiency should therefore, be considered as a factor in the genesis of sexual failure in patients with chronic renal failure undergoing dialysis.

6. HYPERPARATHYROIDISM

Secondary hyperparathyroidism is a common complication of chronic renal failure. Its pathogenesis derives from the interruption of the two functions of the kidney. First a reduced phosphate clearance occurs which then reacts with serum calcium to decrease the level of ionized calcium, and secondly the normal hydroxylation of 25-hydroxycholecalciferol to 1-25-dihydroxycholecalciferol, which is the active metabolite of vitamin D responsible for intestinal transport of calcium, is interrupted. Both these events cause increased levels of PTH with subsequent resorption of calcium from bone in an attempt to maintain the critical levels of this cation. In some patients who had undergone parathyroidectomy to alleviate their hyperparathyroidism, a resumption of normal sexual potency was observed, a proportional relationship existing between the degree of impotence and the intensity of secondary hyperparathyroidism (Massry et al., 1977).

In addition, a relationship between PTH, testosterone and LH titers was demonstrated by administering 1-25-dihydroxycholecalciferol to a group of impotent patients undergoing hemodialysis. Among these patients, approximately 50% showed a decrease in the PTH levels, while testosterone and gonadotropin levels increased; in about 25% of the patients an improvement in sexual potency was noted. The suppression of parathyroid activity can lead to a normalization of blood levels of the sex hormones and improved sexual potency in patients undergoing hemodialysis.

This PTH effect may be mediated by calcium acting directly on the hypothalamus and testes (Massry et al., 1977). Calcium ions act as second intracellular messengers; the modification of their concentration in the cytosol can alter the normal regulatory mechanisms of exocrine and endocrine secretions, neurotransmitter secretions and the action of hormones (Rasmussen, 1974).

7. PROLACTIN EXCESS

Prolactin (HPr) is frequently increased in uremic patients receiving intermittent hemodialytic treatment (Hagen et al., 1976; Nagel et al., 1973). The origin of this increase has not yet been clearly established. An association between an increase in prolactin and the appearance of gynecomastia has not been established. Testicular atrophy in mice has been noted after transplantation of prolactin-secreting tumors (Fang et al., 1974). However, there is lack of agreement on this observation, both in mice (Bartke et al., 1977) and in humans (Carter et al., 1978).

Whether HPr can suppress the activity of the mammalian testis still remains controversial. It appears that increased HPr levels in patients undergoing chronic hemodialysis are not responsible for the observed impotence (Nagel et al., 1973).

8. EFFECTS OF PHARMACOLOGICAL AGENTS

Patients with 'nephrosis lipoidea' or nephrotic syndrome 'minimal lesion' have frequently been sub-

jected to cyclophosphamide treatments. It has been notes that sterility is an important side effect of cyclophosphamide treatment (Fairly et al., 1972). Characteristics of testicular involvement include reduction in the numer of spermatozoa in seminal fluid after 3 weeks, followed by azoospermia after 4 months. These alterations may persist even after suspension of treatment but the effects are dose-dependent.

Testicular biopsy may reveal the absence of spermatogenesis, often with the presence of only Sertoli cells.

Other pharmacological agents such as azathioprine have not produced substantial side-effects of this type.

9. CONCLUSIONS

Testicular alterations, both functional and morphological, are very frequently manifested in males with chronic renal failure in the uremic stage. In these patients, the almost constant presence of reduced libido and impotence are found. Histological examination of the testicle reveals arrested spermatogenesis and serum levels of testosterone are reduced. Serum gonadotropins increase in response to both reduced testicular function and diminished renal clearance.

The origin of these disturbances is ascribed principally to the accumulation of uremic toxins, resulting from altered renal function, which inhibit both testosterone production and spermatogenesis. However, other factors may contribute to the testicular insufficiency: hyperparathyroidism (excess parathyroid hormone being among the causes of impotence), prolonged protein and caloric malnutrition and harmful effects of certain pharmacological agents such as cyclophosphamide.

Hemodialytic treatment, although resulting in improvement of the uremic condition, does not correct the testicular disturbances; on the contrary, following dialysis these disturbances may become accentuated, both functionally and histologically. Only the transplant of a well-functioning kidney will restore normal gonadal function after approximately 6-10 months. Immunosuppressive therapy does not inhibit the return to normal spermatogenesis.

REFERENCES

Antoniou LD, Shalboub RJ, Sudhakar R, Smith JC Jr (1977) Reversal of uraemic impotence by zinc. Lancet 29 Oct.: 895.

Bartke A, Smith MS, Michael SD, Peron FG, Dalterio S (1977) Effects of experimentally-induced chronic hyperprolactinemia on testosterone and gonadotropin levels in male rats and mice. Endocrinology 100: 182.

Broyer M, Kleinknecht C, Loirat C, Marti-Henneberg C, Roy MP (1972) Maturation osseuse et development pubertaire chez l'enfant et l'adolescent en dialyse chronique. Proc Eur Dial Transpl Assoc IX: 181.

Cameron JS, Ogg GS (1977) Sterility and cyclophasphamide. Lancet 27 May: 1174.

Carter JN, Tyson JE, Tolis G, Van Vliet S, Faiman C, Friesen HG (1978) Prolactin-secreting tumours and hypogonadism in 22 men. N Engl J Med 299: 847.

Chen JC, Vidt DG, Zorn EM, Hallberg MC, Wieland RG (1970) Pituitary-Leydig cell function in uremic males. J Clin Endocrinol Metab 31: 14.

Distiller LA, Morley JE, Sagel J, Pokroy M, Rabkin R (1975) Pituitary-gonadal function in chronic renal failure: the effect of luteinizing hormone-releasing hormone and the influence of dialysis. Metabolism 24: 711.

Drukker W, Schouten WA, Alberts C (1968) Report on regular dialysis treatment in Europe. Proc Eur Dial Transpl Assoc V 3.

Fang VS, Refetoff S, Rosenfield RL (1974) Hypogonadism induced by a transplantable prolactin-producing tumor in male rats: hormonal and morphological studies. Endocrinology 95: 991.

Giordano C (1963) Use of exogenous and endogenous urea for protein synthesis in normal and uremic subjects. J Lab Clin Med 62: 231.

Giovannetti S (1964) Low nitrogen diet in severe chronic uremia: clinical experience of 20 months duration. Proc Eur Dial Trans Assoc 1: 147.

Guevara A, Vidt D, Hallberg MG, Zorn EM, Pohlman C, Wieland RG (1969) Serum gonadotropin and testosterone levels in uremic males undergoing intermittent dialysis. Metabolism 18: 1062.

Holdsworth S, Atkins RC, De Kretser DM (1977) The pituitary-testicular axis in men with chronic renal failure. N Engl J Med 296: 1245.

Lim SV, Fang VS (1975) Gonadal dysfunction in uremic men. A study of the hypothalamo-pituitary-testicular axis before and after renal transplantation. Am J Med 58: 655.

Lindsay RM, Boyle IT, Luke RG, Kennedy AC (1968) The endocrine status of the regular dialysis patient. Proc Eur Dial Transpl Assoc V: 230.

Massry SG, Goldstein DA, Procci WR, Kletzky OA (1977) Impotence in patients with uremia: a possible role for parathyroid hormone. Nephron 19: 305.

Mehls O, Ritz E, Gilli G, Kreusser W (1978) Growth in renal failure. Nephron 21: 237.

Mies R, Baeyer HV, Figge H, Finke K, Winkeimann W (1975) Investigations on pituitary and Leydig cell function in chronic hemodialysis and after renal transplantation. Klin Wschr 53: 611.

Nagel TC, Freinkel N, Bell RH, Friesen H, Wilber JF, Metzger BE (1973) Gynecomastia, prolactin and other peptide hormones in patients undergoing chronic hemodialysis. J Clin Endocrinol Metab 36: 428.

Paulsen CA (1974) The testes. In: Williams RH, ed. Textbook of endocrinology, 5th edn, p 361. Philadelphia: W.B. Saunders.

Phadke AG, MacKinnon KJ, Dossetor JB (1970) Male fertility in uremia: restoration by renal allografts. Can M Assoc J 28: 607.

Rager K, Bundschu H, Gupta D (1975) The effect of HCG on testicular androgen production in adult men with chronic renal failure. J Reprod Fertil 42: 113.

Rasmussen H (1974) Parathyroid hormone, calcitonin and calciferols. In: Williams RH, ed. Textbook of endocrinology, 5th edn. p 660. Philadelphia: W.B. Saunders.

Sawin CT, Longcope C, Schmitt WG, Ryan RJ (1973) Blood levels of gonadotropins and gonadal hormones in gynecomastia associated with chronic hemodialysis. J Clin Endocrinol Metab 36: 988.

Stewart-Bentley M, Gans D, Horton R (1974) Regulation of gonadal function in uremia. Metabolism 23: 1065.

Teschan PE (1970 On the pathogenesis of uremia. Am J Med 48: 671.

Vermeulen A, Verdonck L, Van der Straeten M, Orie M (1969) Capacity of the testosterone binding globulin in human plasma and influence of specific binding of testosterone on its metabolic clearing rate. J Clin Endocrinol Metab 29: 1470.

17. ANDROLOGICAL PROBLEMS IN GASTROINTESTINAL DISORDERS

L.J. Cole and R. Bacchus

Sexual dysfunction may appear as a systemic or extra-intestinal manifestation of primary gastro-intestinal disease, or it may complicate systemic disease with prominent gastrointestinal features. Nutritional disorders and catabolic states of diverse etiology may by complicated by disturbed sexuality. Patients with malignant disease not infrequently present with temperamental instability and depression which may affect sexual behavior adversely. Disturbed sexuality also accompanies a variety of endocrine disorders in which gastrointestinal symptomatology may be present.

1. NUTRITIONAL DISORDERS

1.2. Malnutrition

In a comprehensive review (Klatskin, 1947) of the nutritional status and sexual activity in 300 American prisoners of war released following internment in Japanese prison camps for 2-3 years during World War II, gynecomastia was found in 48, usually after prolonged malnutrition. In one third, however, it became evident shortly after return to a normal diet. The breast enlargement was more often bilateral and associated with spontaneous pain in six, secretion in seven and tenderness in 46. In many, the immediate effect of a normal diet was to exacerbate the gynecomastia, with subsequent improvement and cure in most, after 5 months. Hepatomegaly or hepatocellular dysfunction, or both, were encountered in one third of the cases. Palmar erythema and spider nevi were found in a significant number of patients. The problem was complicated in some men by a history of viral hepatitis. However, in those without such a history, malnutrition appeared to be the only evident cause

for the hepatic abnormalities. Complete loss of libido was common even in the absence of gynecomastia. Testicular atrophy was present in one third of the men. Secondary sex characteristics remained normal. Endocrine studies in patients with gynecomastia revealed low urinary 17-ketosteroid levels, estrogens in the low normal range and normal FSH and corticoids. Postulated mechanisms for the gynecomastia have included impaired hepatic inactivation of estrogens due to malnutrition and depression of testicular function either by malnutrition directly, or consequent to suppression of pituitary gonadotropins by starvation. With improved nutrition, pituitary gonadotropin secretion recovered.

1.2. Zinc deficiency

Zinc, an essential nutrient for animals and plants, functions as a constituent of metalloenzymes. Animal proteins (meat, fish, dairy products) are rich in zinc and since the zinc content of most foodstuffs is similar to their iron content, combined deficiencies may ensue. Individuals on protein-restricted or vegetarian diets are likely to develop low plasma zinc levels (Sandstead, 1967). The normal serum zinc is 90-120 μg/100 ml. High concentrations of zinc occur in the epididymis, seminal vesicles and prostate of rat and man; however, seminal fluid has the highest zinc concentration. In the experimental animal, zinc deficiency results in failure of growth, weight loss, changes in the skin and hair, testicular atrophy, impaired fertility, susceptibility to abortion and an increased incidence of congenital malformations (Burch and Sullivan, 1976). Degenerative changes induced by zinc deficiency in the testicular tubules of rats are rapidly reversed by zinc administration

(Jameson, 1976). Teratogenic effects related to zinc deficiency have not yet been definitely encountered in men.

Zinc deficiency occurs in a variety of diseases including malnutrition, chronic inflammation, chronic liver disease and neoplasms. The clinical features of zinc deficiency include anorexia, weight loss, decreased olfactory acuity, perverted taste and delayed wound healing. The fully developed syndrome is most evident in growing children when retarded growth and hypogonadism in males may be prevalent (Ronaghy, 1974). Although no laboratory test is absolutely diagnostic of zinc deficiency, serum and urinary zinc levels are usually low. However, a low serum zinc, per se, does not necessarily imply zinc deficiency. The clinical state and a determination of retinol binding protein will aid in diagnosis. Finally, confirmation of the diagnosis may require an adequate therapeutic trial of elemental zinc.

In young boys, a syndrome of dwarfism, hypogonadism, iron deficiency anemia and in some cases hepatosplenomegaly, has been investigated in Iran (Prasad et al., 1963) and Egypt (Prasad et al., 1963; Sandstead, 1967). The patients' physical characteristics in the fully developed syndrome included underdevelopment, sparse fine facial axillary and pubic hair, and retarded genital and secondary sexual development. Diminished zinc levels were found in the plasma, hair, sweat and red blood cells. The iron and zinc deficiencies were related to a predominantly wheat-based diet rich in phytate, which, in combination with these metals, led to their malabsorption. Geophagia, a common habit in these dwarfs, was regarded as a possible contributing factor to the development of these deficiencies, resulting from the combination of iron and zinc with clay. Treatment with supplemental oral elemental zinc produced weight gain and striking acceleration in growth and sexual maturation.

Sandstead (1967) noted the resemblance of the hypogonadal dwarfs to patients with hypopituitarism. Decreased ACTH reserve was demonstrated. The relationship of zinc to pituitary function has recently been reviewed (Henkin, 1976). These studies in experimental animals suggest that the gonadal changes result primarily from the effects of zinc deficiency on the release of pituitary gonadotropins.

Some doubt has been cast on these observations (Coble et al., 1966). They re-examined the Egyptian subjects studied and treated over three years previously. The boys had attained a height similar to their healthy peers and exhibited normal sexual maturation, but their plasma zinc levels remained unchanged. Furthermore, low plasma zinc levels were detected in normally developed random subjects. Nevertheless, the present state of our knowledge indicates that adequate zinc is necessary for normal growth and male sexual maturation (Burch and Sullivan, 1976). An evaluation of zinc metabolism may be of value in cases of unexplained fertility.

1.3. Anorexia nervosa

Anorexia nervosa is a disorder of unknown etiology, occurring predominantly in young females and characterized by profound anorexia, cachexia and amenorrhea. However, it does occur in males. It is interesting that in one review of 31 male patients with anorexia nervosa, no evidence of an abnormal personality pattern was encountered (Beumont et al., 1972). The fear of gaining weight leads to self-induced starvation associated with bizarre behavior directed towards losing weight. On examination patients may appear depressed, weepy, hostile and agitated with marked hyperactivity.

Coincident with starvation, there is a loss of libido and potency which return to normal with weight gain. Emaciated males exhibit decreased testicular function as reflected by lowered urinary testosterone levels. Impaired testicular function secondary to malnutrition has been reported by several investigators (Zubiran et al., 1953), who found involutionary changes in most testicular elements, accompanied by low levels of urinary gonadotropins. As nutrition improved, most laboratory indices quickly returned to normal except for LH and FSH which may not attain normal levels for 6-12 months. The changes in androgen metabolism may result from hepatic dysfunction consequent to malnutrition (Boyar and Bradlaw, 1977). Detailed studies have confirmed the presence of hypothalamic dysfunction which may lead to functional impairment of the pituitary gland. The recorded abnormalities in this situation are partial diabetes insipidus, disturbed thermal regulation,

delayed TSH release after TRF, delayed LH and FSH release after LRH, lack of diurnal cortisol variation and elevated GH levels (Vigersky, 1977). All of these may be related to the effects of starvation (Mecklenburg et al., 1974).

The diagnosis must be made on the basis of positive psychiatric evidence and distinct indications that the malnutrition results from inadequate food intake. Implicit in the diagnosis is the exclusion of other psychiatric disorders (e.g. schizophrenia) and organic disease associated with marked weight loss (especially hypopituitarism), and primary gastrointestinal disorders, including malabsorption syndromes and systemic diseases.

1.4. Malabsorption syndromes

The clinical features of the malabsorption syndromes are the complex result of inadequate food intake (because of anorexia), increased enteric loss and intestinal malabsorption of nutrients per se. Such patients may present with gastrointestinal symptoms, manifestations of specific nutrional deficiencies, or systemic features including weakness, weight loss, retarded growth and sexual development. Symptomatology in particular cases can be subtle and the patient may appear relatively well.

In children, adolescents and adults in the active reproductive age group, gonadal dysfunction has been noted in the generalized primary malabsorption syndrome (celiac sprue) and in inflammatory bowel disease, especially Crohn's disease. Celiac sprue or gluten-sensitive enteropathy, is a malabsorptive disorder of the small intestine in which the histological abnormalities and the associated clinical features are reversed by gluten withdrawal (Kalser, 1976).

Panhypopituitarism may accompany the marked malnutrition of celiac disease, resembling the consequences of starvation. Decreased gonadal function is usually the earliest evidence manifested by loss of libido, thinning of axillary and pubic hair and in severe cases, testicular atrophy. Diminished urinary gonadotropins have been reported (Perloff et al., 1954). Infertility in male celiac patients has been reversed by treatment with a gluten-free diet (Merianos, 1975). The response to gluten withdrawal was confirmed by repeated seminal fluid analysis and successful conception (Baker and Read, 1975).

Low serum zinc values have been found in some patients with malabsorption syndromes including celiac disease, dermatitis herperiformis and regional enteritis (Crohn's disease). A marked increase in the urinary zinc level may follow oral zinc therapy (Jameson, 1976). Adolescents with retarded growth and sexual maturation associated with Crohn's disease may respond well to zinc supplementation.

2. LIVER DISEASE

2.1. Viral hepatitis

This common infectious disease of the liver results in an acute diffuse hepatic inflammation. The symptoms of the condition are variable systemic upset, gastrointestinal manifestations and abnormal liver function tests reflecting predominantly hepatocellular impairment (Sherlock, 1975). Gynecomastia and spider angiomas are uncommon complications of acute viral hepatitis (Glider and Haagland, 1946). Refeeding gynecomastia occurs during recovery from hepatic decompensation.

2.2. Chronic active hepatitis

Chronic active hepatitis is a chronic progressive liver disease with superimposed episodes of active hepatitis, frequently associated with or terminating in hepatic cirrhosis. The etiology remains obscure, although viral infection and autoimmune mechanisms have been suggested. The disease is most frequent in women but males may be affected. There is evidence not only of liver disease, but also of multisystem involvement. Endocrine changes commonly found in adolescent and young adult patients include cushingoid features, obesity, and gynecomastia in males (Schiff, 1969).

2.3. Hepatic cirrhosis

Cirrhosis is a chronic diffuse disease of the liver characterized by widespread hepatic fibrosis and nodular regeneration. Cirrhosis is the end-stage of many types of liver injury. Despite the morphological classification, the tissue changes are similar. Portal, micronodular cirrhosis is typical of end-stage alcoholic liver disease (Sherlock, 1975).

Cirrhosis may exist with a normal or almost normal liver profile. In the absence of an untreatable coagulopathy, the diagnosis may be confirmed by percutaneous liver biopsy or peritoneoscopy.

The endocrine changes in cirrhotic men include gynecomastia, loss of pectoral and axillary hair, feminine distribution of pubic hair, loss of libido, impotence and testicular atrophy. Oligospermia is common. The prostate is small and prostatic hypertrophy rare (Martini, 1975). Testicular biopsies reveal a diffuse reduction in the germinal elements of the seminiferous tubules and peritubular fibrosis although the Leydig cells appear normal. The endocrine manifestations are most frequent in alcoholic cirrhosis. There does not appear to be a consistent correlation between the incidence of the endocrine abnormalities and the degree of hepatic dysfunction (Green, 1977). Patients with well-compensated cirrhosis may have a normal reproductive capacity (Sherlock, 1975). Gynecomastia may also be seen in patients recovering from hepatic failure during high protein feeding. It may then be associated with an increase in testicular size, return of libido and regrowth of hair with a male distribution. Such gynecomastia has been regarded as a masculinizing effect and is usually transient, simulating refeeding gynecomastia in emaciated persons.

Hypogonadism is manifested by a low plasma testosterone level due to decreased testosterone production by the testes. There is an increase in the concentration of sex hormone binding globulin and a decrease in the amount of free testosterone. Feminization has not yet been adequately explained. There is no clear evidence of an increased concentration of biologically active estrogens. The total plasma estradiol concentrations are minimally elevated in a significant number of cirrhotic men while the free plasma estradiol concentration is marginally raised in only a minority of subjects. The slight correlation between gynecomastia and total plasma estradiol concentration is absent in many patients (Green, 1977). Breast tissue in male cirrhotics may be unusually sensitive to circulating estrogens. Raised plasma levels of the weak estrogen estrone, are frequently found in cirrhotic men but these do not correlate consistently with gynecomastia. In several studies of male cirrhotics increased conversion of androgens to estrogens has

been demonstrated, viz. testosterone to estradiol and androstenedione to estrone (Green et al., 1976). These changes do not seem to be directly related to disturbed hepatic metabolism.

In a review of 150 patients with liver disease of diverse etiology, 12% had unexplained hyperprolactinemia (Morgan et al., 1978). This was not related to the sex of the patient, the type or severity of the liver disease or the presence of gynecomastia. Serum prolactin levels have been shown to rise in response to hyperestrogenemia. Contradictory observations are recorded regarding the rise in prolactin secretion following alcohol ingestion (in both men and women) presumably resulting from a direct effect on the hypothalamic pituitary pathway (Van Thiel, 1975). Prolactin cells are present in a greater percentage of male cirrhotics than in normal male controls (Jung, 1972). However, serum prolactin levels are more often normal in the male cirrhotic, which correlates with the absence of galactorrhea in these patients. Most cirrhotic males with hypogonadism have normal plasma gonadotropins. This has been attributed to a double defect, primary gonadal failure and hypothalamic- pituitary suppression. The relationship between the clinical endocrinopathy and the observed hormonal abnormalities is not yet clear and awaits further elucidation (Mowat et al., 1976; Van Thiel et al., 1974).

Hemochromatosis

The designation hemochromatosis is reserved for iron overload associated with tissue damage, usually cirrhosis. Idiopathic or hereditary hemochromatosis is a distinct primary familial iron storage disease. Increased iron stores, though most marked in the liver, commonly occur also in the pancreas, gastrointestinal tract, heart and endocrine glands. Excessive iron deposition may be found in younger asymptomatic relatives of patients with this disease. The term 'bronzed diabetes' refers only to the endstage of the disease (Sherlock, 1975).

Hemochromatosis is encountered most frequently in middle-aged males, presenting in the fully developed syndrome with evidence of hepatic cirrhosis (often compensated), diabetes mellitus, oral and cutaneous slate grey pigmentation, cardiomyopathy and arthropathy. Pigmentation may

be absent. Carbohydrate intolerance may precede cirrhosis and may be evident only on glucose tolerance testing (Feller et al., 1977).

An elevated serum iron level and decreased serum iron binding capacity are suggestive but not diagnostic. The diagnostic feature is the demonstration of abnormal amounts of stainable iron in tissue biopsies and a quantitative estimation of liver iron content (Edwards et al., 1977).

Hypogonadism is common, presenting with loss of libido, impotence, loss of secondary sexual hair, testicular atrophy and atrophic skin. Infantilism and sexual hypoplasia are noted in children (Perkins et al., 1965). Significant iron deposition is uncommon in the testes and is more frequently found in the pituitary. Pituitary dysfunction is common in advanced hemochromatosis, manifested by low levels of gonadotropins as well as blunted growth hormone and cortisol responses to hypoglycemia. Pituitary hypofunction is the main cause of the hypogonadal features (Walsh et al., 1976). Diabetic autonomic neuropathy may be an additional cause of impotence in some patients.

2.5. Androgenic steroids

Only the 17-α-alkylated androgenic steroids (e.g. oxymethalone, methyltestosterone, methandrostenolone) appear to be hepatotoxic. Prolonged therapy (usually with large doses) has been associated with a number of undesirable and potentially dangerous sequelae.

The development of gynecomastia in some athletes has been attributed to the conversion of such agents to estrogens (Frasier, 1973). Hepatotoxic effects have included mild or moderate abnormalities of liver function tests, e.g. elevations of SGOT, SGPT, alkaline phosphatase and BSP retention, with or without jaundice. A spectrum of histological changes has been observed in the liver: liver cell necrosis, intrahepatic cholestasis, hyperplasia, and neoplastic transformation. The hepatic abnormalities are usually reversible but fatal hepatic failure has occurred.

Isolated reports of peliosis hepatis resulting from the use of androgens have appeared (Bagheri and Boyer, 1974). In this condition, the liver is studded with blood-filled cyst-like spaces communicating with the liver sinusoids and intrahepatic veins. The

lesion has been regarded as a complication of hepatic necrosis. Peliosis hepatis is a potential source of serious intraperitoneal hemorrhage.

Experimental and epidemiologic studies in animals indicate that an androgenic environment favors the development of hepatocellular carcinoma, in the absence of primary liver disease (Andrevont, 1952). At least 25 cases of primary liver tumors (adenoma and hepatocellular carcinoma) complicating androgen therapy have been recorded (Farrell et al., 1975). The androgen-induced tumors are histologically indistinguishable from true hepatocellular carcinoma. Many of the tumors were α-fetoprotein negative, lasted over 4-7 years and regressed following cessation of hormonal treatment without a fatal termination. Metastasis was reported in only one case.

The liver function profile and serum α-fetoprotein are not dependable diagnostic modalites in this situation. Regular isotopic liver scanning, combined with ultrasonography, especially when hepatomegaly is detected, may be more useful parameters. The results may then dictate cessation of androgen therapy, with the expectation that the hepatic lesions will stop growing or regress. Percutaneous liver biopsy may be very dangerous in this setting. Intra-abdominal hemorrhage may complicate necrosis and hemorrhage in a hepatic adenoma.

3. ECTOPIC ENDOCRINE SYNDROMES

Ectopic endocrine syndromes result from the ectopic secretion of hormones by tumors arising from cells which do not normally secrete the hormone. Such neoplasms may be endocrine or non-endocrine tumors (Rees and Ratcliffe, 1974) and a single tumor may secrete both native and ectopic hormones. Early diagnosis by hormone assay may lead to a curative resection or to palliative endocrine therapy (Omenn, 1970).

3.1. Isosexual precocity and hepatoma

Sexual precocity has been associated with ectopic gonadotropin secretion by hepatoma and hepatoblastoma in male children between 7 months and $7\frac{1}{2}$ years of age. The clinical findings include hepato-

megaly, accelerated growth and maturation, enhanced muscular development, facial acne, deep voice, sparse axillary and pubic hair, slight testicular enlargement and an enlarged penis with frequent erections. Testicular biopsy discloses Leydig cell hyperplasia and slight tubular enlargement, but no evidence of spermatogenesis. The increased stroma and number of glands in the prostate indicate precocious maturation. Hormonal studies have demonstrated markedly increased urinary testosterone levels, increased urinary estrogens, high levels of serum LH and slightly increased urinary gonadotropins (McArthur et al., 1973). The syndrome is limited to the male sex.

The hepatomegaly may be asymmetrical and associated with an abnormal liver profile, particularly elevation of the serum alkaline phosphatase. In other instances, the liver function tests and the serum α-fetoprotein are normal. Definitive diagnosis may be achieved by isotopic liver scanning, hepatic angiography and percutaneous liver biopsy.

3.2. Adrenal rest tumors of the liver

These are uncommon neoplasms often encountered as incidental small solitary lesions which rarely become malignant. Grossly, they resemble a hepatic adenoma or metastatic nodule. Rarely, they have been associated with clinical endocrinopathy in children between 9 months and 7 years of age, presenting with sexual precocity and Cushing's syndrome. A 5-year-old male with pernicious peptic ulcer disease and recurrent severe gastrointestinal hemorrhage simulating the Zollinger-Ellison syndrome was found to have a small adrenal rest tumor at the hilum of the liver on post-mortem examination (Hyams et al., 1960).

3.3. Gynecomastia

Gynecomastia may be a presenting or complicating feature of ectopic hormone production by carcinomas of the stomach, colon, pancreas or liver which elaborate a hormone with gonadotropic or estrogenic activity. The gynecomastia may be painful and bilateral. It may precede the clinical evidence of the tumor by many months (Marcus and Korenman, 1976) and may be the only endocrine abnormality in a patient with hepatoma in the

absence of cirrhosis. Successful resection of the tumor may be followed by rapid relief from pain and resolution of the gynecomastia over a period of six months. Gynecomastia has been associated with retardation of sexual maturation in primary liver cell carcinoma hypersecreting chorionic gonadotropin (Kew et al., 1977). Secondary sex characteristics may develop normally after resection of the tumor.

3.4. Feminization associated with ectopic chorionic gonadotropin

Ectopic production of human chorionic gonadotropin by non-trophoblastic neoplasms of the gastrointestinal tract has been observed with carcinomas of the stomach, small bowel, colon, pancreas and liver. It is most frequent with pancreatic and stomach carcinomas and hepatoma. Because of the paucity of information on testicular histology in males with non-testicular tumors, a small focus of active or burned out choriocarcinoma in the testes cannot be absolutely excluded (Fine et al., 1972). Tumors of the gastrointestinal tract, particularly, may show transitions from primary adenocarcinomas to trophoblastic elements. The simultaneous occurrence of both cell types has been documented in such tumors (McKechnie and Fechner, 1971).

Primary choriocarcinoma of the gastrointestinal tract is rare. It may present with gynecomastia, pigmentation of the areolae and genitalia, gastrointestinal hemorrhage, dysphagia, etc., depending on the primary site and local complications. The urine is positive for gonadotropins. Hyperplasia of Leydig cells has been found on testicular biopsy. The gynecomastia is attributed to increased estrogen production by Leydig cells consequent to high gonadotropic levels. Metastatic involvement of the liver is common.

4. MISCELLANEOUS CONDITIONS

4.1. Carcinoid syndrome

Carcinoid tumors are neoplasms of enterochromaffin cells developing most frequently in the gastrointestinal tract, although they may originate in other sites, particularly the bronchial epithelium.

They are locally invasive but may metastasize to regional lymph nodes and the liver.

The syndrom is most often associated with metastatic (liver) extra-appendiceal carcinoid originating in the terminal ileum. Large non-metastasizing carcinoids may also induce the carcinoid syndrome. Less frequently, the responsible lesion is a bronchial carcinoid. In the latter situation, an increased incidence of endocrinopathies is recorded, i.e. pleuriglandular adenomatosis. The syndrome is related to the secretion by the tumor of a variety of biologically active substances, particularly serotonin.

It appears most often in middle age and exhibits a prolonged course. The clinical features include episodic flushing, bronchoconstriction, manifestations due to intestinal hypermotility, endocardial involvement and an enlarged firm liver. Most patients exhibit an increased urinary excretion of 5-hydroxyindole acetic acid, the metabolite of serotonin (Kowlessar, 1973).

Gonadal dysfunction is common in male patients with the carcinoid syndrome. The majority complain of decreased libido and potency. The testes and secondary sexual characteristics are normal. Peyronie's disease may develop, manifested by painful angulation of the penis during erection and intercourse. In some patients the serum testosterone level may be decreased and the serum LH elevated. The serum FSH is usually normal. There is no apparent correlation between the levels of urinary 5-hydroxyindoleacetic acid and the serum LH. On the basis of experimental and clinical evidence, it has been suggested that the hyperserotonemia may be partly responsible for the gonadal disturbance. This may be related to effects of serotonin on the central nervous system as well as on the vascular supply of the penis. Hyperserotonemia may modulate the secretion of hypothalamic releasing hormones by its action on the median eminence leading to the elevated serum LH (Feldman et al., 1974). Impaired sexual function is common in patients with malignant disease but the mechanism for this disturbance has not been elucidated.

4.2. Cystic fibrosis

Cystic fibrosis (mucoviscidosis) has been considered to be the most frequent lethal disease of childhood. It is currently regarded as an inborn error of metabolism characterized by a generalized exocrinopathy related to disturbed function of mucous glands. Excessive accumulations of viscid mucous secretion lead to the formation of concretions, ductular obstruction, inflammatory changes and fibrosis. The principal clinical features are pancreatic exocrine insufficiency and diffuse obstructive bronchopulmonary disease. In the milder forms of the disease, patients may not become symptomatic until their teen years or later. With early effective management, survival to adult life is becoming more common (Stern et al., 1977). The best diagnostic test is the demonstration of elevated sodium and chloride concentrations in the sweat, by pilocarpine iontophoresis in a localized area (Shwachman and Grand, 1973).

Most males with cystic fibrosis are infertile because of azoospermia and biochemically abnormal seminal fluid. Sterility in these patients is related to mechanical obstruction of the transport of spermatozoa, because of developmental mesonephric abnormalities affecting the vas deferens. An alternative hypothesis suggests that these alterations may be due to the underlying inborn metabolic disturbance (Agnese, 1968).

Although on examination the external genitalia and secondary sex characteristics are often normal, the appearance of the latter may be delayed. In some series, common findings have included abnormally small testes (uni- or bilateral) incomplete development of the epididymis and inability to palpate the vas. Abnormalities of the seminal vesicles and ejaculatory ducts are described. In surgically explored patients, the vas could not be identified (Kaplan et al., 1968). While spermatogenesis may be normal, more commonly diminished spermatogenesis and abnormal sperm forms are encountered. A few patients exhibit testicular atrophy and peritubular fibrosis. Seminal fluid analysis reveals reduced volume, azoospermia, increased acidity, diminished fructose concentration and elevated concentrations of citric acid and acid phosphatase. The elevated citric acid and acid phosphatase suggest that the ejaculate may be mainly of prostatic origin. Hormonal values are normal in non-debilitated patients (Taussig, 1972).

Isolated males with cystic fibrosis may possess normal seminal fluid and father normal children.

These findings raise the possibility of different genetic forms of the disease (Blank and Mendoza, 1976).

4.3. Inflammatory bowel disease

4.3.1. Idiopathic ulcerative colitis. Idiopathic mucosal ulcerative colitis is a primary diffuse mucosal inflammation of the rectum and colon of unknown etiology occurring in both sexes and at all ages, especially in the second and third decades. The disease presents with abdominal cramps, bloody diarrhea with mucopus and variable constitutional upset. In individual patients, a variety of colonic and extracolonic complications may ensue. In children, the disease tends to be more severe and more frequently involves the whole colon. The diagnosis is established by stool examination, endoscopy and barium enema.

4.3.2. Regional enteritis. Regional enteritis or Crohn's disease is a non-specific chronic, recurrent granulomatous inflammation of undetermind etiology involving typically but not exclusively the distal ileum. Although it may occur at any age, the disease is most common in youth. Pathologically, the disease is a transmural necrotizing ulcerative inflammation, penetrating and perforating in its behavior. These features account for the frequency of fistulization and abscess formation. Transmural fibrosis leads to stricture formation and luminal stenosis. The disease may remain localized or spread proximally and distally to involve any area of the alimentary canal including colon, rectum, and anus. A segmental distribution of lesions with skip areas of normal intervening bowel is characteristic. The principal clinical manifestations are diarrhea, abdominal pain, fever and weight loss. Local and extraintestinal complications are frequent. The diagnosis rests on clinical awareness of the various presentations, endoscopy, and radiologic studies of the entire gastrointestinal trace (Donaldson, 1973).

Delayed growth and sexual maturation are common in children and adolescents with inflammatory bowel disease especially regional enteritis. The first indications of these disorders may be a cessation of linear growth which may or may not be associated with failure to gain weight or with weight loss. When the disease begins in the prepubertal years, dwarfism of 'intestinal infantilism' may result (Logan et al., 1938), characterized by marked retardation of growth and gonadal development with poorly developed secondary sex characteristics. Retarded growth and sexual maturation may be noted for several years before the gastrointestinal manifestations become evident. Gastrointestinal symptoms may be minimal or absent and are often attributed to psychological problems.

These changes have been related to malnutrition and the suppressive effects of steroid therapy. There are no deficiencies of circulating growth hormone or somatomedin and no other specific endocrine abnormalities have been demonstrated in the pathogenesis of growth retardation in inflammatory bowel disease. Furthermore, growth failure may continue during remissions (Gryboski and Spiro, 1978). Zinc deficiency has been demonstrated in some patients and zinc therapy may lead to a spurt of growth and sexual maturation (Sandstead, 1967).

4.4. Peptic ulcer

The incidence of peptic ulcer and its complications is much higher in males. In a review of 404 peptic ulcer patients, the reproductive capacity was reduced by 25% compared with 1000 controls, irrespective of sex. There was a higher incidence of childless marriages and a smaller number of children in each family. The significance of these findings is not clear (Kubickova and Vesely, 1974).

4.5. The irritable bowel syndrome

The irritable bowel syndrome or gastrointestinal response to stress is probably the commonest cause of abdominal misery. It is primary functional colonopathy manifested by abdominal pain, constipation, diarrhea, bloating, flatulence, mucus in the stools, dyspepsia and symptoms and signs of vasomotor instability. It may closely mimic organic disease. Afflicted patients are often tense, anxious, frustrated and depressed. Over 70% of these patients reportedly exhibit psychiatric features, manifested by constant fatigue, agitation, decreased interest in usual activities, impaired concentration, recurrent thoughts of suicide and diminished sex drive (Young et al., 1976).

The usual features of impotence, associated with decreased libido in affective disorders, include ejaculatio praecox and erectile dysfunction associated with retained morning erection. Such patients may present complaining of decreased potency. Only after careful questioning are the gastrointestinal symptoms and associated psychiatric features disclosed.

The responsible mechanism may be hypothalamic dysfunction and associated autonomic disturbances in the areas of appetite, sleep, mood regulation and sex drive (Gruen, 1978).

4.6. Carcinoma of the pancreas

The effect of pancreatic cancer on mental function and emotional control is well documented (Perlos and Faillace, 1964). Patients with carcinoma of the pancreas typically present with jaundice with or without abdominal pain and systemic deterioration. However, they may appear with mental or emotional aberrations including depression simulating mental illness (Savage and Noble, 1954). Loss of libido in such situations may not be unusual and may be related to neuroendocrine dysfunction.

4.7. Amyloidosis

The amyloidoses are disease of obscure etiology, characterized by accumulations of an amorphous eosinophilic extracellular protein-polysaccharide complex in tissues. Secondary amyloidosis may occur in a generalized form associated with recognized predisposing disorders. In the absence of known predisposing disease it is regarded as primary amyloidosis. The common sites of involvement are the liver, spleen, kidneys, adrenals, gastrointestinal tract and heart. Peripheral neuropathy in patients with systemic amyloidosis results from infiltration or compression of the nerve by amyloid deposits (Cohen, 1967). Diagnostic biopsies may be obtained from gingiva, stomach, small bowel, rectum, liver and peripheral nerves.

Primary familial amyloidosis with polyneuropathy is endemic to several regions of Portugal. It affects young people in their twenties and thirties, presenting with polyneuropathy of the lower limbs, sphincteric disturbances, abdominal pain, constipation, diarrhea, malabsorption and impotence (Monteiro, 1973). In the heredofamilial type with urticaria and nephropathy, loss of libido is common (Muckle and Wells, 1962). Amyloid deposits may be found in the testes.

5. POST-OPERATIVE GONADAL DYSFUNCTION

The normal male sexual response involves libido, erection and ejaculation. Erection depends on sacral parasympathetic stimuli travelling through the inferior hypogastric plexus to the pelvic viscera. Such stimuli produce vascular dilation and engorgement of penile vessels. Interruption of this pathway abolishes erectile function. Ejaculation depends on the integrity of the sympathetic nerve supply to the internal genitalia. Damage to the inferior hypogastric plexus or lumbar sympathectomy may abolish ejaculatory function. Both of these neural pathways lie close to the rectum and may therefore be interrupted in pelvic dissection (Whitelaw and Smithwick, 1951). The latter is particularly liable to occur in the treatment of rectal cancer where wide dissection is employed to remove the related lymphatic drainage. If damage to the pelvic autonomic nerves is avoided by careful surgical technique, disturbed sexual function becomes unlikely or transient (Brooke, 1956).

5.1. Ileostomy and colostomy

Approximately 86,000 ostomies are performed annually in the United States and most of these are permanent. These operations fashion an artificial opening or stoma on the anterior abdominal wall for the discharge of intestinal contents from the terminal ileum or colon. The usual indications for ileostomy and total colectomy are complicated, intractable, non-specific inflammatory bowel disease and multiple polyposis. Low-lying cancer of the rectum frequently requires abdomino-perineal resection and a descending colostomy.

The ostomy per se does not affect sexual function. The loss of continence may be associated with a sense of dirtiness, personal inadequacy and a destroyed image of body perfection. Fear, ignorance, inability to accept or adjust to the stoma and failure to learn how to live with and care for the ostomy and appliance, all have an important

bearing on post-operative sexual performance. In many patients, decreased sexual activity is more often related to the psychosocial upheaval and depression (Wirsching et al., 1975).

Bilateral damage to the pelvic autonomic nerves results in impotence. With improved surgical technique for removal of the rectum, only transient sexual dysfunction can be anticipated. Many other factors may be involved in post-operative male sexual dysfunction, viz. age, previous sexual pattern, control of the disease, stress of major surgery, malnutrition, accidental ligation of the vas, epididymo-orchitis complicating catheterization, reflex ejaculation and unrelated hypogonadism (Davis and Jelenko, 1975).

5.2. Sexual dysfunction after aorto-iliac surgery

Atherosclerotic aorto-iliac occlusive disease with associated thrombosis may lead to complete aortic obstruction. The resultant constellation of findings has come to be known as the Leriche syndrome. The clinical features include low back pain with gluteal claudication, absent femoral pulses, atrophy of the lower limbs and erectile dysfunction consequent to an impaired blood supply to the penis. The diagnosis is confirmed by aortography. Resection of the aortic bifurcation and insertion of a prosthetic graft are frequently effective in alleviating the syndrome.

Pre-operatively, approximately 24% of patients with abdominal aortic aneurysm and 29% with aorto-iliac stenosis and claudication, suffer from sexual dysfunction. Following aneurysmectomy approximately 50% become impotent (Van Broodhoven, 1977). In occlusive disease, postoperative erectile dysfunction is uncommon, but abnormal ejaculatory function occurs in 20%. The latter may be reduced to 11% and potency preserved by special precautions (May et al., 1969).

5.3. Rectal fistula

Male sterility due to a fistula between the rectum and the common ejaculatory ducts may result from an unusual developmental gastrointestinal anomaly. In a 23-year-old male, anal atresia and a rectovesical fistula had been corrected surgically. At the age of 16 years, masturbation resulted in ejaculation through the anus. Libido and other sexual functions were normal. Because of satisfactory sexual performance and a happy marriage, surgical treatment was refused. Artificial insemination using semen obtained after a cleansing enema resulted in a pregnancy (Abramovici et al., 1972).

6. DRUG-INDUCED GONADAL DYSFUNCTION

Gonadal dysfunction and feminization complicating drug therapy in gastrointestinal disease are usually pharmacologic side-effects of the medications.

6.1. Anticholinergics

The antimuscarinic agents inhibit the actions of acetylcholine on postganglionic cholinergic nerve terminals as well as on smooth muscles without cholinergic innervation. Such parasympatholytic drugs may be useful adjuncts in therapeutic regimens for a variety of gastrointestinal disorders. The lack of selectivity in the action of these drugs makes it difficult to achieve significant effects without concomitant side-effects. By interfering with autonomic innervation these drugs may cause diminished potency. Libido is not affected (Goodman and Gilman, 1975).

6.2. Cimetidine (Tagamet)

Cimetidine is a potent H_2 receptor antagonist, which markedly suppresses basal and stimulated gastric hydrochloric acid secretion. This has led to widespread use of this agent in the treatment of peptic ulcer disease, reflux esophagitis, and the marked gastric hypersecretion in the Zollinger-Ellison syndrome due to a gastrinoma (McCarthy, 1978). Experimentally, Leydig cell tumours have been found in the testes of rats on long-term therapy, but the significance of this uncommon finding has not been clarified (Hirschowitz, 1977).

Gynecomastia, an infrequent complication, may appear within 2-8 months of starting treatment and may disappear despite continued therapy. The breast becomes enlarged, painful and tender. Some patients have mild hepatocellular dysfunction re-

flected in elevations of the serum transaminase and alkaline phosphatase. The plasma prolactin levels may be remarkably elevated without gynecomastia (Delle Fane et al., 1977). Such changes might result from the suppressed release of hypothalamic prolactin inhibitory factor or a direct effect on the pituitary gland. Reversible impotence has been seen after 2 weeks of cimetidine therapy (Wolfe, 1979).

6.3. Spironolactone

Spironolactone, an aldosterone antagonist, has been extensively used for the treatment of hypertension, decompensated cirrhosis with ascites and edema. Its action as a competitive antagonist to aldosterone is apparently mediated by binding to the kidney cytosol mineralo-corticoid receptor. The chronic administration of this diuretic in moderate or high dosage may be complicated by gynecomastia and impotence.

The gynecomastia has been attributed to alterations in the estrogen-testosterone ratio leading to estrogenic breast stimulation and ductal tissue proliferation. Peripherally, spironolactone raises estradiol levels by increasing the peripheral conversion of testosterone to estradiol. Through increasing the metabolic clearance of testosterone, it lowers the circulating blood level of the androgen. Finally, the antiandrogenic effect of spironolactone may be due to its inability to inhibit binding of testosterone to specific receptor sites (in cytosol and on plasma proteins) thus enhancing its metabolic inactivation and diminishing its effect on target tissue (Rose et al., 1977). Spironolactone therapy may be the commonest cause of gynecomastia in patients with decompensated liver disease.

6.4. Metoclopramide (Maxeran)

Metoclopramide is a chlorbenzamide derivative with proven efficacy in the management of selective gastrointestinal problems. It appears to activate intramural cholinergic neurons resulting in an increased release of acetylcholine. The drug is currently enjoying widespread use as an antiemetic in the treatment of reflux esophagitis and in selected patients with impaired gastric emptying due to gastric hypomotility (Pinder et al., 1976). Chronic use of the drug may be complicated by galactor-

rhea, consequent to prolactin stimulation. Marked elevations of serum prolactin have been noted in males following intravenous administration of metoclopramide. The drug appears to antagonize the dopamine mediated hypothalamic secretion of prolacting inhibitory factor (McCallum et al., 1976).

6.5. Phenothiazines

Many of these drugs are currently used in gastroenterologic practice for the treatment of alcoholic hallucinosis, nausea, vomiting, hiccups, selected cases of anorexia nervosa and chronic anxiety states. The drugs affect all levels of the nervous system including the extra-pyramidal pathways. In the hypothalamus, they antagonize the secretion of prolactin inhibitory factor. Through their ability to enhance prolacting release, their use may be complicated by the development of gynecomastia and galactorrhea. Possibly by andrenergic blockade, phenothiazines may interfere with ejaculation without effecting erectile function (London, 1975).

6.6. Colchicine

Colchicine binds to tubulin, the dimer of which the microtubules are composed. Its effect on cell movement and the mitotic apparatus may thus be related to interference with microtubule assembly. In most instances no serious side-effects have been encountered with colchicine. However, patients on chronic colchicine therapy have exhibited chromosomal non-disjunction and azoospermia (Merlin, 1972). It has been suggested that the medication be stopped 3 months before intended conception; however, colchicine use by parents has not been associated with abnormalities in the offspring.

6.7. Alcohol

Although alcohol in small doses may temporarily increase libido by relaxing inhibitions, the depressant effects of large amounts lead to weakened sexual responses. 'It provokes the desire, but it takes away the performance' (Shakespeare, Macbeth, Act II). Both short-term (1 month) and chronic alcoholism may be associated with decreased libido and impotence (Green, 1977). Short-term consumption of alcohol in normal men is accompanied by a fall

in plasma testosterone associated with increased hepatic metabolism and increased metabolic clearance rate of the hormone from the plasma. Both plasma testosterone and the protein binding of the plasma testosterone are decreased. No consistent changes have been observed in the serum LH level. These findings have been attributed to the suppression of both testicular and hypothalamic pituitary function by alcohol. In chronic (non-cirrhotic) alcoholics, the plasma hormone binding globulin is markedly elevated reducing the free plasma testosterone below normal. However, many have only a slightly lowered free testosterone and raised plasma gonadotropins (Green, 1977). Chronic alcoholism may directly impair spermatogenesis by inhibiting the testicular conversion of retinol to retinal, an essential step for spermatogenesis in animals (Van Thiel et al., 1975). Despite these observed effects in animals, their importance in man has not yet been clearly established.

6.8. Analgesics

Continuous daily ingestion of large doses of analgesic drugs (especially phenacetin and acetaminophen) produce testicular atrophy and inhibition of spermatogenesis in experimental animals. A review of records of men hospitalized with analgesic abuse indicated that very few fathered children while on large daily doses of such drugs (Boyd, 1970).

6.9. Cannabis (T.H.C.)

Smoking marijuana is reportedly associated with increased sexual activity attributed to the active ingredient of the hallucinogen, tetrahydrocannabinol. Gynecomastia has been reported in chronic marijuana users. T.H.C. stimulates the development of breast tissue in the rat, attributed to the structural similarity between T.H.C. and estradiol. Chronic intensive use of marijuana has been associated with low plasma testosterone levels without effect on prolactin secretion (Kolodny et al., 1974). In a review of idiopathic gynecomastia in American soldiers, no association was observed between the use of cannabis and idiopathic gynecomastia (Cates and Pope, 1977).

7. THE GAY BOWEL SYNDROME

A large number of men participate in homosexual activity, the incidence in unmarried men being estimated at approximately 37%. In 1977, the male homosexual population of the United States exceeded one million men. Homosexuality has become a major factor in the spread of sexually transmitted diseases. The spectrum of gastrointestinal problems encountered in this population has been referred to as the 'Gay Bowel Syndrome' (Kazal et al., 1976). Sexually transmitted diseases are now regarded as the commonest communicable diseases in the industrialized world. A tactful, discreetly taken sexual history is important to determine whether the pattern of sexual behavior includes orogenital, anolingual or rectal intercourse. Exclusive heterosexuality cannot be assumed even in the married man.

7.1. Venereal disease

The classical venereal diseases, gonorrhea, syphilis, chancroid and lymphogranuloma venereum, account for only a small proportion of sexually transmitted diseases. Many patients acquire a variety of other specific and non-specific genital infections, e.g. scabies, pediculosis, warts, candidiasis and herpes simplex. Further complications related to homosexual activity include hemorrhoids, anal fissure and non-specific proctitis. Traumatic lacerations of the rectum have followed fist fornication or sexual gratification achieved by the partner's hand inserted in the rectum (Sohn and Robilotti, 1977).

A high incidence of gonorrheal and syphilitic pharyngeal and anorectal infection is found in homosexual men. Early diagnosis is important not only for the treatment of the patient, but to prevent dissemination of the disease. The followup examination and investigation of contacts thus become very important (Catteral, 1975).

Gonorrheal pharyngitis may be relatively asymptomatic or manifested by sore throat with erythema and exudate. Gonorrheal proctitis presents with anal soreness, painful defection, purulent anal discharge and at times blood streaked diarrhea. Proctosigmoidoscopy reveals a red, edematous, friable mucosa and tenacious creamy mucopus in the

lumen. The diagnosis is established by Gram stain and culture of material from pharyngeal or rectal swabs (Owen, 1972).

Extragenital chancres may be located on the lip, tongue, pharynx and in the anorectal region, appearing as a painless ulcer or erosion. They have been misdiagnosed as anal fissures or piles. The diagnosis rests on the use of dark field examination to demonstrate *Treponema pallidum* in material from lesions. Blood serology may not become positive for several weeks. Secondary syphilis may present with oral mucous patches, or an erythematous maculopapular eruption on the trunk, limbs, palms and soles. In the perianal area, condylomata lata are common and highly infectious. Symphilitic proctitis results in painful defecation, tenesmus, and diarrhea which may be blood-streaked. On proctoscopy, the mucosa is edematous and inflamed with mucous patches, erosions or ulcerations. The diagnosis is established by dark field examination of material from the lesions, rectal biopsy and positive blood serology (Nazemi et al., 1975).

7.2. Enteric infections

An increasing incidence of sexually transmitted enteric pathogens is becoming evident in homosexually active males. These include *Entamoeba histolytica, Dientamoeba fragilis, Amoeba buetschilii* (Kean, 1976), *Giardia* (Meyers et al., 1977), *Shigella* (Drusin et al., 1976), *S. typhi* (Dritz and Braff, 1977), *E. vermicularis* and viral hepatitis B (Szmuness et al., 1975). They may produce no symptoms or cause gastrointestinal complaints such as abdominal pain, constipation, diarrhea, flatulence, anal pain, rectal discharge and bleeding, the features of malabsorption or jaundice. Clinically, they may closely mimic the manifestations of inflammatory bowel disease or functional enterocolonopathy.

Asymptomatic and promiscuous carriers are important reservoirs of infection. In the absence of a relevant travel history (or despite it) these infections are not infrequently acquired via fellatio, oroanal sexual practice and rectal intercourse with foreign visitors or carriers in the local population. Investigations include stool cultures, examination of fresh stools for ova and parasites, appropriate serological tests, proctosigmoidoscopy and gastrointestinal roentgenograms. The high incidence of promiscuity in homosexual men and the sexual behavior of bisexual individuals leads to the transmission of these diseases not only to the homosexual community but to the heterosexual group as well.

7.3. Virus B Hepatitis

Hepatitis B antigen has been found in saliva and semen (Heathcote, 1974). The transmission of virus B hepatitis by sexual intercourse and kissing has been alluded to repeatedly. An unusually high prevalence of HBs antigen and antibody has been found in the serum of male homosexuals (Coleman et al., 1977). Promiscuity is much commoner in male homosexuals than in the general population. HBsAg has not been found in feces. Salivary transmission is probably a major means of non-parenteral spread of type B hepatitis. A high incidence of hepatitis B infection in male homosexuals has been noted mainly in those whose sexual activities include rectal intercourse. The high carrier rate of hepatitis B in these males provides a basis for the high risk of sexually transmitted HB infections in male homosexuals (Villarejos et al., 1974). Such infections may lead to non-icteric viral hepatitis, icteric hepatitis or the carrier state.

8. CONCLUDING REMARKS

In the absence of organic disease, male sexual dysfunction is frequently attributed to a psychological disturbance. It is important, however, to avoid becoming 'one tract minded'. The physician must study such patients thoroughly, being very vigilant of the stigmata of organic disease. He or she must be alert to gastrointestinal symptoms in patients with andrological disorders to ferret out gonadal disturbances in people with primary gastrointestinal disease as well as those afflicted by systemic disease with prominent involvement of the alimentary tract.

Impaired sex drive or decreased libido may accompany debilitating illness, malnutrition, or hepatocellular dysfunction, or follow drug administration. Erectile dysfunction may complicate chronic alcoholism, parasympatholytics or abdomino-

perineal surgery. impaired ejaculation may follow abdominal aortic surgery, lumbar sympathectomy and drug therapy for gastrointestinal disorders (Betts, 1975).

An accurate record of sexual complaints should be part of a thorough medical history. Medical students and physicians must develop a technique and means of establishing rapport so that patients will discuss problems of sexual behavior freely. This would inevitably lead to the accumulation of a body

of knowledge for further study. Physicians dealing with problems of sexuality must become aware of the potential hazards of current sexual behavior and their public health implications.

In the past 25 years, our knowledge of sexuality has made eminent advances. A thorough investigative approach along physical as well as psychological lines will lead to earlier correct diagnosis and hopefully to more effective management.

REFERENCES

Abramovici H et al. (1972) Sterility due to a fistula between the rectum and ejaculatory ducts. Am J Obstet Gynecol 114: 6.

Agnese PA, diSant (ed.) (1968) Fertility and the young adult with cystic fibrosis. New Engl J Med 279: 103.

Andrevont HB (1952) Studies on the occurrence of spontaneous hepatomas in mice of strains C-3H and CBA. J Natl Cancer Inst 11: 581.

Bagheri SA, Boyer JL (1974) Peliosis hepatitis associated with androgenic-anabolic steroid therapy. A severe form of hepatic injury. Ann Intern Med 81: 610.

Baker PG, Read AE (1975) Reversible infertility in male coeliac patients. Br Med J 2: 316.

Betts TA (1975) Disturbances of sexual behaviour. J Clin Endocrinol Metab 4: 619.

Beumont PJV et al. (1972) The occurrence of the syndrome of anorexia nervosa in male subjects. Psychol Med 2: 216.

Blank RR, Mendoza EM (1976) Fertility in a man with cystic fibrosis. JAMA 235: 1364.

Boyar RM, Bradlaw HL (1977) Studies on testosterone metabolism in anorexia nervosa. In: Vigersky RA, ed. p 271. Anorexia nervosa. New York: Raven Press.

Boyd EM (1970) Testicular atrophy from analgesic drugs. A possible factor in chronic abdominal pain syndromes. J Clin Pharmacol July.

Brooke BN (1956) Outcome of surgery for ulcerative colitis. Lancet ii: 532.

Burch RE, Sullivan JF (1976) Clinical and nutritional aspects of zinc deficiency and excess. Med Clin North Am 60: 675.

Cates W, Pope JN (1977) Gynecomastia and cannabis smoking. Am J Surg 134: 613.

Catteral RD (1975) Sexually transmitted disease of the anus and rectum. Clin Gastroenterol 4: 659.

Coble YD et al. (1966) Zinc levels and blood enzyme activities in Egyptian male subjects with retarded growth and sexual development. Am J Clin Nutr 19: 415.

Cohen AS (1967) Amyloidosis. New Engl J Med 574: 000.

Coleman JC et al. (1977) Hepatitis B antigen and antibody in a male homosexual. Br J Vener Dis 53: 132.

Davis LP, Jelenko C (1975) Sexual function after abdomino-perineal resection. South Med J 68: 422.

Delle Fane GF et al. (1977) Gynecomastia with cimetidine. Lancet i: 1319.

Donaldson RM Jr (1973) Regional enteritis. In: Sleisenger MH, Fordtran JS, eds. Gastrointestinal disease, pp 886-908. Philadelphia: W.B. Saunders.

Dritz SK, Braff EH (1977) Sexually transmitted typhoid fever. New Engl J Med 296: 1359.

Druesen LM et al. (1976) Shigellosis – another sexually transmitted disease. Br J Vener Dis 52: 348.

Edwards CI et al. (1977) Hereditary hemochromatosis. New Engl J Med 297: 7.

Farrell GC et al. (1975) Androgen induced hepatoma. Lancet i: 430.

Feldman JM et al. (1974) Alterations of pituitary-gonadal function in carcinoid syndrome. Am J MEd Sci 268: 4.

Feller ER et al. (1977) Familial hemochromatosis. New Engl J Med 296: 1422.

Fine G et al. (1972) Primary extragenital choriocarcinoma in the male subject. Am J Med 32: 776.

Frasier SD (1973) androgens and athletes. Am J Dis Child 125: 479.

Gilder H, Hoagland CL (1946) Gynecomastia in acute viral hepatitis. Proc Soc Exp Biol Med 61: 62.

Goodman LS, Gilman A (1975) Antimuscarinic drugs. In: Pharmacological basis of therapeutics, 5th edn pp 514-532. Toronto: Macmillan.

Green JRB (1977) Mechanism of hypogonadism in cirrhotic males. Gut 18: 843.

Green JRB et al. (1976) Plasma estrogens in men with chronic liver disease. Gut 17: 426.

Gruen PH (1978) Endocrine changes in psychiatric diseases. The brain and the endocrine systems. Med Clin North Am 62: 285.

Gryboski JD, Spiro HM (1978) Prognosis in children with Crohn's disease. Gastroenterology 74: 807.

Heathcote J (1974) Hepatitis-B antigen in saliva and semen. Lancet i: 71.

Henkin RI (1976) Trace metals in endocrinology. Med Clin North Am 60: 4.

Hirschowitz BI (1977) Histamine H-2 receptor antagonists. Ann Intern Med 87: 373.

Hyams V et al. (1960) Adrenal rest tumour of the liver. Am J Surg 99: 960.

Jameson S (1976) Zinc deficiency in malabsorption states. Acta Med Scand Suppl 593.

Jung Y, Russfield AB (1972) Prolactin cells in the hypopophysis of cirrhotic patients. Arch Path 94: 265.

Kalser MH (1976) Coeliac sprue. In: Bockus HL, ed. Gastroenterology, 3rd edn, vol 2, pp 245-284. Philadelphia: W.B. Saunders.

Kaplan E et al. (1968) Reproductive failure in males with cystic fibrosis. New Engl J Med 279: 65.

Kazal HL et al. (1976) The gay bowel syndrome. Ann Clin Lab Sci 6: 184.

Kean BH (1976) Venereal amebiasis. NY State Med J 76: 930.

Kew MC et al. (1977) Feminization in primary liver cancer. New Engl J Med 296: 1084.

Klatskin G et al. (1947) Gynecomastia due to malnutrition. I. Clinical studies. Am J Med Sci 213.

Kolodny RC et al. (1974) Depression of plasma testosterone levels after chronic intensive marijuana use. New Engl J Med 290: 872.

Kowlessar OD (1973) Carcinoid tumors and the carcinoid syndrome. In: Sleisenger MH, Fordtran JS, eds. Gastrointestinal disease. Philadelphia: W.B. Saunders.

Kubickova A, Vesely KT (1974) Fertility and reproduction in patients with duodenal ulcer. J Reprod Fertil 36: 311.

Logan AH et al. (1938) Intestinal infantilism as a result of regional enteritis. Mayo Clin Proc 13: 335.

London DR (1975) Medical aspects of hypogonadism. Clin Endocrinol Metab 4: 597.

Marcus R, Korenman SG (1976) Estrogens and the human male. Ann Rev Med 27: 357.

Martini GA (1975) Extrahepatic manifestations of cirrhosis. Clin Gastroenterol 4: 439.

May AG et al. (1969) Changes in sexual function following operations on the abdominal aorta. Surgery 65: 41.

McArthur JW et al. (1973) Sexual precocity attributable to ectopic gonadotropin secretion by hepatoblastoma. Am J Med 54: 390.

McCallum RW et al. (1976) Metoclopramide stimulates prolactin secretion in man. J Clin Endocrinol Metab 42: 1148.

McCarthy DM (1978) Experience with cimetidine in the Zollinger Ellison syndrome and other hypersecretory states. Gastroenterology 74: 453.

McKechnie JC, Fechner RE (1971) Choriocarcinoma and adenocarcinoma of the esophagus with gonadotropin secretion. Cancer 27: 694.

Mecklenburg RS et al. (1974) Hypothalamic dysfunction in patients with anorexia nervosa. Medicine 53: 147.

Merianos P (1975) Reversible infertility in male coeliac patients. Br Med J 1: 316.

Merlin HE (1972) Azoospermia caused by colchicine. Fertil Steril 23: 180.

Meyers JD et al. (1977) *Giardia lamblia* infection in homosexual men. Br J Vener Dis 53: 54.

Monteiro JG (1973) The digestive system in familial amyloidotic polyneuropathy. Am J Gastroenterol 60: 47.

Morgan MY et al. (1978) Serum Prolactin in liver disease and its relation to gynecomastia. Gut 193: 170.

Mowat NAG et al. (1976) Hypothalamic-pituitary-gonadal function in men with cirrhosis of the liver. Gut 17: 345.

Muckle TJ, Wells M (1962) Urticaria, deafness and amyloidosis. Q J Med 31: 235.

Nazemi MM et al. (1975) Syphilitic proctitis in a homosexual. JAMA 231: 389.

Omenn GS (1970) Ectopic polypeptide hormone production by tumors. Ann Intern Med 72: 136.

Owen RL (1972) Rectal and pharyngeal gonorrhea in homosexual men. JAMA 220: 1315.

Perkins KW et al. (1965) Idiopathic hemochromatosis in children. Am J Med 39: 118.

Perloff WH et al. (1954) Functional hypopituitarism in coeliac disease. JAMA 155: 1307.

Perlos AP, Faillace LA (1964) Psychiatric manifestations of carcinoma of the pancreas. Am J Psychiatr 121: 182.

Pinder RM et al. (1976) Metoclopramide, a review of its pharmacological properties and clinical use. Drugs 12: 81.

Prasad AS et al. (1963) Zinc metabolism in patients with the syndrome of iron deficiency anemia, hepatosplenomegaly, dwarfism and hypogonadism. J Lab Clin Med 61: 537.

Rees LH, Ratcliffe JG (1974) Ectopic hormone production by non-endocrine tumors. Clin Endocrinol (Oxf) 3: 263.

Ronaghy (1969) Controlled zinc supplementation for malnourished schoolboys. Am J Clin Nutr 22: 1279.

Rose LI et al. (1977) Pathophysiology of spironolactone-induced gynecomastia. Ann Intern Med 87: 398.

Sandstead HH (1967) Human zinc deficiency, endocrine manifestations and response to treatment. Am J Clin Nutr 20: 422.

Savage C, Noble D (1954) Cancer of the pancreas simulating psychogenic illness. J Nerv Men Dis 120: 62.

Schiff L (1969) Diseases of the liver, 3rd edn. Philadelphia: J.B. Lippincott.

Sherlock S (1975) Diseases of the liver and biliary system, 5th edn. Oxford: Blackwell Scientific.

Shwachman H, Grand RJ (1973) Cystic fibrosis. In: Sleisenger NH, Fordtran JS, eds. Gastrointestinal disease. Philadelphia: W.B. Saunders.

Sohn N, Robilotti JG (1977) The gay bowel syndrome. A review of colonic and rectal conditions in 200 male homosexuals. Am J Gastroenterol 67: 478.

Stern RC et al. (1977) Cystic fibrosis diagnosed after the age of 13. Ann Intern Med 87: 188.

Szmuness W et al. (1975) On the role of sexual behaviour in the spread of hepatitis B infection. Ann Intern Med 83: 489.

Taussig LM (1972) Fertility in males with cystic fibrosis. New Engl J Med 287: 586.

Van Thiel DH et al. (1974) Hypogonadism in alcoholic liver disease – evidence for a double defect. Gastroenterlogy 67: 1188.

Van Thiel DH et al. (1975) Plasma estrone, prolactin, neurophysis and sex steroid binding globulin in chronic alcoholic men. Metabolism 24: 1015.

Van Thiel DH, Lester R (1976) Alcoholism: its effect on hypothalamic pituitary gonadal function. Gastroenterology 71: 318.

Vibersky R. (1977) Anorexia nervosa. New York: Raven Press.

Villarejos VM et al. (1974) The role of saliva, urine and feces in the transmission of type B hepatitis. New Engl J Med 26: 1375.

Walsh CH et al. (1976) A study of pituitary function in patients with hemochromatosis. J Clin Endocrinol Metab 43: 866.

Whitelaw GP, Smithwick RH (1951) Some secondary effects of sympathectomy with particular reference to disturbance of sexual function. New Engl J Med 245: 121.

William DC et al. (1977) Sexually transmitted enteric pathogens in a male homosexual population. NY State J Med 77: 2050.

Wirsching M et al. (1975) Results of psychosocial adjustment to long-term colostomy. Psychother Psychosom 26: 245.

Wolfe MM (1979) Impotence on cimetidine treatment. New Engl J Med 300: 94.

Young SJ et al. (1976) Psychiatric illness and the irritable bowel syndrome. Gastroenterology 70: 162.

Zubiran S et al. (1953) Endocrine disturbances in chronic human malnutrition. Vitam Horm 11: 97.

18. ANDROLOGICAL DISORDERS IN HEMATOLOGY

H. GOLDENBERG and L.M.C. GOLDENBERG

The purpose of this chapter is to explore what little is known about andrologic influences on blood and the hematopoietic system as well as the reciprocal andrologic changes consequent to hematologic disorders. The latter are of much greater clinical concern and better understood and so accordingly constitute the bulk of the chapter. The gonadal manifestations of hematological disorders occurring in the human male may be subclinical or cause overt abnormalities of spermatogenesis, steroidogenesis or both. Both proven as well as speculative mechanisms of pathogenesis are discussed.

1. HEMATOLOGICAL MANIFESTATIONS OF GONADAL DISORDERS OF THE MALE

1.1. Androgens and erythropoiesis

The hematological changes which occur in disorders of the endocrine organs may result from deficiency or excess of one or more of the hormones. The endocrine system plays a distinct role in red-cell formation, regulating the rate of erythropoiesis rather than exercising absolute control. The hematological effects of the endocrine disorders are thus relatively slight in degree in comparison with the gross abnormalities which result from deficiencies of such substances as iron, vitamin B_{12} and folic acid, which are essential for normal erythropoiesis. Thus, with diseases of the gonads, the changes in the blood are often not prominent clinical features; however, there is no doubt that the sex hormones exert an influence upon erythropoiesis. It is well recognized that the hemoglobin concentration, red-cell count and packed cell volume are, on the average, significantly higher in adult males than in adult females, although in prepubertal children there is no sex difference.

A large amount of evidence has accumulated from animal experiments and from clinical studies indicating that androgens have the property of increasing red-cell production (Fried and Gurney, 1968; Naets and Wittek, 1966). The administration of androgens to eunuchoid men without evidence of pituitary disease results in significant rises in hemoglobin concentration and red-cell count. On withdrawal of therapy the blood findings revert to their previous level (McCullagh and Jones, 1942). Cases of hypopituitarism with hypogonadism have been recorded, in which anemia resistant to therapy with liver, iron and thyroid, responded well to treatment with testosterone (Watkinson et al., 1947). High doses of androgens increase red-cell production in patients with advanced carcinoma of the breast (Kennedy and Gilbertson, 1957). Following discontinuation of treatment, the red-cell values slowly revert to their pre-treatment levels. In these patients the improvement in the blood during testosterone therapy was not closely correlated with general clinical improvement. No changes were noted in the leucocytes or platelets.

In contrast to the stimulatory effect of androgens on erythropoiesis, estrogens tend to reduce red-cell production. Clinically, it is recognized that males treated with estrogens for carcinoma of the prostate have, on the average, hemoglobin concentrations and red-cell counts similar to those of normal females.

Androgens have now been utilized in the treatment of bone marrow failure for about 20 years, following the initial report of Shahidi and Diamond (1961), that testosterone produced remission in children with aplastic anemia. Androgens in pharmacologic amounts were subsequently found to stimulate erythropoiesis in adults with myelofibrosis and myeloid metaplasia, hypoplastic anemia

J. Bain and E.S.E. Hafez (eds.), Diagnosis in andrology, 241-253. All rights reserved.
Copyright © 1980 by Martinus Nijhoff Publishers bv, The Hague/Boston/London.

and various types of refractory anemia (Gardner, 1978; Sanchez-Medal, 1971).

The initial enthusiasm for the effectiveness of androgen therapy has now, however, been replaced by the realization that patients with severe aplastic anemia rarely if ever respond successfully to such treatment (Camitta et al., 1977). Such patients require a careful physiological evaluation of residual erythropoietic foci to help assess the severity of the aplasia and thus to predict the response to androgen therapy. In severe cases of aplasia, with absence of such foci, one may anticipate no response to androgen therapy.

With the advent of successful bone marrow transplantation in aplastic anemia the response to androgen therapy has been re-evaluated. A large prospective study designed to determine the efficacy of androgens for the treatment of severe aplastic anemia revealed the ineffectiveness of these agents (Camitta and Thomas, 1978). In contrast, this study showed that histocompatible bone marrow transplantation significantly improved hematological recovery and survival. Alternative methods of treatment must therefore be carefully evaluated for patients with severe bone marrow aplasia who do not have a compatible sibling marrow donor.

1.2. Autoimmune hemolytic anemia associated with seminoma

Following the introduction of the Coombs' antiglobulin test, the association between autoimmune hemolytic anemia and neoplasia has been frequently documented, the vast majority occurring in the lymphoproliferative diseases such as chronic lymphocytic leukemia and lymphomas. The hemolytic anemia is characterized by a falling hemoglobin and red-cell count in association with a rising reticulocyte count and the presence of microspherocytes coated with immunoglobulin.

Non-hematopoietic neoplasms are only infrequently associated with autoimmune hemolytic anemia and are epithelial in type with the main exception being ovarian teratoma. There appears to be a clear relationship between teratomatous ovarian cystic tumors and autoimmune hemolytic anemia (Debruyère et al., 1971; Pirofsky, 1969), in the majority of which, removal of the tumor is associated with cessation of hemolysis and dis-

appearance of antibodies.

No testicular teratomas or dermoids have been reported in association with autoimmune hemolytic anemia but seminoma, which shares its germinal origin with ovarian teratomas, has been reported in three cases (Lundberg and Mitchell, 1977). In one patient with a seminoma presenting concurrently with a severe IgC-mediated warm antibody and autoimmune hemolytic anemia, treatment directed against the tumor and the hemolytic process resulted in the complete disappearance of the antibodies. In addition to the production of red cell autoantibody, a monoclonal (IgM/k) cryoglobulinemia and a biologically false positive test for syphilis were also found, all transient immunological phenomena which may have occurred in response to the seminoma. Since seminomas are known to provoke a lymphoid response, at times so brisk as to mimic lymphoma (Johnson, 1972), one may speculate that the autoimmune hemolytic anemia is associated with the lymphoproliferation.

2. GONADAL MANIFESTATIONS OF HEMATOLOGICAL DISORDERS

2.1. Abnormal spermatogenesis

2.1.1. Infertility due to antineoplastic drugs. Antineoplastic agents as a group are clinically effective in treating malignant disease because of their toxicity to rapidly proliferating malignant cells. The clinically useful agents have a greater toxicity for malignant cells than for the normal cells of the tumor bearing host, this selective toxicity being made possible because of a variety of differences between malignant and normal cells. Because these differences may be slight, the margin of safety is often a very narrow one. Many normal tissues have a high proliferative capacity rivaling those of malignant tissues. Such normal tissues, including bone marrow elements, gastrointestinal epithelium, hair follicles and gonads, bear the brunt of toxic effects of certain antitumor agents. With the chronic administration of antineoplastic and immunosuppressive drugs to patients with cancer and nonmalignant conditions, the long-term toxicity of these agents has become the subject of increasing concern.

Sieber and Adamson (1975) have extensively reviewed some of the deleterious toxic effects of cancer chemotherapeutic agents in humans, namely, their ability to induce chromosome damage, infertility, congenital malformations and carcinogenesis.

All three classes of antineoplastic compounds (alkylating agents, antimetabolites, and antitumor antibiotics), which have been studied extensively, are known to induce damage to human chromosomes under both in vitro and in vivo conditions. These abnormalities vary according to the agent and test system used. Combinations of agents or agents plus irradiation also produce cytogenetic damage to human cells to a greater degree than with single-agent chemotherapy. The long-term sequelae of such damage has not yet been ascertained. Should the genetic apparatus of germinal cells be affected in the same way as that of somatic cells, such effects could be far-reaching since they might be transmitted from generation to generation.

Antineoplastic agents, particularly the alkylating compounds which are radiomimetic, exert cytotoxic effects and hence inhibit spermatogenesis. Oligospermia or azoospermia induced by alkylating agents such as chlorambucil has been noted in lymphoma patients. The cytotoxicity is usually dose related. A minimum total dose of 400 mg, is required for germinal cell line damage resulting in azoospermia (Vilar, 1974). Testicular biopsy reveals spermatogenesis to be completely absent with only Sertoli cells lining the tubules and with varying degrees of peritubular fibrosis present. No apparent damage to the interstitial cells or vascular apparatus occurs and the secretion of testosterone remains normal (Sherins and DeVita, 1973). Profound azoospermia has been noted for periods ranging from 1 to 13 months after the last dose of chlorambucil and has only occasionally been reversible (Vilar, 1974). Vinblastine has a similar effect on spermatogenesis, the impairment however, being incomplete (Vilar, 1974). Since this drug does not act on resting cells, a reserve of stem cells is probably available to reestablish the germinal epithelium. There is insufficient information on the possible adverse effects of the antimetabolites and antitumor antibiotics on spermatogenesis.

Similar observations of sterility in males have been reported following the use of cyclophospha-mide in the treatment of postpubertal males with glomerulonephritis and nephrotic syndrome (Sieber and Adamson, 1975). Since the seminiferous tubules are permanently damaged if treatment is prolonged, the increasing use of such cytotoxic agents in nonmalignant conditions in prepubertal males in their reproductive years, should be governed by greater caution.

2.1.2. Infertility due to irradiation. Exposure to X rays, neutrons and radioactive materials can inhibit spermatogenesis by causing germinal cell destruction (Paulsen, 1964). The spermatogonia are quite sensitive to radiation, which produces a maturation arrest of the germinal cells. The antifertility effect of the radiation is thus similar to that caused by the antineoplastic alkylating compounds. This chemical action has therefore been appropriately termed radiomimetic. As with cytotoxic agents, the radiation damage is dose related. Provided the dose is not excessive, spermatogenesis may eventually recover. The maximum dose that allows full recovery is approximately 400-600 R for a radiation source consisting of 250 kV X ray energy. With such a source spermatogenesis may be temporarily damaged by dose levels as low as 15 R (Heller et al., 1966).

In contrast, Leydig cell function is quite resistant to irradiation, the highest tolerated dose probably exceeding 800 R X rays. Since Leydig cell function remains intact, testosterone levels, as well as urinary LH excretion titers, are normal (Paulsen, 1973). FSH levels are increased as a result of damaged spermatogenesis but return to normal when the germinal epithelium is restored.

2.1.3. Vitamin B_{12} deficiency – a cause of infertility? Although pernicious anemia may be associated with infertility in females (Jackson et al., 1967), there are no reports of infertility in males due to vitamin B_{12} deficiency.

Experimental findings, however, suggest that vitamin B_{12} may influence the maturation of human spermatozoa (Watson, 1962). The addition of vitamin B_{12} to stored bull semen used in artifical insemination improved eventual motility and enhanced its degree of fertility (Busch, 1957). Watson (1962) found that when the seminal B_{12} levels were less then serum B_{12} levels, one was likely to find

azoospermia and an increase of spermatozoa with morphological abnormalities, suggesting that vitamin B_{12} may influence the maturation of human spermatozoa. Testicular biopsy of male pernicious anemia patients would, of course, be distinctly helpful in clarifying whether or not a maturation arrest occurs, similar to the megaloblastosis seen in the B_{12} deficient bone marrow.

Although pernicious anemia may be associated with other autoimmune endocrine diseases, no such relationship is known to occur with regard to the testis. Despite extensive information available on experimental autoimmune orchitis a similar natural human autoimmune disease of the testis does not clearly exist.

2.2. Abnormal steroidogenesis

2.2.1. Gonadal dysfunction in sickle cell anemia: associations with zinc deficiency. Impairment of skeletal and sexual maturation in patients with sickle cel anemia has been attributed to hypopituitarism resulting from intravascular thrombosis and pituitary infarction (Daughaday, 1974). However, detailed endocrine evaluation in adults with this disease had not been carried out to support this hypothesis. Prasad et al. (1977), in their studies of zinc metabolism, found this element essential for the development of animals and humans, its deficiency causing growth retardation and hypogonadism. They noted the clinical similarity in patients with sickle cell anemia, reported the occurrence of zinc deficiency in such patients and found improvement in skeletal and sexual development following zinc therapy. They suggested that androgen deficiency may be related to lack of zinc. Since zinc is an important constituent of erythrocytes, the chronic hemolytic state in patients with sickle cell anemia may be responsible for the zinc deficiency.

In a syndrome of iron deficiency anemia, hepatosplenomegaly, dwarfism and hypogonadism reported in Iranian males, the associated zinc deficiency was felt to be due to poor nutritional intakes as well as chronic loss of iron- and zinc-rich blood from parasitic infestations. Oral zinc supplementation appears to result in genital and skeletal growth (Prasad et al., 1977).

Further studies by Abbasi et al. (1976) on patients with sickle cell anemia and androgen defi-

ciency, showed serum LH and FSH levels before and after stimulation with gonadotropic releasing hormones to be consistent with primary testicular failure. The serum testosterone response was sluggish in patients with this disease. The study indicated that the integrity of the hypothalamic-pituitary axis is intact in patients with sickle cell anemia and that androgen deficiency in this disease is a result of primary rather than secondary hypogonadism. The role of zinc in the pathogenesis of testicular failure in sickle cell anemia requires further study.

Zinc levels are measured in plasma, erythrocytes and hair, using an atomic absorption spectrophotometer. In sickle cell anemia, zinc in erythrocytes and hair more accurately reflects the status of chronic zinc nutrition than plasma levels since release of zinc from erythrocytes spuriously raises the plasma level. In sickle cell anemia, erythrocyte and hair zinc concentrations are significantly decreased, and there is a positive correlation between erythrocyte zinc and serum testosterone.

In addition to dysfunction of steroidogenesis in Leydig cells, abnormal spermatogenesis with maturation arrest is evident in testicular biopsies (Follis, 1966; Wong et al., 1973).

Zinc is present in high concentrations in the epididymis, seminal vesicle and prostate of the rat and man (Vallee, 1959). Zinc deficient rats have decreased levels of lactic dehydrogenase, malic dehydrogenase and alcohol dehydrogenase (Prasad et al., 1977). Alcohol dehydrogenase is necessary for retin*ol* formation in liver, retina and testicle. Vitamin A is essential for spermatogenesis, and although it is absorbed and transported in plasma as retin*ol* its oxidation to retin*al* is necessary for activation (Van Thiel & Lester, 1974). Ethanol competitively inhibits testicular retin*al* formation in vitro. Although testicular atrophy in severe alcoholic cirrhosis has long been felt to be consequent to the metabolic inbalance of the liver disease, there is growing evidence to implicate either direct toxicity due to ethanol and/or zinc deficiency. This hypothesis is attractive now that hypogonadism reversed by zinc therapy has been documented in the human models of sickle cell anemia and the syndrome described by Prasad et al. (1977). Careful balance studies have clearly demonstrated that severe alcoholic cirrhosis is a state of chronic zinc deficiency with obligatory zincuria (Vallee, 1959). It appears

then that both alcohol and zinc deficiency may directly affect spermatogenesis synergistically via a biochemical lesion in the vitamin A – alcohol dehydrogenase pathway.

2.2.2. Hypogonadism in hemochromatosis. Hemochromatosis is a disorder of parenchymal cell iron overload characterized pathologically by widespread excessive accumulations of iron (as hemosiderin) in parenchymal tissues with resultant cellular dysfunction. The sex incidence in overt idiopathic hemochromatosis indicates increased male vulnerability, the main reason probably being the protective effects of chronic iron loss in females through menstruation. Clinically, the iron overload results in structural and physiological impairment of hepatic, pancreatic and myocardial tissue. In addition to the more generally recognized features, hemochromatosis may cause hypogonadism. Skin pigmentation, hepatic cirrhosis and diabetes mellitus, which form the classic triad of this disease, should make one suspect the diagnosis.

The diagnosis of hemochromatosis is established by finding an elevation of the serum iron (> 200 μg/100 ml), saturation of the serum iron binding capacity (greater than 90%), and demonstration of increased parenchymal tissue iron stores on liver biopsy. Diagnostic tests with iron chelating agents such as desferrioxamine are useful in demonstrating increased iron stores but are seldom required for diagnosis.

Deposits of hemosiderin also appear in the epithelial cells of the pituitary, adrenal, thyroid and parathyroid glands, with resultant brownish discoloration of these organs. In the pituitary gland, the hemosiderin is limited to the anterior lobe while in the testis iron excess is not found, the deposition being usually small and located in the blood vessels and interstitial connective tissue.

Loss of libido and testicular atrophy are common findings and are considered to be more prominent features of hemochromatosis than of Laennec's cirrhosis while severe portal hypertension and ascites are rarer. The bulk of evidence indicates that the hypogonadism is primarily due to pituitary involvement, as a result of damage due to iron deposition. The serum and urinary gonadotropin levels are depressed and clomiphene and LHRH have subnormal responses in this condition (Tour-

niaire et al., 1974). Other investigators (Simon et al., 1972), however, have suggested that the hypogonadism of hemochromatosis is due to primary testicular failure claiming that the blood gonadotropin levels tend to be elevated. Since iron excess is not found in the affected gonads this conclusion requires experimental confirmation.

If testosterone deficiency exists it can be managed with androgen replacement therapy. The impotence may be more difficult to manage if it is due to the autonomic neuropathy of the associated diabetes. With removal of excessive iron deposits by repeated phlebotomy, improvement of the skin pigmentation, cirrhosis and diabetes may occur but little or no effect on the hypogonadism has been reported (Williams et al., 1969).

2.3. Combined abnormalities of spermatogenesis and steroidogenesis (destructive lesions of the testis)

2.3.1. Testicular replacement by leukemia and lymphoma. Leukemia and lymphoma are the most common neoplasms to metastasize to the testis, yet clinical evidence of testicular involvement in these conditions is rare. Interest in this situation has been stimulated since the introduction of chemotherapy, by the appearance of testicular involvement in acute leukemia of childhood often developing during hematologic remission. Such involvement is apparently increasing in frequency and is now by far the most common type of testicular infiltration by hematopoietic neoplastic disease.

In a large autopsy series, Givler (1969) found microscopic testicular infiltration to be most common in acute leukemia (64.3% of 140 males), less in chronic leukemia (22.4% of 76 males), least in non-Hodgkin's lymphoma (18.6% of 102 males) and absent in all of 44 males with Hodgkin's disease. Of the acute leukemias, the vast majority of cases were lymphoblastic in type, while in the chronic forms, one quarter were lymphocytic in type, the remainder granulocytic. The lymphomas were predominantly undifferentiated, either lymphoblastic, histiocytic or mixed cell type. Two children with lymphomatous testicular involvement had the features of Burkitt's lymphoma. In all types of leukemia and lymphoma, testicular involvement at autopsy was usually associated with widespread and extensive infiltration elsewhere.

Hemorrhage, thrombosis and infarction of the testicle may occur as complications of extensive local infiltration, and add to the destructive process. To affect adversely male reproduction, testicular structures need be significantly destroyed.

All varieties of leukemia occur more often in men than in women, the sex disparity being greatest in chronic lymphocytic leukemia where the male-to-female ratio is greater than 2 to 1 (Rundles, 1977). Hodgkin's disease, too, has a predilection for the male sex, the M/F ratio being 3/2. The exact role of the sex hormones in the etiology of the leukemias and lymphomas has never been defined. In chronic lymphocytic leukemia there are no known basic sex differences in lymphocyte physiology, in immune responsiveness or in the natural course of the disease once it develops. The exposure to leukemogenic agents is presumably equal in both sexes.

Testicular disease in childhood acute lymphoblastic leukemia (ALL). Following the development of effective systemic chemotherapy for the control of childhood ALL, the latent features of extramedullary involvement and its implications were revealed. With the achievement of ever increasing durations of hematological remission, the importance of extramedullary involvement increases proportionately.

Central nervous system leukemia, the most common form of extramedullary relapse became a major obstacle in the control of childhood leukemia in the 1960s, supposedly because the blood-brain barrier makes the meninges a sanctuary from chemotherapy. With eradication of meningeal disease and improvement in prognosis owing to the use of intrathecal drugs and cranioaxial irradiation, the problem of testicular leukemia now looms ahead.

Testicular relapse in childhood leukemia was rarely recognized before 1960. The suggestion that the increased clinical recurrence reflects improvement in leukemia therapy and more prolonged survival (Givler, 1969), is borne out in a recent survey in which the frequency of testicular involvement was distinctly related to the duration of survival (Hustu and Aur, 1978). As with CNS leukemia, testicular involvement occurs more often in the setting of relapsing disease, developing after initial remission induction and during hematological bone marrow remission.

The frequency of testicular involvement during the course of the disease ranges from 8 to 16%, contrasting with the microscopic occurrence of infiltration variously reported in 27-92% of autopsied cases (Hustu and Aur, 1978), far more frequent than appreciated clinically at the bedside. Others have confirmed the presence of microscopic extramedullary leukemic disease often in multiple sites in patients with 'complete hematological remission', the testicular involvement only reflecting the systemic process (Simone, 1974).

Clinically, the child presents with testicular enlargement, often asymptomatic and unnoticed by the patient or parents. Although the enlargement is usually unilateral, biopsy often confirms the presence of bilateral disease (Finklestein et al., 1969).

Other factors appear to influence testicular relapse in addition to the increased incidence as longer remissions from bone marrow and meningeal disease have been achieved. A high initial blood leukocyte count (greater than 20,000) at the time of diagnosis of leukemia has been considered to be a bad prognostic sign (Zuelzer and Flatz, 1960), suggesting that testicular relapse is related to the degree of extramedullary involvement, presumably due to earlier dissemination of the leukemic process. Following the introduction of immunological typing, it now appears that T-cell ALL with typical anterior mediastinal masses can infiltrate the testis with a high frequency (Hustu and Aur, 1978).

The postulate that a blood-gonad barrier exists (Finklestein et al., 1969), making the testis a pharmacologic sanctuary analogous to the central nervous system, has no anatomical or physiological basis. The main factor influencing testicular relapse appears to be the cessation of chemotherapy, most cases occurring within one year of stopping treatment (Medical Research Council, 1978).

Because of the high frequency of bilateral disease, the probable existence of other sites of extramedullary leukemia, and the demonstrated value of irradiation in clinically controlling local disease, radiotherapy rather than surgery seems to be the treatment of choice with this local complication, with doses of 1200 rads or more being recommended (Stoffel et al., 1975). Routine biopsy of both testes and early prophylactic irradiation may be as beneficial as early therapy of the central nervous system before the appearance of neurolo

gical manifestations (Nesbit et al., 1977). Other data (Hustu and Aur, 1978), however, suggest that patients with unilateral involvement confirmed by bilateral testicular biopsies should receive radiation treatment to the involved side only. The present policy of these authors is to do bilateral testicular biopsies regardless of the clinical impression before chemotherapy is discontinued. A radiation dose of 1200 rads is apparently capable of producing sterility for an uncertain period but it does not impair normal male maturation, suggesting that spermatogonia are more sensitive to irradiation than are the Leydig cells (Stoffel et al., 1975).

Even with control of the local disease, it is clear that systemic therapy has been inadequate but immediate intersification of systemic chemotherapy may delay hematological recurrence as it has in CNS relapse. Most authors at present recognize that clinical testicular relapse is not simply an indicator that the testis is a true sanctuary site but rather a clue to the presence of systemic disease or foreshadows further recurrence at other sites and thus bodes unfavorably for adequate and prolonged control of the leukemic process (Editorial, Lancet, 1978).

Testicular disease in acute non-lymphoblastic leukemia (including acute myeloblastic leukemia (AML), acute myelomonocytic leukemia, monocytic leukemia and erythroleukemia). To date the incidence of extramedullary leukemic relapse in childhood has been highest in acute lymphoblastic leukemia, although relapses have been reported with meningeal involvement and testicular infiltration in childhood acute myeloblastic leukemia (Sullivan and Hrgovcic, 1973). It appears that the major determinant for extramedullary involvement is the duration of the disease rather than the cell type. As the survival duration improves in AML, the incidence of involvement in the 'pharmacologic sanctuaries' may increase. Conceivably, in the future, prophylactic irradiation of 'sanctuary organs' combined with chemotherapy may be indicated to prolong leukemia-free remissions, as is being carried out in acute lymphoblastic leukemia.

Chronic leukemias. In the chronic leukemias, testicular infiltration is of a minor degree and noted only microscopically at autopsy. This involvement is simply a reflection of the generalized infiltration throughout the body.

Malignant lymphoma of the testis. Lymphoma of the testicle as a primary tumor is rare and may not even exist as a distinct entity. Testicular lymphoma is part of disseminated disease and may appear as a precocious local development. Testicular tumor is thus generally associated with a poor prognosis, 69-84% of patients dying of disseminated tumor within 2 years of orchiectomy (Gowing, 1976; Kiely et al., 1970). It is only in retrospect that, after being without evidence of recurrence for some years, a malignant lymphoma of the testis may be accepted as primary.

Although the testicular tumor is often followed by generalized involvement of lymph nodes and extranodal sites, the development of a leukemic blood picture is rare (Gowing, 1976). The frequent association of cutaneous and nasopharyngeal involvement with malignant lymphoma of the testis has been stressed (Altman and Winkelmann, 1960; Kiely et al., 1970), the association of purple-red nodular or ulcerated cutaneous lesions with enlargement of one or both testes indicating probable lymphoma. Twenty percent of cases of nasopharyngeal lymphoma are associated with a similar lesion of the testis.

Of metastatic tumors affecting the testis, lymphoma appears to be the most frequent (Kiely et al., 1970). Malignant lymphoma of the testis, unlike testicular neoplasms of germ cell origin, affects men older than 50 years in 80% of cases (Gowing, 1976) and is the commonest testicular neoplasm of elderly males (Abell and Holtz, 1968). Also, in contrast to germ cell tumors, lymphoma of the testis has no special propensity to develop in cryptorchid testes (Kiely et al., 1970).

The usual history is that of a painless, testicular swelling of several weeks' or months' duration, steadily increasing in size, with a definite tendency to affect both testes, either synchronously or more usually consecutively. Although lymphomas comprise only about 5% of all testicular malignancies, approximately 50% of patients with bilateral tumors have lymphoma (Gowing, 1976).

On gross examination, the body of the testis is usually hard within the distended tunica vaginalis.

The cut surface may be either homogenous or lobulated, grey or buff-coloured. There is no encapsulation, and extension into the epididymis and spermatic cord occurs frequently. Histopathologically almost all testicular neoplasms due to malignant lymphoma are of the poorly differentiated, immature type, either lymphoblastic or histiocytic (Gowing, 1976; Kiely et al., 1970). Tumors with the histopathologic criteria of Hodgkin's disease are rare, as are those due to well differentiated small, mature lymphocytes (Gowing, 1976). A nodular follicular pattern is not seen. The pattern of infiltration is characteristically one of diffuse penetration into the tissue spaces, producing wide separation of the normal components of the region, but usually without complete obliteration of the basic architecture, a picture similar to that seen with leukemic infiltration of various origins.

Gonadal involvement is a prominent feature of Burkitt's lymphoma being more common in the ovary than the testis. In African patients, gonadal involvement was a main presenting clinical feature in 3.8% of 373 males in 38% of 183 females, while at autopsy, the gonads were involved in 7 of 11 females and in 6 of 60 males (Wright, 1967). In studies of Burkitt's lymphoma in the United States testicular involvement at autopsy was noted in 9 of 22 males (Dorfman, 1965; Wilkinson et al., 1967).

Treatment consists primarily of orchiectomy and post-operative radiotherapy to the regional lymph nodes in those cases considered, by virtue of careful staging procedure, to be 'primary' or clinically localized to the testis at time of diagnosis. When dissemination occurs chemotherapy may be of some value.

Plasmacytoma of the testis. Plasmacytoma of the testis is extremely rare, about two dozen cases having been reported, presenting as painless testicular tumors (Gowing, 1976; Levin and Mostofi, 1970).

Careful investigation usually reveals the plasmacytoma to be an extramedullary manifestation of widespread multiple myeloma, but on occasion, however, the precocious development of a testicular lesion may precede clinical recognition of the underlying neoplastic process. The unsuspected diagnosis is made after orchiectomy and under these conditions may be confused clinically and histologically with a primary germ cell tumor of the testis or malignant lymphoma. An unusual case of testicular plasmacytoma occurring in the absence of hematological, radiological or immunoglobulin abnormalities, has been described in a patient who was free of myeloma one year following orchiectomy (Steinberg, 1975).

As with malignant lymphoma of the testis, most cases of testicular plasmacytoma occur in men older than 50 years of age, are frequently bilateral and have an especially poor prognosis, survival being rarely more than 2 years after diagnosis. Pathologically, too, the gross and microscopic characteristics of the tumor may resemble those of malignant lymphoma. The stroma between the seminiferous tubules is flooded with myeloma cells and the tubules are compressed (Levin and Mostofi, 1970).

Extramedullary lesions in multiple myeloma occur in up to 75% of autopsied cases (Hayes et al., 1952), most often in the liver, spleen, and lymph nodes. These organs are rich in reticuloendothelial elements, while the testis with meager tissue of that type is involved in only 1-3% of patients with multiple myeloma.

The treatment is that of the underlying neoplastic disease.

2.3.2. Other infiltrative disorders
Myeloid metaplasia. Extramedullary hematopoiesis (myeloid metaplasia) of the testis associated with myelofibrosis has been reported (Küchemann, 1969).

Histiocytosis. Although diabetes insipidus is a well known feature of histiocytosis X due to posterior pituitary involvement, panhypopituitarism associated with histiocytosis has also been reported (Ezrin et al., 1963). The testes, however, are rarely affected in histiocytosis X. Mild infiltration of the tunica vaginalis and interlobar septums of the testes were noted in one case reported (Shafer, 1949). An unusual variant of histiocytosis has been described in a child clinically presenting with bilateral testicular tumors, lymphadenopathy, hepatomegaly, and rheumatoid arthritis, but with no bone involvement (Azoury and Reed, 1966). The testes in this case were firm and rubbery and microscopically revealed immature tubules widely separated by large histiocytes.

Amyloidosis. Amyloid associated with aging has been found at autopsy located in senile plaques of the brain, in the aorta and in the endocrine organs including the pancreas and testes. Deposits in the testis are not prominent in either the primary or secondary types of amyloidosis (Franklin, 1977). However, in addition to generalized secondary amyloidosis involving the pituitary, amyloid deposits in the pituitary of a patient with multiple myeloma has been reported (Barr and Lampert, 1972).

2.4. Miscellaneous disorders

2.4.1. Vasculitis and testicular involvement. Necrotizing inflammation of the blood vessels gives rise to many clinical syndromes caused by immunologic phenomena mostly of unknown etiology. Because the clinical pictures may be pleomorphic they have been classified on a histological basis.

In periarteritis the lesions, involving the large muscular arteries, are widespread throughout the body, their size, extent and location dictating the severity of the clinical symptoms. Although often suspected in adult patients presenting with multiple system disease and a clinically compatible syndrome, periarteritis nodosa often eludes easy diagnosis. Histologic examination of tissue is the ultimate criterion for proper diagnosis and for distinction from the other vasculitides. Although the best sources for histological examination are clinically involved tissues such as tender cutaneous and subcutaneous nodules or muscles, blind muscle biopsy may give positive information in only one-third of patients (Maxeiner et al., 1952).

Because of the frequent finding of angiitis in the testis at autopsy, testicular biopsy has been recommended (Dahl et al., 1960). In their review of post mortem material, these authors found significant morbid changes in the testes in 41 of 44 male patients with all types of angiitis. Such abnormalities included specific arterial lesions in 86%, recent and healed infarcts, diffuse parenchymal obliteration, focal degeneration of testicular tubules, hematomas and hemorrhage. Smaller than normal testes were noted in one-fourth of patients. Because of the rarity of testicular signs and symptoms in other generalized diseases (including systemic lupus erythematosis), careful search for testicular pain, tenderness or swelling or a decrease in size of one or both testes in suspected cases may help establish the diagnosis clinically. Dahl et al. (1960) estimate that a histologic diagnosis of angiitis can be made in one-fifth of male patients with this disease. They suggest that testicular biopsy be considered in appropriate cases in which clinical testicular abnormality is present in a patient suspected of having vasculitis but who does not have skin or muscular lesions available for biopsy.

Hypersensitivity vasculitis (small vessel vasculitis) is the most frequent type of vasculitis with the inflammation and necrosis involving arterioles, venules and capillaries. Clinically this produces hemorrhagic and exudative lesions and microinfarcts rather than the ischemia and infarction seen with the larger artery involvement of periarteritis nodosa.

Hypersensitivity vasculitis may present clinically as Henoch- Schönlein purpura (anaphylactoid purpura), a vascular disorder with purpura as a striking feature. It is frequently associated with abdominal pain and bleeding and evidence of joint and renal involvement. It is more common in children during the first decade with males affected twice as often as females. In a series of 20 cases reviewed by Sahn and Schwartz (1972), of which 13 were males, five had testicular swelling while two of these had associated testicular pain. Six other cases of testicular swelling in Henoch-Schonlein purpura have been reported (Lipsitz et al., 1973). In the setting of a classical picture of Henoch-Schonlein purpura, the diagnosis is usually easily made, but with an atypical presentation, testicular torsion has been erroneously considered leading to unnecessary surgical exploration (Lipsitz et al., 1973).

Presumably the microangiopathic lesions of thrombotic thrombocytopenic purpura may involve the testes, as well as the most common sites, but not to any clinically significant degree.

2.4.2. Priapism. Priapism, a striking pathophysiologic condition characterized by persistent painful penile erection occurring apart from sexual excitement is a very unusual condition, with at least 20% of all cases being secondary to a hematologic disorder, such as sickle cell anemia or leukemia (Kinney et al., 1975). The incidence is less than 1% in the latter group, and occurs predominantly in

CML, and very rarely in CLL (Beckler and Mitchell, 1965) and the acute leukemias (Vadakan and Ortega, 1972; Veenhof et al., 1973). The mechanism of production is not clear although obstruction to venous drainage of the corpora cavernosa, by sludging of blood as in sickle cell anemia and leukemia has been considered. Only the corpora cavernosa are affected, the spongiosum and glans remaining flaccid.

An uncommon complication of sickle cell anemia, the painful symptoms result from local tissue anoxia secondary to mechanical occlusion of the vascular system by a 'log jam' of sickled erythrocytes, without thrombus formation, the corpora cavernosa being engorged with irreversibly sickled erythrocytes. In the leukemias priapism is generally associated with a marked leucocytosis, the pathogenesis being ascribed to the sludging effect of the leukemic cells with or without thrombosis. A nervous origin is unlikely since narcotics and general anaesthesia do not abolish it.

Numerous therapeutic measures have been proposed, usually acting locally and non-specifically and generally unrelated to the underlying pathophysiologic process occurring in the above hematologic disorders. Generally improvement of priapism is associated with a significant decrease of the peripheral leukocyte count in the leukemias or a reduction in the number of obstructing sickled cells, thus allowing better drainage of the obstructed corpora cavernosa. In the leukemias the treatment of choice is the rapid use of intensive cytotoxic chemotherapy to lower rapidly the blood counts before attempts at surgical intervention with corpora cavernosum shunt or aspiration (Schreibman et al., 1974). In sickle cell anemia improvement by diluting obstructing sickled cells with transfused normal red blood cells has been noted.

3. CONCLUSION

That androgens exert a stimulatory effect on hematopoiesis is now well established, yet detailed insight into the precise mulecular and biochemical mechanism is still lacking. In contrast to the androgenic influences on the blood and hematopoiesis which are usually very mild, there is much greater clinical relevance to the impact which various hematologic disorders may have on both spermatogenesis and steroidogenesis. These are schematically summarized in Fig. 1. These is little evidence to suggest that androgens are useful in the treatment of severe marrow hypoplasia, especially now that the era of tissue typing and immunosuppression has made marrow transplantation a greater reality. Much is now known of the adverse effects of chemical agents and irradiation upon spermatogenesis.

Little is known about the molecular influences which vitamin B_{12} deficiency may have on spermatogenesis. A study of testicular biopsy in infertile males with pernicious anemia or other forms of B_{12} deficiency may shed light on the associated infertility. Now that reversible hypogonadism has been demonstrated in some zinc deficiency states such as certain cases of sickle cell anemia it is of interest to speculate whether the low serum zinc levels in pernicious anemia are of pathogenetic significance and whether zinc supplementation might enhance fertility in these patients. Similarly, zinc therapy for the infertility seen in severe alcoholic cirrhosis and severe inflammatory bowel disease, both associated with zinc deficiency, may be helpful. Pertinent clinical studies have yet to be reported on this problem.

Testicular biopsy has become an important tool in identifying subclinical relapse in acute lymphoblastic leukemia. As chemotherapeutic remissions progressively lengthen with newer regimens used in adult acute myeloblastic leukemia, one can speculate that testicular biopsy may be used to identify asymptomatic extramedullary hematopoietic relapse in an effort to extend survival further. Biopsy is also of use in the diagnosis of mass lesions of the testis due to infiltrative hematologic disorders as well as the vasculitides when the diagnosis is suspected in the absence of clinically involved skin or muscle but with a gross testicular abnormality. Contrary to popular belief, blind testicular biopsy in the absence of clinical involvement will be positive for polyarteritis in at best 20% of true cases. These data are based on autopsy studies only.

There appear to be several exciting discoveries and advances on the horizon regarding the interactions between the gonadal and hematologic systems of the male.

SCHEMATIC SUMMARY OF HEMATOLOGIC DISORDERS CAUSING:

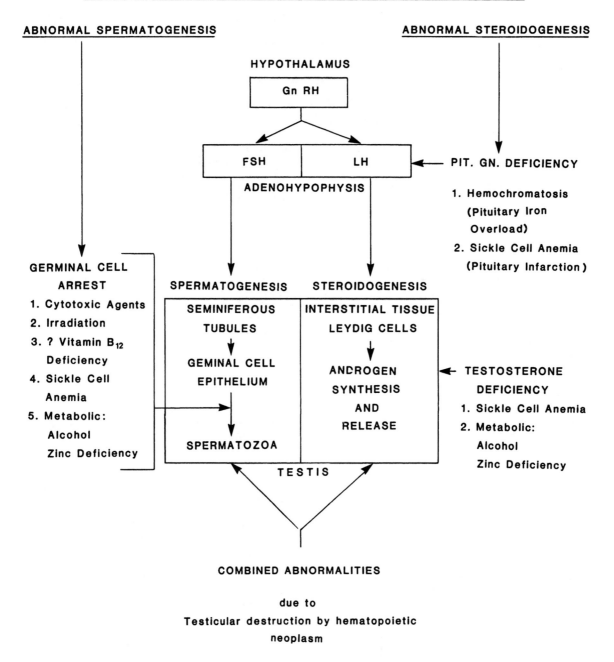

Figure 1. Schematic summary of hematologic disorders causing abnormal spermatogenesis an abnormal steroidogenesis.

REFERENCES

Abbasi AA, Prasad AS, Ortega J, Congco E, Orberleas D (1976) Gonadal function abnormalities in sickle cell anemia. Studies in adult male patients. Ann Intem Med 85: 601.

Abell MR, Holtz F (1968) Testicular and paratesticular neoplasms in patients 60 years of age and older. Cancer 21: 852.

Altman J, Winkelmann RK (1960) Lymphosarcoma of the skin and testis. Arch Dermatol 82: 943.

Azoury FJ, Reed RJ (1966) Histiocytosis. Report of an unusual case. New Engl J Med 274: 928.

Barr R, Lampert P (1972) Intrasellar amyloid tumor. Acta Neuropathol 21: 83.

Beckler L, Mitchell A (1965) Priapism. Surg Clin N Am 45: 1522.

Camitta BM, Thomas ED (for the International Aplastic Anemia Study Group) (1978) Severe aplastic anemia: a prospective study of the effect of androgens or transplantation on hematological recovery and survival. In: Clinics in haematology, Vol 7, p 587. London: W.B. Saunders.

Camitta B, Thomas ED, Nathan D, Santos G, Gordon-Smith E, Rappeport E (1977) Severe aplastic anemia: effect of androgens on survival. Blood 50: 313 (Suppl 1).

Dahl EV, Baggenstoss AH, DeWeerd JH (1960) Testicular lesions of periarteritis nodosa, with special reference to diagnosis. Am J Med 28: 222.

Daughaday WH (1974) The adenohypophysis. In: Williams RH, ed. Textbook of Endocrinology, p 550 Philadelphia: W.B. Saunders.

Debruyère M, Sokal G, Devoitille JM et al. (1971) Autoimmune hemolytic anemia and ovarian tumor. Br J Haematol 20: 83.

Dorfman RF (1965) Childhood lymphosarcoma in St. Louis, Missouri, clinically and histologically resembling Burkitt's tumor. Cancer 18: 418.

Editorial (1978) Testicular infiltrates in childhood leukemia: harbour or harbinger? *Lancet* 11: 136.

Ezrin C, Chaikoff R, Hoffman H (1963) Panhypopituiarism caused by Hans-Schüller-Christian disease. Can Med Assoc J 89: 1290

Finklestein JZ, Dyment PG, Hammond GD (1969) Leukemic infiltration of the testes during bone marrow remission. Pediatrics 43: 1042.

Follis RH Jr (1966) The pathology of zinc deficiency. In: Prasad AS, ed Zinc metabolism, p 129. Springfield, Ill.: Charles C. Thomas.

Franklin EC (1977) In: Williams WJ, Beutler E, Erslev AJ, Rundles RW, eds. Hematology, p 1137. New York: McGraw-Hill.

Fried W, Gurney CW (1968) The erythropoietic-stimulating effects of androgens. Ann N Y Acad Sci 149: 356.

Gardner FH (1978) Androgen therapy of aplastic anemia. Clin Hematol 7: 571.

Givler RL (1969) Testicular involvement in leukemia and lymphoma. Cancer 23: 1290.

Gowing NFC (1976) Malignant lymphoma of the testis. Br J Urol (Suppl) 36: 85, 1964. Also in: Pugh RCB, ed. Pathology of the testis, p 334. Oxford: Blackwell.

Hayes DW, Bennett WA, Heck FJ (1952) Extra-medullary lesions in multiple myeloma: review of literature and pathologic studies. Arch Pathol 53: 262.

Heller CG, Wootton P et al. (1966) Proc 6th Pan-American Congr Endocrinol. Amsterdam: Excerpta Medica Foundation Int Congr Ser 112.

Hustu HO, Aur RJA (1978) Extramedullary leukemia. In: Simone JV, ed. Clinics in hematology, Vol 7 No. 2, p 313. London: WB Saunders.

Jackson I, Doig WB, McDonald G (1967) Pernicious anemia as a cause of infertility. Lancet 11: 1159.

Johnson DE (1972) Testicular tumors, p 70 New York: Medical Examination Publishing.

Kennedy BJ, Gilbertson AS (1957) Increased erythropoiesis induced by androgenic-hormone therapy. New Engl J Med 256: 719.

Kiely JM, Massey BD Jr, Harrison EG Jr, Utz DC (1970) Lymphoma of the testis. Cancer 26: 847.

Kinney TR, Harris MB, Russell MO et al. (1975) Priapism in association with sickle hemoglobinopathies in children. J Pediatr 86: 241.

Küchemann K (1969) Complete testicular necrosis with extramedullary hematopoiesis and infiltration of megakaryocytes in a case of osteomyelosclerosis. Verh Dtsch Ges Pathol 53: 373.

Levin HS, Mostofi FK (1970) Symptomatic plasmacytoma of the testis. Cancer 25: 1193.

Lipsitz PJ, Orkin LA, Tarasuk A (1973) An unusual surgical manifestation of Schonlein-Henoch purpura. J Pediatr Surg 8: 437.

Lundberg WB, Mitchell MS (1977) Transient warm autoimmune hemolytic anemia and cryoglobulinemia associated with seminoma. Yale J Biol Med 50: 419.

Maxeiner SR Jr, McDonald JR, Kirklin LW (1952) Muscle biopsy in diagnosis of periarteritis nodosa: evaluation. S Clin N Am 32: 1225.

McCullagh EP, Jones R (1942) Effects of androgens on the blood count of men. J Clin Endocrinol 2: 243.

Naets JP, Wittek M (1966) Mechanism of action of androgens on erythropoiesis. Am J Physiol 210: 315.

Nesbit M, Ortega J, Donaldson M, Hittle R, Hammond D, Weiner J (1977) Prevention of testicular relapse by prophylactic radiation (XRT) in childhood acute lymphoblastic leukemia (ALL) (abstract). J Proc Am Soc Clin Oncol 18: 317.

Paulsen CA (1964) In: Carlson WD, Gassner FX, eds. In: Effects of ionizing radiation on the reproductive system. New York: Macmillan, p 305.

Pirofsky B (1969) Autoimmunization and the autoimmune hemolytic anemias Chap 10, p 229. Baltimore Williams & Wilkins.

Prasad AS et al. (1977) In: Brewer GJ, Prasad AS, ed S. Zinc metabolism. New York: AR Liss.

Medical Research Council (1978) Working Party on Leukemia in Childhood: testicular disease in acute lymphoblastic leukemia in childhood. Br Med J 1: 334.

Rundles RW (1977) In: Williams WS, Beutler E, Erslev AJ, Rundless RW, eds. Hematology, 2nd edn, p 1006. New York: McGraw-Hill.

Sahn DJ, Schwartz AD (1972) Schonlein-Henoch syndrome: observations on some atypical clinical presentations. Pediatrics 49: 614.

Sanchez-Medal L (1971) The hemopoietic action of androstanes. In: Brown EB, Moore CV, eds. Progress in hematology, vol 7. New York: Grune & Stratton.

Schreibman SM, Gee TS, Grabstald H (1974) Management of priapism in patients with chronic granulocytic leukemia. J Urol 111: 786.

Shafer EL (1949) Nonlipid reticulo-endotheliosis: Letterer-Siwe's disease: report of 3 cases. Am J Pathol 25: 83.

Shahidi NT, Diamond LK (1961) Testosterone-induced remission in aplastic anemia of both acquired and congenital types. New Engl J Med 264: 953.

Sherins RJ, DeVita VT (1973) Effects of drug treatment for lymphoma on male reproductive capacity. Studies of men in remission after therapy. Ann Intern Med 79: 216.

Sieber SM, Adamson RH (1975) Toxicity of antineoplastic agents in man: chromosomal aberrations, antifertility effects, congenital malformations, and carcinogenic potential. In: Klein G, Weinhouse S, eds. Advances in cancer research, Vol 22, p 57. New York: Academic Press.

Simon M, Franchimont P, Marie N, Ferrand B, Van Cauwenberge H, Bowel M (1972) Studies of somatotropic and gonadotropic pituitary function in idiopathic hemochromatosis (31 cases). Eur J Clin Invest 2: 384.

Simone JV (1974) Acute lymphocytic leukemia in childhood. Semin Hematol 11: 25.

Steinberg D (1975) Plasmacytoma of the testis. Report of a case. Cancer 36: 1470.

Stoffel TJ, Nesbit ME, Levitt SH (1975) Extramedullary involvement of the testes in childhood leukemia. Cancer 35: 1203.

Sullivan MP, Hrgovcic M (1973) Extramedullary leukemia. In: Sutow WW, Vietti TJ, Fernbach DJ Eds. Clinical pediatric oncology p 227. St. Louis: Mosby.

Tourniaire J, Feure M, Mazenod B, Posin G (1974) Effects of clomiphene citrate and synthetic LHRH on serum luteinizing hormone (LH) in men with idiopathic hemochromatosis. J Clin Endocrinol Metab 38: 1122.

Vadakan VV, Ortega J (1972) Priapism in acute lymphoblastic leukemia. Cancer 30: 373.

Vallee BL (1959) Biochemistry, physiology and pathology of zinc. Physiol Rev 39: 443.

Van Thiel DH, Lester R (1974) Editorial: sex and alcohol. New Engl J Med 291: 251.

Veenhof CHN, van der Meer J, Goudsmit R (1973) Successfully treated priapism in acute myeloblastic leukemia complicating Hodgkin's disease. Acta Med Scand 194: 349.

Vilar O (1974) Effect of cytostatic drugs on human testicular function. In: Mancini RE, Martini L, eds. Male fertility and sterility, p 423. London: Academic Press.

Watkinson G, McMenemy WH, Evans G (1947) Hypopituitarism, hypogonadism and anemia. Lancet I: 631.

Watson AA (1962) Seminal vitamin B_{12} and sterility. Lancet II: 644.

Wilkinson HA III, Hutchins GM, Hartmann WH (1967) Occurrence of African lymphoma syndrome in Baltimore, Maryland. Johns Hopkins Med J 121: 21.

Williams R, Smith PM, Spicer EJF, Barry M, Sherlock S (1969) Venesection therapy in idiopathic hemochromatosis. QJ Med 38: 1.

Wong T-W, Straus FH, Warner NE (1973) Testicular biopsy in the study of male fertility: 1. Testicular causes of infertility. Arch Pathol 95: 151.

Wright DH (1967) The gross and microscopic pathology of Burkitt's tumor. In: Burchenal JH and Burkitt DP, eds. Treatment of Burkitt's Tumor, p 14. New York: Springer-Verlag.

Zuelzer WW, Flatz G (1960) Acute childhood leukemia: a ten-year study. Am J Dis Child 100: 886.

SUBJECT INDEX

without infertility may reflect a disorder at the pituitary, hypothalamic, or gonadal level. The term sexual infantilism encompasses short stature together with evidence of sexual immaturity. This may result from genetically determined disorders, e.g. midline defects with pituitary deficiency, or environmentally caused lesions such as zinc deficiency with consequent gonadal defects, or from a combined etiology as in inherited sickle-cell anemia with hypozincemia.

Excessive weight, unusual obesity, atypical distribution of adipose tissue merit special note in the assessment of individuals with suspected andrological disorders. For example, in the Prader-Willi syndrome, striking obesity, developing beyond infancy, is associated with short stature, severe hypogonadism, cryptorchidism and infertility (DeFraites et al., 1975; Katcher et al., 1977). Furthermore, in the autosomal recessively inherited Laurence-Moon-Bardet-Biedl syndrome, excessive obesity involving the trunk and proximal portions of the limbs, is associated with retinitis pigmentosa, hypogonadism and infertility, postaxial polydactyly, deafness and renal hypoplasia (Alton and McDonald, 1973; Ammann, 1979). Conversely, recent weight loss may suggest the onset of diabetes mellitus.

The amount and distribution of body hair are also significant in determining the extent and duration of the hypogonadic condition, in anticipating the onset of puberty, and in ascertaining the nature of the andrological disorder. For example, despite widespread evidence of sexual maturation, with adequate masculinization, only scanty beard hair growth is often observed in adults with pseudo-vaginal perineoscrotal hypospadias (PPSH) - a disorder of defective synthesis of dihydrotestosterone due to 5-α-reductase deficiency.

Assessment of the sense of smell is, of course, significant particularly if the diagnosis of Kallmann's syndrome is contemplated.

Examination of the genitalia is obviously invaluable.

It is significant to note whether the testes are in the scrotum, have failed to descend (cryptorchid) or are extopically placed. The size, shape and symmetry of the scrotal sac as well as the quality and pigmentation of its skin and the completeness of fusion of its halves are all noteworthy features which are of help in identifying the particular genetic entities with specific andrological implications. In Noonan's syndrome one or both testes may be undescended (Collins and Turner, 1973; Noonan, 1968) whereas in male pseudohermaphroditism, cryptorchidism is prevalent (Goldstein and Wilson, 1974). In Reifenstein's syndrome, on the other hand, the testes are frequently scrotal though the two scrotal halves (derivatives of the labioscrotal folds) are only imperfectly, if at all, fused (Fig. 1a) (Shokeir, 1978).

The size, consistency and tenderness of the testes may also serve as a guide to the diagnosis. Small, firm, non-tender testes are the characteristic, though not invariable, finding in Klinefelter's XXY syndrome, whereas in many other forms of hypogonadism, the testes are usually small, soft and tender.

The presence, site and appearance of hypospadias which may be an isolated anomaly or a component of a more diverse and wide-spread syndrome, are valuable findings in establishing the possible existence and nature of the genetic disorder. In the telecanthus-hypospadias syndrome variable degrees of penile hypospadias are noted (Fig. 1b) (Shokeir, 1978) whereas dihydrotestosterone deficiency is attended with perineoscrotal hypospadias, along with bifid scrotum and small phallus (Fig. 1c) (Shokeir, 1978). The hypospadias in incomplete testicular feminization syndrome (ITFS) (Winterborn et al., 1970), complete and partial male pseudohermaphroditism (Fig. 1d) (Lubs et al., 1959), Reifenstein's syndrome, and Rosewater's syndrome (Rosewater et al., 1965), though variable, is penoscrotal, scrotal or perineal in location.

The absence of the prostate and seminal vesicles, as can be ascertained by rectal examination, is usually a manifestation of failure either in testosterone production or in the response of the Wolffian duct to testosterone during fetal life.

Funduscopic examination may indicate changes in the optic discs often seen in pituitary tumors.

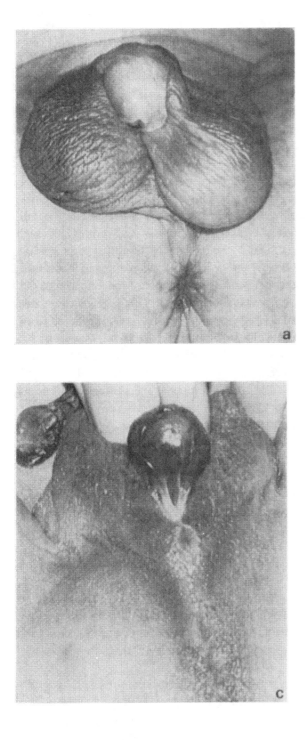

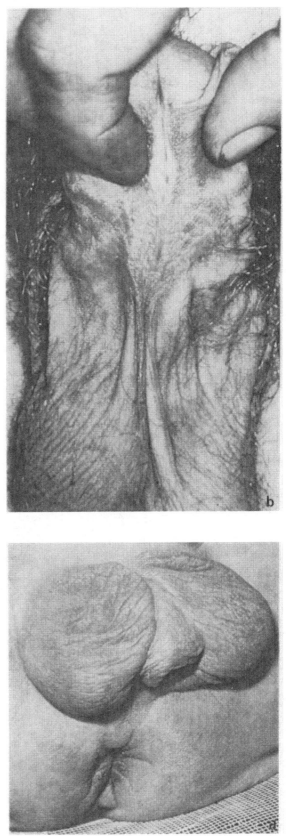

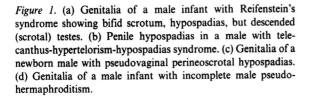

Figure 1. (a) Genitalia of a male infant with Reifenstein's syndrome showing bifid scrotum, hypospadias, but descended (scrotal) testes. (b) Penile hypospadias in a male with tele-canthus-hypertelorism-hypospadias syndrome. (c) Genitalia of a newborn male with pseudovaginal perineoscrotal hypospadias. (d) Genitalia of a male infant with incomplete male pseudo-hermaphroditism.

2. CYTOGENETIC EVALUATION

2.2. Sex chromatin

2.2.1. X chromatin body. Nuclei of somatic cells containing more than one X chromosome display one or more X chromatin bodies. The number of these bodies equals the number of X chromosomes minus 1. In normal males with an XY sex chromosome constitution, therefore, no X chromatin bodies are discerned in the nuclei of their cells. In a normal female with an XX sex chromosomal make-up, one X chromatin body is seen in each of a certain proportion of the nuclei of their cells. In Klinefelter's XXY syndrome (Fig. 2), one X chromatin body is seen with a frequency similar to

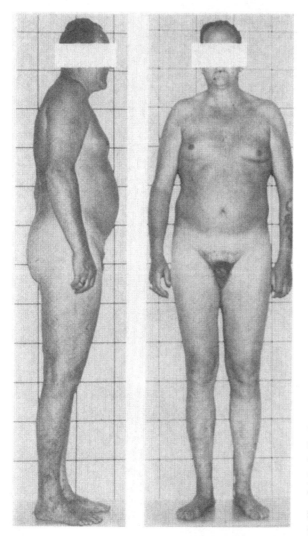

Figure 2. Front and profile of a man in his forties with Klinefelter's XXY syndrome.

that of females in cell nuclei (Fig. 3a). The X chromatin body or bodies represent genetically functionally inactivated X chromosomes – there being only one functionally active X chromosome per each cell nucleus regardless of the individual's sex (Fig. 3b and c).

2.2.2. Y chromatin body. The Y chromatin body is also detectable in cell nuclei containing Y chromosomes, albeit by a special staining method, namely quinacrine staining and fluorescence. When observed, the number of the Y bodies in the cell nucleus equals the number of Y chromosomes (Fig. 3d). The Y body, which fluoresces with special brilliance in UV light following quinacrine mustard staining, is made up of most of the long arm of the Y chromosome (Pearson, 1970). The genetic material is largely hetero-chromatin and is believed to be genetically functionally inactive (cf. X chromatin body). Thus by combining quinacrine staining and fluorescence to conventional staining of epithelial cells scraped from mucous membranes (e.g. buccal smear), adequate information can be furnished about the sex chromosomes.

The use of this technique, which capitalizes on the intense fluorescence of the end of the long arm of the Y chromosome, has permitted not only easy recognition of the Y chromosome but has also exposed its polymorphism among various males.

3. CHROMOSOME EVALUATION

3.1. Lymphocytes

By stimulating circulating lymphocytes with phytohemagglutinin, a universal mitogen, these cells can be incited to undergo mitotic division within 48-

The division process is arrested by the addition of colchicine which effectively halts the segregation of chromosomes. The dividing chromosomes still held together by their centromeres are discernible by light microscopy using oil immersion objective lens. They are then best visualized during the metaphase stage of mitosis because of their tightly coiled thickened state. A hypotonic solution ensures dispersion of the chromosomes and enables their staining is the conventional stain which defines the gross morphology of chromosomes including their size and shape, centromeres and their positions and presence of constrictions along the length of the chromosomes or satellites at their ends (Fig. 4a). Though effective in determining the total number of chromosomes, placing them in groups, and disclosing breaks, major deletions or additions (duplications), orcein staining is usually incapable of precisely identifying individual chromosomes or segments thereof.

The advent of newer staining procedures has enabled unambiguous identification of individual chromosomes and has made feasible the detection of even subtle structural alterations. Furthermore, the application of these techniques revealed the presence of many morphological variants in otherwise largely unremarkable individuals. The possible functional significance of these structural variants has remained mostly elusive.

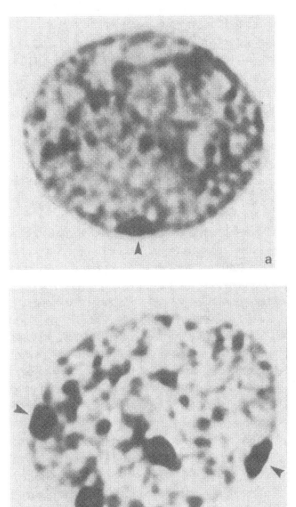

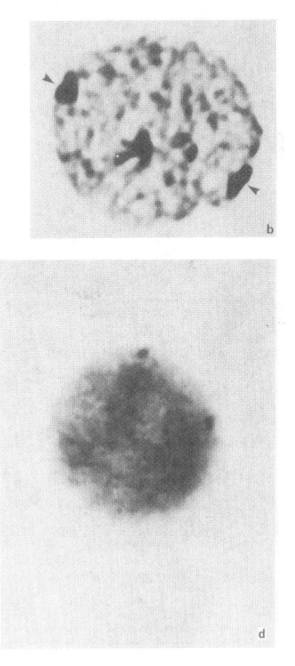

Figure 3. (a) Buccal smear nucleus from a male with Klinefelter's XXY syndrome showing one X chromatin body. (b) Buccal smear nucleus from a male with XXXY syndrome showing two X chromatin bodies. (c) Buccal smear nucleus from a male with XXXXY syndrome showing three X chromatin bodies. (d) Buccal smear nucleus from a male with XYY syndrome showing two brilliant fluorescent Y bodies.

3.1.1. Fluorescent staining (Q-banding). The introduction of this technique is credited to Caspersson et al. (1970). The preparations are treated with quinacrine mustard (hence the term Q-banding) and examined using ultraviolet (UV) fluorescence (Fig. 4b).

3.1.2. Trypsin-Giemsa staining. Q-banding has been superseded by a technique equally or more reliable,

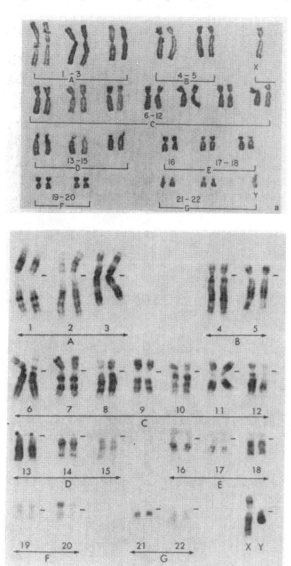

namely treating the chromosome preparation with the enzyme, trypsin, followed by staining with Giemsa (G-banding) (Schnedl, 1971, 1973; Seabright, 1971). The resulting appearance is characteristic in having alternating dark and light bands (Fig. 5a).

The dark G-bands correspond to the fluorescent Q-bands and both represent heterochromatic material which is believed to be functionally less active or inactive. Conversely, the light bands in trypsin-Giemsa stained chromosome preparations, which correspond to the less fluorescent bands in quinacrine staining, are euchromatic and represent functionally active DNA. Despite the superiority of G-banding techniques, fluorescence remains particularly useful in identifying the Y chromosome, in particular the distal portion of its long arm, which tends to stain with special brilliant fluorescence. Indeed the Y chromosome is thereby demonstrable in interphase nuclei, a useful adjunct to buccal smear examination (Fig. 3d). Similarly the inactive X chromosome as in the XX female or Klinefelter XXY male, stains with intense fluorescence, albeit less than that of the Y chromosome.

The application of banding techniques to chromosomal preparations has virtually supplanted orcein staining. A report of a normal karyotype in the absence of an evaluation of banded chromosomes should be viewed with great scepticism.

3.1.3. C-banding. Considerable interest has long been entertained in the centromere zones of various chromosomes, regarding both their morphological characteristics and possible functional significance. However, the use of conventional stains has provided only a limited opportunity for detailed visualization of the centromeric regions. This is now possible because of the introduction of a specific staining technique – designated C (for centromere) banding (Fig. 5b) (Sumner, 1972). It appears to depend on the presence of constitutive heterochromatin which is located opposite the centromeres and is probably composed of repetitive adenine/thymine (A-T) rich DNA. C-banding has disclosed the physical features of the centromeres, revealed the presence of structural variants and permitted the assessment of their frequency. It has also shed light on the potential functional role of the centromeric areas and their possible involve-

Figure 4. (a) Orcein stained chromosomal preparation, a karyotype, of a normal male (note unusually long Y chromosome – a normal variant). (b) A karyotype of a normal male, with the chromosomal preparation stained with quinacrine and examined by ultraviolet fluorescent microscopy. The chromosomes reveal the characteristic Q-bands. Note in particular the brilliantly fluorescent long arms of the Y chromosome.

ment in the regulatory mechanism for control of genetic expression. Furthermore, by providing a tool for precise definition of the centromeres and their adjacent areas, their implication in the phenomena of non-disjunction and anaphase lag could be probed, and the relevant theories tested. It is, of course, these phenomena which account for the observed aneuploidy such as that seen in Klinefelter's XXY syndrome and XYY syndrome, and both the consequence of non-disjunction, or in the XO female Turner syndrome which could result from either non-disjunction or anaphase lag, during the meiotic division in the parental gonads.

3.1.4. R-banding. As pointed out, the intensively fluorescent Q-bands correspond to the darkly stained G-bands and both represent heterochromatic areas of the chromosomes. the light bands seen with trypsin-Giemsa staining or lightly fluorescent areas on Q-banding, however, can be shown to advantage by the technique of R-(reversed) banding. The technique is particularly useful in defining the ends of the chromatids which are always positively stained (Fig. 6), and is therefore valuable in morphological analysis of chromosomes especially their length and centromere index. T-(terminal) banding is a derivative of the R-banding which focuses on the terminal portion of the chromatids. These are the segments that are most readily demonstrable either after Giemsa staining or fol-

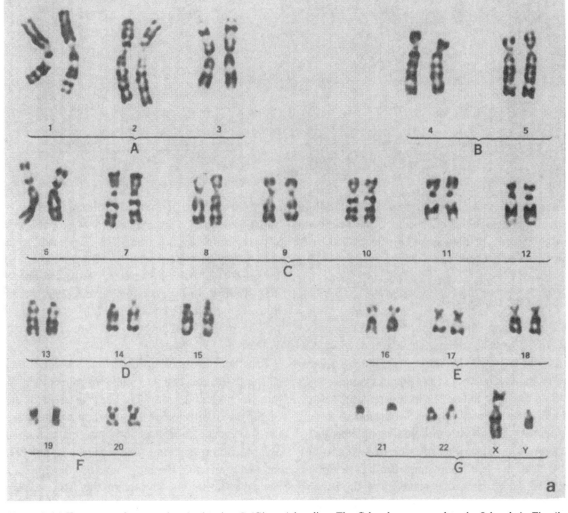

Figure 5. (a) Karyotype of a normal male showing G-(Giemsa) banding. The G-bands correspond to the Q-bands in Fig. 4b. Both G-bands and Q-bands represent heterochromatic areas. (b) (*See next page.*) A normal female karyotype showing C-(centromeric) banding.

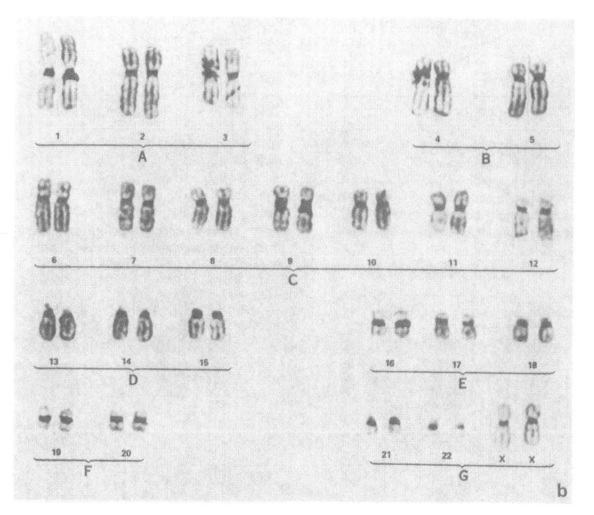

lowing the application of acridine orange. Minor structural variations which affect the telomeres can be thereby best studied (Lejeune et al., 1973, Dutrillaux and Lejeune, 1971).

3.2. Somatic tissues

Cells other than blood lymphocytes are also amenable to cytogenetic studies. The major purpose is to detect chromosomal mosaicism (i.e. the presence of two or more cell lines in the same individual – each with its own and different chromosomal make-up), and to determine its extent. For instance, a male zygote with XY sex chromosomal complement may undergo a division whereby one of two progeny cells loses the Y chromosome through anaphase lag. The sex chromosome make-up of the embryo will thus be XY/XO myxoploid. the resulting phenotype in the newborn may significantly depart from normal (Fig. 7).

Skin, including genital skin, offers an extensive and topologically diverse source of somatic cells with high division potential. The fibroblasts in the skin biopsy specimens tend to outgrow the epithelial cells. Their chromosomes can be best visualized and studied during the metaphase stage of the mitotic division of the cultured cells. This stage is usually attained in a few weeks of culture of the skin explant.

Fragments from other tissues and viscera, if their cells possess or can be made to re-acquire the mitotic potential, may be likewise treated and investigated with a view to ascertaining the make-up of their chromosomes both in terms of number and individual structure. The tendency is, however, for the connective tissue to outgrow the epithelial elements during the culture of the tissue explant with the eventual preponderance of fibroblasts and fibroblast-like cells at the expense of the parenchymatous component when the specimen is obtained, for instance, from a viscus.

3.3. Gonadal and germinal tissues

Biopsy specimens from the testes may be studied both for their stromal and germinal components. When the germinal cells are examined meiotic division may be directly monitored and possible anomalies ascertained. Unfortunately, however, on culturing testicular tissue fragments, the stromal elements with their rich fibroblast content may sometimes outgrow the germinal constituents, interfering with the study of the latter's chromosomes.

3.4. Spermatozoa

A technique which enables direct analysis of human spermatozoal chromosomes has recently been developed. The technique aims at reactivation of the spermatozoa and involves in vitro insemination of zona-free hamster (*Mesocricetus auratus*) eggs with capacitated human spermatozoa. Following their entry into the hamster egg, human spermatozoa form normal pronuclei which condense into readily analyzable chromosomes. These remain cytologically distinct from those of the hamster for a certain interval. In fixed preparations, the chromosomes from human spermatozoa can be stained by the

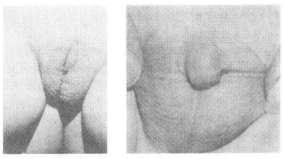

Figure 7. Ambiguous genitalia in an infant with XY/XO sex chromosomal mosaicism.

standard available procedures and are analyzable with the same accuracy as the chromosomes from somatic cell preparations. Apart from these technical advantages, this approach obviates the need for testicular biopsy in non-azoospermic males. It has rendered feasible the detection and study of aneuploidy and the appearance and function of heterochromatin, particularly constitutive heterochromatin (Rudak et al., 1978).

4. BIOCHEMICAL EVALUATION

Quantitative assay of testicular and adrenal steroid hormones, pituitary gonadotropins and hypothalamic LHRH constitutes a powerful tool in the assessment of andrological disorders. Furthermore, qualitative evaluation and quantitative assay of androgen receptors in the cytosol of cellular preparations of potentially responsive end-organs have provided another facet to the evaluation of suspected end-organ unresponsiveness (Aiman et al., 1979; Walsh, 1979). Specific enzyme determinations, e.g. 5-α-reductase, and serum electrolytes may shed light on specific inherited disorders characterized by hypogonadism with or without endocrine imbalance.

5. RADIOLOGICAL EVALUATION

Assessment of bone age and specialized radiological investigations such as contrast studies (e.g. genitourinary or selective angiography) are useful in evaluating selected patients with suspected andrological disorders.

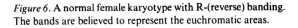

Figure 6. A normal female karyotype with R-(reverse) banding. The bands are believed to represent the euchromatic areas.

The preceding two sections (4) and (5) are more fully covered in other chapters in this volume.

6. CONCLUDING REMARKS

The role of genetic disorders and chromosomal anomalies in the genesis of hypogonadism, both structural and functional, as well as infertility is receiving increasing recognition. Such etiologies account for a substantial proportion of andrological disorders seen in clinical practice. For instance, Klinefelter's XXY syndrome with a frequency of 1:500 among liveborn males, is perhaps the single most common cause of hypogonadism when it is associated with infertility. Furthermore, more patients with inherited disorders, such as cystic fibrosis, now survive infancy and childhood. This has largely been brought about by rising awareness of the importance and frequency of genetically determined disease, earlier diagnosis due to improved investigative methods, and the prompt institution of therapeutic measures which are often highly effective in controlling the disease process, or reversing or minimizing its most deleterious manifestations. As a result, an increasing number of young men affected with genetic conditions which would not have permitted survival or function in the past now seek medical attention for the andrological problems connected with their original illnesses. The infertility which is virtually universal among patients (males) with cystic fibrosis provides a typical example of this situation.

Moreover, there has been a steady decrease in the frequency of damage to the testes and genitalia resulting from infection, trauma, unshielded exposure to radiation and other environmental insults. Further decrease is anticipated; for instance, the advent of mumps immunization and its near universal adoption in recent years promises to reduce substantially the occurrence of mumps orchitis with major sequelae on gonadal function. Although the prevalence of gonorrhea may not have dropped significantly lately, it probably no longer constitutes as big a cause of permanent andrological disability as it once did. Undoubtedly this welcome development has resulted largely from the widespread availability and efficacy of specific antibiotic therapy. Similar, albeit more dramatic, developments occurred with regards to syphilis.

With the progressive decline in the magnitude of environmentally determined andrological disorders, those with genetic etiologies have assumed an ever greater importance. Genetic and chromosomal evaluation of a patient presenting with hypogonadism, infertility, impotence or other manifestations suggestive of andrological disorders should be an integral part of the assessment. Moreover, it should not be looked upon as a last resort and postponed until more conventional methods of investigations have failed to yield the necessary information and suggested a reasonable approach for management.

Another area in which genetic and chromosomal assessment of ostensibly normal adult males is emerging as a useful approach is that of artificial insemination using donor sperm (AID). It is imperative that a potential donor for AID should receive a critical genetic appraisal including family history evaluation to rule out possibly transmitted genetic disease, particularly those that are dominantly inherited. Furthermore, chromosome studies including detailed karyotypic analysis is a mandatory prelude to the acceptance of a candidate as a donor. This will ensure that chromosomal rearrangements, particularly balanced translocations are excluded. Although such rearrangements are usually phenotypically unremarkable they may be transmitted to the offspring, with relatively high frequency, in an unbalanced fashion, with drastic phenotypic anomalies. It is regrettable that such obvious and fairly simple examination is neglected in the majority of instances of selection of donors for AID, as shown in a recent survey in the United States (Behrman, 1979; Curie-Cohen et al., 1979).

In this chapter I have attempted to review, from the point of view of clinical practitioners, the possible role of genetic evaluation including chromosomal analysis in assessing individuals with suspected andrological disorders. The lack of familiarity of many physicians with the principles and techniques of genetics has posed an obstacle to the application of these powerful tools to the practice of medicine including the new and burgeoning field of andrology. I trust that in some measure this chapter will have contributed to surmounting this difficulty.

ACKNOWLEDGMENT

The author gratefully acknowledges the kind courtesy of Dr. C.C. Liu in providing Figs. 4b and 6.

REFERENCES

Aiman J, Griffin JE, Gazak JM, Wilson JD, MacDonald PC (1979) Androgen insensitivity as a cause of infertility in otherwise normal men. N Engl J Med 300: 223.

Alton DJ, McDonald P (1973) Urographic findings in Laurence-Moon-Biedl syndrome. Radiology 109: 659.

Ammann F (1979) Investigations cliniques et génétics sur le syndrome de Bardet-Biedl en Suisse. J Genet Hum 18 (Suppl): 1.

Behrman SJ (1979) Artificial insemination and public policy – editorial. N Engl J Med 300: 619.

Caspersson T, Zech L, Johansson C, Modest DJ (1970) Identification of human chromosomes by DNA-binding fluorescent agents. Chromosoma 30: 215.

Collins E, Turner G (1973) The Noonan syndrome. J Pediatr 83: 941.

Curie-Cohen M, Luttrell L, Shapiro S (1979) Artificial insemination by donor in the United States. N Engl J Med 300: 585.

DeFraites EB, Thurmon TF, Farhadian H (1975) Familial Prader-Willi syndrome. In: Bergsma D (ed.) Genetic forms of hypogonadism, pp 123-6. New York: National Foundation March of Dimes.

Dutrillaux B, Lejeune J (1971) Sur une nouvelle technique d'analyse du caryotype humain. CR Acad Sci [D] (Paris) 272: 2638.

Goldstein JL, Wilson JD (1974) Hereditary disorders of sexual development in man. In: Motulsky AG, Lenz W (eds.) Birth defects, pp 165-73. Amsterdam: Excerpta Medica.

Ham RG (1963) An improved nutrient solution for diploid chinese hamster and human cell lines. Exp Cell Res 29: 515.

Ham RG (1965) Clonal growth of mammalian cells in chemically defined synthetic medium. Proc Natl Acad Sci USA 53: 288.

Katcher ML, Bargman GJ, Gilbert EF, Opitz JM (1977) Absence of spermatogonia in the Prader-Willi syndrome. Eur J Pediatr 124: 257.

Kaufman M, Straisfeld C, Pinsky L (1976) Male pseudoherma-phroditism presumably due to target organ unresponsiveness to androgens. Deficient 5-alpha-dihydrotestosterone binding in cultured skin fibroblasts. J Clin Invest 58: 345.

Lejeune J, Dutrillaux B, Rethore MO, Prieur M (1973) Comparaison de la structure fine des chromatides d'Homo sapiens et de Pan troglodytes. Chromosoma 43: 423.

Lubs HA Jr, Vilar O, Bergenstal DM (1959) Familial male pseudohermaphroditism with labial testes and partial feminization: endocrine studies and genetic aspects. J Clin Endocrinol 19: 1110.

Noonan JA (1968) Hypertelorism with Turner phenotype. A new syndrome with associated congenital heart disease. Am J Dis Child 116: 373.

Pearson PL (1970) A fluorescent technique for identifying human chromatin in a variety of tissues. Bull Eur Soc Hum Genet 4: 35.

Rosewater S, Gwinup G, Hamwi GJ (1965) Familial gynecomastia. Ann Intern Med 63: 377.

Rudak G, Jacobs PA, Yanagimachi R (1978) The chromosome constitution of the human spermatozoa: a method for direct chromosome analysis. Am Soc Hum Genet Prog Abs 92A.

Schnedl W (1971) Banding pattern of human chromosomes. Nature New Biol 233: 93.

Schnedl W (1973) Giemsa banding techniques. In: Caspersson T, Zech L (eds.) Chromosome identification, pp 34-7, Academic Press, New York.

Seabright M (1971) A rapid banding technique for human chromosomes. Lancet ii: 971.

Shokeir MHK (1978) Genetic aspects of male infertility. In: Bain J, Hafez ESE and Barwin BN (eds.) Progress in reproductive biology, andrology: basic and clinical aspects of male reproduction and infertility, pp 70-103, Basel: Karger.

Sumner AT (1972) A simple technique for demonstrating centromeric heterochromatin. Exp Cell Res 75: 304.

Walsh PC (1979) A new cause of male infertility. N Engl J Med 300: 253.

Winterborn MH, France NE, Raiti S (1970) Incomplete testicular feminization. Arch Dis Child 45: 811.

3. SEXUAL AMBIGUITY AT BIRTH*

P. SAENGER, L.S. LEVINE, S. PANG and M.I. NEW

The condition of ambiguous genitalia in a newborn is a difficult disorder to manage. The decision of sex assignment has lifelong consequences for the child and the entire family. Pediatricians should arrive at a judicious choice of sex assignment not hastily but only after prudent use of modern diagnostic procedures and in some cases after consultation with geneticists, surgeons, psychiatrists and other physicians. This chapter first gives a brief review of the regulatory processes of sex determination in man; then pathophysiological mechanism are discussed in detail. Only anomalies that are present in the newborn are reviewed.

1. NORMAL DEVELOPMENT

1.1. Genetic basis and role of H-Y antigen in primary sex determination

A gene or set of genes on the Y chromosome causes the indifferent embryonic gonad to develop as a testis. A fetal ovary develops in the absence of a Y chromosome (Jost, 1970). In mammals female development represents the inherent tendency of the fetus, and maleness has to be constantly enforced against this innate tendency. The testis is the only significant source of fetal androgen. Therefore, castrated embryos develop as phenotypic females regardless of gonadal sex (Jost, 1970). Embryos with the chromosomal constitution 45,X also develop ovaries with follicles, which are sometimes still present at birth (Singh and Carr, 1966). However, in older children and adults whose karyotype

is 45,X primary follicles have vanished from the ovaries, leaving only streaks of fibrous tissue. It appears therefore that a 46,XX karyotype is a prerequisite for the maintenance of follicles. It is unclear at present whether the X chromosome contains genes for an ovary-inducing antigen.

The testis-organizing plasma membrane protein through which the Y chromosome plays its pivotal role in mammalian sex differentiation has been termed H-Y antigen (Ohno, 1977; Wachtel, 1977). Evidence for a Y-situated H-Y gene is provided by the demonstration of a double dose of H-Y antigen in the cells of human males with two Y chromosomes (Wachtel et al., 1975). Mapping studies have shown that the H-Y gene is probably on the short arm of the Y chromosome, near the centromere (Koo et al., 1977b).

The role of H-Y antigen is limited to the induction of the male gonad; subsequent fetal masculinization is due to secretion of androgens by the fetal Leydig cells in the fetal gonad. If H-Y antigen is indeed the primary determinant of testicular development, then expression of this cell surface component in man should be accompanied by development of at least rudimentary testes (Wachtel et al., 1976).

To date this hypothesis has been supported by cases of abnormal gonadal or phenotypic differentiation. True hermaphrodites who have testicular tissue and whose karyotype is 46,XX demonstrate the presence of H-Y antigen (Saenger et al., 1976); patients with testicular feminization syndrome (46, XY) are also H-Y positive (Koo et al.,

*Abbreviations: Aldo, aldosterone; Δ⁴,Δ⁴-androstenedione; CAH, congenital adrenal hyperplasia; B, corticosterone; F, cortisol; DHEA, dehydroepiandrosterone; DS, dehydroepiandrosterone sulfate; DOC, desoxycorticosterone; S, desoxycortisol; DHT, dihydrotestosterone; E/A, etiocholanolone/androsterone; HCG, human chorionic gonadotropin; 17-OH, 17-hydroxycorticoids; 17-OHP, 17-hydroxyprogesterone; 3-β-HSD, 3-β-hydroxysteroid dehydrogenase; 17-HSD, 17-hydroxysteroid dehydrogenase; 17-KS, 17-ketosteroids; MPH, male pseudohermaphroditism; T, testosterone; THF, tetrahydrocortisol; TH, true hermaphroditism.

J. Bain and E.S.E. Hafez (eds.), Diagnosis in andrology, 31-52. All rights reserved.
Copyright © 1980 by Martinus Nijhoff Publishers bv, The Hague/Boston/London.

1977a). The 'inducer substance' for testicular or-
ganogenesis proposed by Jost appears to be H-Y
antigen. This antigen is the first plasma membrane
or cell surface protein to which a specific organo-
genesis function has been assigned (Ohno, 1977)
(Fig. 1).

1.2. Morphologic processes in primary sex determi-
nation

Until the 12 mm stage (at approximately 42 days of
gestation), the gonads of the male and female are
morphologically indistinguishable. During the 7th
week of fetal life the differentiation of the initially
bipotential gonad begins. During this process the
undifferentiated gonad is being shaped from three
elements:
1. a thickened area of coelomic epithelium (germinal epithelium);
2. the mesenchymal cell mass on the urogenital
ridge which also contains mesonephric elements;
3. gonadal primordial cells.

These primordial germ cells have migrated from the
posterior endoderm of the yolk sac through the
mesenchyme of the mesentery to the gonadal ridges.
The germ cells can be distinguished in the 12- to 17-
day-old human embryo. These germ cells are larger
than somatic cells and are characterized histo-
chemically by a high glycogen content and high
alkaline phosphatase activity (Jirásek, 1976, p. 52).

By about 42 days, 300-1300 primordial germ cells
have reached the indifferent gonad. There, cells will
later become either spermatogonia or ova.

The coelomic epithelium gives rise to seminiferous
tubules or primary ovarian follicles. The mesenchymal cell mass forms Leydig cells in the male and
granulosa cells in the female. The mesonephric
elements finally differentiate into the rete testis,
septa and tunica albuginea and tunica vaginalis in
the male and into theca cells, interstitial cells and
rete ovarii in the female.

The transformation of the indifferent gonad into
the embryonal testis occurs in the 7-week-old embryo as soon as the migration of the primordial

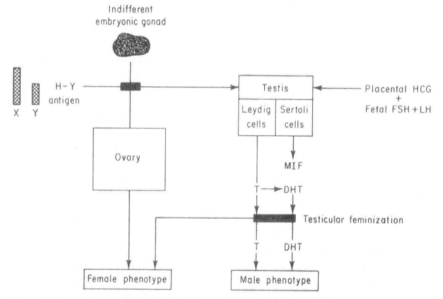

Figure 1. Mammalian sex determination. In normal XX embryos the indifferent embryonic gonad
becomes an ovary and further development is female. In XY embryos H-Y antigen blocks female
development by inducing the gonad to differentiate as a testis. Sertoli cells of the newly formed
testis secrete Müllerian inhibition factor (MIF) which prevents differentiation of Müllerian
derivatives (Fallopian tubes, uterus and cephalad portion of the vagina). Testicular Leydig cells
secrete testosterone which induces differentiation of Wolffian derivatives (vasa deferentia, seminal
vesicles and epididymides). Some of the testosterone is converted enzymatically into dihydrotestosterone; this induces orderly differentiation of penis and scrotum in the same tissues that would
otherwise give rise to clitoris, labia minora and labia majora. The testicular feminization mutation
blocks responsiveness to androgens; this leads to development of a female phenotype (but does not
affect Müllerian duct regression) in the H-Y+ chromosomal male. Adapted from Wachtel and
Ohno (1979).

germ cells from the yolk sac to the gonadal ridge is completed.

In the XY gonadal ridge, under the influence of the Y chromosome, the contact between primordial cells and resident somatic cells is made earlier and leads to formation of seminiferous tubules rather than follicles (Ohno, 1976).

Leydig cells appear at about day 60; their appearance signifies the beginning of fetal testicular development (Jirásek, 1977). By 14-18 weeks Leydig cells make up more than half the volume of the testis (Pelliniemi and Niemi, 1969). This coincides with the peak HCG release. Soon thereafter the number of Leydig cells decreases and by 27 weeks the seminiferous tubules are separated by only a narrow interstitium containing few Leydig cells. Several weeks after birth Leydig cells are not visible histologically; they reappear at puberty (Jirásek, 1977).

The development of the fetal ovary follows a much slower time course. By 20 weeks of fetal age, more than three months after the start of testicular development, ovarian germ cell population reaches a peak of approximately 7 million germ cells. This population declines in the second half of pregnancy to 2 million at term as a result of cessation of mitotic activity and atresia (Baker, 1963) (Fig. 2).

1.2.1. Hormone secretion of the fetal gonad and its role in internal and external genital differentiation. The fetal testis secretes two substances: steroidal androgens from the Leydig cells and a non-steroidal antiMüllerian hormone from the Sertoli cells (Blanchard and Josso, 1974).

The chemical structure of the factor responsible for Müllerian duct regression is not yet known. It is most likely a high molecular weight glycoprotein (200-320,000 daltons) (Josso et al., 1977). Secretion of the antiMüllerian hormone begins shortly after testicular differentiation and lasts into the perinatal period (Donahoe et al., 1977); however, the Müllerian duct is responsive to the antiMüllerian hormone only during a short critical period during fetal testicular differentiation (Josso et al., 1977).

Testosterone and dihydrotestosterone are the two most important fetal androgens. A testosterone crystal can replace the masculinizing influence of the testis, but cannot inhibit Müllerian duct development. Jost showed that when a crystal of testosterone is implanted adjacent to the fetal rabbit ovary, the differentiation of the male ducts was stimulated on that side only (for review see Jost, 1972). This lateralization suggests that for the differentiation of male ducts, higher local concentrations of androgens are required than for the differentiation of external genitalia and the urogenital sinus. Wilson (1973) showed in elegant experiments, also using the fetal rabbit as a model, that immediately before and during the critical period of male ductal differentiation the Wolffian ducts and their derivatives were rich in a specific testosterone binding protein. Soon after completion of Wolffian differentiation this binding protein was no longer detectable. Wolffian duct differentiation is probably not sensitive to circulating androgens. These animal data may explain why females with virilizing congenital adrenal hyperplasia show no Wolffian differentiation though their external genitalia may be markedly virilized. This is in striking contrast to the urogenital sinus and the genital tubercle which are sensitive to circulating androgens and also have the additional ability to convert testosterone to dihydrotestosterone, its 5-α-reduced product. These structures acquire this enzyme even before testicular testosterone secretion has begun. Therefore, the tenet that testosterone induces the 5-α-reductase enzyme is not valid (Siiteri and Wilson, 1974).

Testicular testosterone formation in the human embryo begins at about the 8th week of fetal life and reaches a maximum at 17-21 weeks (Siiteri and Wilson, 1974). This pattern coincides closely with that for differentiation of the male urogenital tract, and the maximum placental HCG release (Clements et al., 1976). Testosterone *and* dihydrotestosterone stimulate the growth of the genital tubercle, induce the fusion of the urethral and labioscrotal folds and prevent the separation of the vagina from the urogenital sinus by inhibiting the growth of the vesicovaginal septum. In the female, after the 12th fetal week, fusion of the labioscrotal folds can no longer be induced hormonally. Clitoral hypertrophy, however, can be caused by androgens at any time during fetal life or even postnatally.

1.2.2. Development of the genital ducts. Both Müllerian and Wolffian ducts exist simultaneously as primordia in the 7-week-old fetus. The Müllerian ducts serve as the anlagen of the uterus, Fallopian tubes and the upper part of the vagina, whereas the mesonephric or Wolffian ducts have the potential of differentiating further into the epididymis, vas deferens, seminal vesicles, and the ejaculatory duct of the male. Regression of the Müllerian ducts begins in the 50- to 60-day-old human embryo (Fig. 2). Remnants of the Müllerian ducts may persist as hydatids of Morgagni on the cranial pole of the testis (Jirásek, 1976, p. 97). Persistence of Müllerian ducts as a clinical entity (persistent oviduct syndrome) has been described (see below). One commonly encountered structure, the utriculus masculinus or prostaticus which is frequently present in normal males is derived from the entodermal urogenital sinus and therefore is probably not a Müllerian duct remnant (Jirásek, 1976, p. 99).

1.2.3. Differentiation of the external genitalia. Until the eighth week the external genitalia of both sexes are identical and are capable of differentiation in either direction. The common primordial anlagen are: the urogenital tubercle, the urogenital swellings, and the urogenital folds. The paired urogenital folds surround a urogenital slit. In the female fetus at age 65 days the urogenital tubercle becomes the clitoris, the urogenital swellings the labia majora, and the urogenital folds the labia minora. In the male, under the influence of testosterone and dihydrotestosterone, the urogenital tubercle becomes the corpora cavernosa and the glans penis. The urogenital folds, the shaft of the penis, and the urogenital swellings fuse in midline to form a scrotum. This process begins in male fetuses 65 days old and is completed in the 14-week-old fetus (Jirásek et al., 1968). Leydig cell stimulation in later fetal life is under the control of the fetal pituitary (Figs. 2 and 3).

2. ABNORMAL DEVELOPMENT

2.1. Abnormal gonadal differentiation presenting as sexual ambiguity at birth

2.1.1. Mixed gonadal dysgenesis (Y-gonadal dysgenesis). This descriptive term is used to describe individuals with a 45,X line and at least one additional line containing a Y chromosome. Independent of the tissue distribution of the various cell lines, the ambiguity of the genitalia ranges from normal female external genitalia to normal male genitalia (Davidoff and Federman, 1973).

Like other forms of mosaicism, a 45,X/46,XY karyotype is the result of mitotic nondisjunction or anaphase lag. Structural rearrangments of the Y chromosome occur frequently (Morillo-Cucci and German, 1971). Of nine patients reported by Morishima and Grumbach (1969), one was a phenotypic female, one had normal male genitalia and the remaining seven had ambiguous genitalia. Stigmata of Turner's syndrome are frequently present.

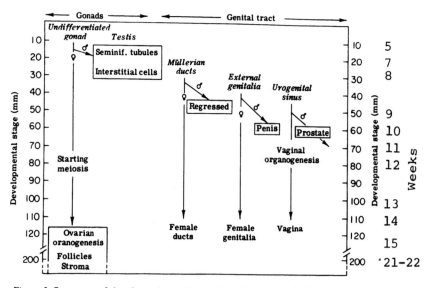

Figure 2. Summary of the chronology of sexual development in the human fetus according to fetal crown-rump length (ordinates). Adapted from Jost et al. (1973).

There is a spectrum in the differentiation of the gonad: from bilateral streaks to bilateral dysgenetic testes; asymmetric combinations of streak and testis and streak and dysgenetic gonad occur as well. The streak gonad in this syndrome contains ovarian stroma but no follicles, just as in Turner's syndrome. Gonadal complement and phenotype may depend on the preponderance of a particular cell line, XO or XY, within the gonad during the crucial period of sexual differentiation. The local action of the testicular hormones, testosterone and anti-Müllerian hormone may explain the asymmetry in ductal development seen in these patients.

Most 45,X/46/XY individuals with ambiguous or female external genitalia have Müllerian derivatives and at least a rudimentary uterus (Federman, 1967). On the side containing the streak gonad a Fallopian tube is usually present. In a case reported by De Grouchy et al. (1963), with the karyotype 45,X/ 46,XY bilateral testes and no uterus were present. This observation lends support to the hypothesis that Müllerian inhibitory factor, when released from the embryonal testis, may act locally in mixed gonadal dysgenesis.

Sex assignment in these patients in the newborn period is guided by the presentation of the external genitalia. Regardless of the sex assignment, a detailed endocrine evaluation including HCG stimulation should be carried out in all patients with a 45,X/46,XY karyotype to evaluate the endocrine

function of the streak or testis. HCG stimulation serves as a valuable test for detection of cryptic testis tissue (Levine and New, 1971). In our ex-

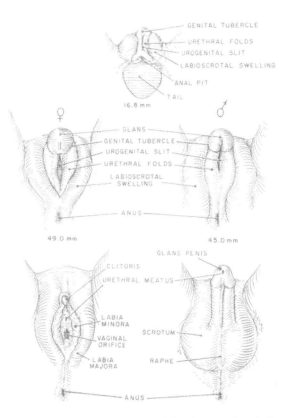

Figure 3. Differentiation of male and female external genitalia from indifferent primordia. Male development will occur only in the presence of androgenic stimulation during the first 12 fetal weeks. From Grumbach MM and Van Wyk JJ (1974).

Table 1. Spectrum of findings in mixed gonadal dysgenesis.

Subject	Sex of rearing	Age	Karyotype	External genitalia	Gonads	Uterus present	Serum testosterone (ng/dl)		FSH/LH (ng/ml)
							BASELINE	AFTER HCG	
1	Male	6 yr	46 XY/45XO	Normal male	(R) testis (L) streak	+	blank/blk*	89.7 +	0.5/2.9
2	Female	1 month	46 XY,q+/ 45 XO	Enlarged clitoris, bifid scrotum, separate urethral and vaginal opening	(R) streak (L) testis	+	12/11*	43	1.8/1.0
3	Male	11 yr	46 XY/45 XO	3rd degree hypospadias	(R) streak (L) testis	+	–	137+	–
4	Male	15 yr	45 XO/ 46 XY/ 47 XYY	3rd degree hypospadias	(R) streak (L) testis	+	230/177*	420+	1.0/1.7
5	Female	15 yr	45 XO/ 46 XY	Normal female	Bilateral streaks	+	27/10*	30	>50/11

* Serum testosterone in the baseline and after dexamethasone suppression.

+ Normal HCG response for male.

perience with five patients aged between 11 months and 15 years of age, a significant testosterone rise following HCG stimulation was seen in three. Subsequent laparotomy in all five patients confirmed the presence of testicular tissue in four. One patient with entirely normal female external genitalia was found to have bilateral streak gonads (Table 1).

Streak gonads as well as testes should probably be removed from 45,X/46,XY individuals reared as females since non-malignant gonadoblastomas or dysgerminomas occur in about 15-20% of 45,X/46,XY individuals. The tumor risk is probably somewhat less in patients with bilateral streak gonads (Simpson, 1976, p. 187). In patients reared as males an attempt should be made to mobilize the undescented testis into the scrotum. Once externalized, the gonad can be more easily examined for the presence of tumor.

2.1.2. True hermaphroditism (TH). In the true hermaphrodite, ovarian and testicular tissue coexist. Abnormal differentiation of external and internal genitalia is also observed and may make sex assignment difficult. Of 300 or more cases that have been described in the literature, approximately 80% of the karyotypes have been 46,XX, 10% have been 46,XY and the remaining 10% consisted of various mosaics. The gonadal development has been reviewed by van Niekerk (1974, p. 15) (see Table 2).

In the majority of patients the ovarian and testicular portions are arranged in an end-to-end fashion allowing clear cut differentiation between the two of them.

The fetal testis of TH can suppress development of the adjacent Fallopian tube, but it does not usually suppress the development of the uterus

Table 2. Gonadal distribution in 302 true hermaphrodites as reported in the world literature.

Type of distribution	Percentages
Ovary-testis	30
Ovotestis-ovary	29
Ovotestis-ovotestis	19
Ovotestis-testis	10
Ovotestis-?	4
Others	8
Total	100

Adapted from van Niekerk (1974, p. 15).

(Federman, 1967). Cyclical stimulation leads eventually to uterine bleeding at menarche, a most disturbing event in those patients with TH assigned the male sex at birth. The testicular tissue in TH is defective in the secretion of both androgens and antiMüllerian hormone as evidenced by inadequate virilization of the external genitalia and the failure of inhibition of Müllerian ducts. However, we could not document the androgen deficiency postnatally in a 2½-year-old patient we recently studied (Saenger et al., 1976). The patient showed a response in serum testosterone comparable to that observed in normal prepubertal boys (Fig. 4).

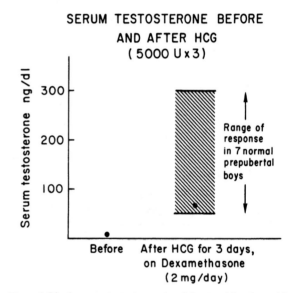

SERUM TESTOSTERONE BEFORE AND AFTER HCG (5000 U x 3)

Figure 4. Rise in serum testosterone in a 2.6-year-old patient with TH, in response to HCG stimulation compared to response of seven normal prepubertal boys. From Saenger et al. (1976, p. 1236).

In a newborn with genital ambiguity, normal 17-hydroxyprogesterone and androgen secretion, and a karyotype 46,XX, TH is the most likely diagnosis.

Once the diagnosis of TH is established the decision of sex assignment should be based upon the appearance of the external genitalia. It is generally advisable to rear the patient as a female because an adequate functional vagina is more easily established than a functional penis (van Niekerk, 1974, p. 153). If the gonad has an end-to-end arrangement of ovary and testis, the ovarian part can be spared, as suggested by van Niekerk (1974, p. 154). In most instances, however, an ovotestis must be removed in toto. A uterus is present in the majority of THs.

If patency of the cervical canal is established, the uterus may remain in situ. At puberty breast development and virilization may occur if the ovotestis is in place. Menstruation occurs in approximately 2/3 of those who have a uterus (Simpson, 1976, p. 250).

The etiology of TH is unclear. There is probably undetected chimerism or mosaicism in TH with a 46,XY karyotype. In 46,XX TH, several possible etiologies have been advanced (Ferguson-Smith, 1966; Wachtel et al., 1976):

a. sex chromosome mosaicism;
b. X-Y interchange;
c. Y-autosome translocation;
d. single gene mutation.

Immunologic detection of H-Y antigen in patients with 46,XX TH suggests that in many individuals the postulated X-Y interchange or a Y-autosome translocation indeed takes place (Fig. 5). The additional observation of two patients with a minute additional band on the short arm of one of the X chromosomes further supports this theory (Wachtel et al., 1976). Other factors, such as single gene mutations, may be responsible for some cases of TH. H-Y serology may thus be an important adjunct to the endocrinologic evaluation of intersex patients. The data of Wachtel et al. (1976) and Saenger et al. (1976) support the interpretation that a Y-chromosomal translocation too small for cytologic detection accounts for testicular differentiation in true hermaphrodites with a 46,XX karyotype.

2.2. Abnormal ductal differentiation

2.2.1. Persistent oviduct syndrome. Patients with persistent oviduct syndrome (persistent Müllerian structures) present with inguinal hernia or cryptorchidism and are diagnosed during surgical repair of these conditions. These patients are phenotypically normal males who have well-developed male external genitalia and relatively well-developed testicular morphology. Internally, however, they possess persistent Müllerian structures in addition to their male ducts. Their karyotype is 46,XY. This condition has been termed 'hernia uteri inguinali'. A deficiency of Müllerian inhibitory factor or an end organ unresponsiveness provides the best explanation for this condition. Since there is a normal male phenotype, fetal testosterone and dihydrotestosterone secretion are probably normal. The condition is inherited either as a sex-limited autosomal recessive or as a sex-linked recessive condition and familial cases have been reported. (Brook et al., 1973; Weiss et al. 1978). Treatment should consist of the removal of as much as possible of the Müllerian structures without damaging testes, epididymes or vasa deferentia.

2.2.2. Vaginal aplasia and atresia. Aplasia of the Müllerian ducts lead to absence of the uterine corpus, absence of the uterine cavity and absence of the upper portion of the vagina. A short 1-2 cm blind-ending vagina, derived from the ectodermal urogenital sinus, is usually present. This presentation is sometimes termed the Rokitansky-Kuster-Hauser syndrome (Simpson, 1976, p. 342). Primary amenorrhea is the presenting complaint. Urological and skeletal anomalies are frequently associated with this condition.

In vaginal atresia, on the other hand, the contribution of the urogenital sinus to vaginal development is lacking. The lower portion of the vagina is replaced by fibrous tissue above which normal pelvic structures are present. Although hydrocolpos

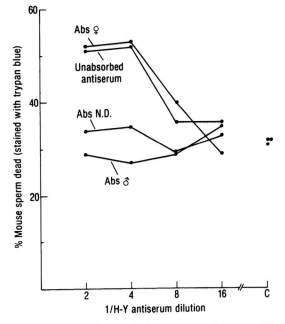

Figure 5. Cytotoxicity tests on mouse sperm with mouse H-Y antiserum absorbed with leukocytes from females (XX) and males (XY) and leukocytes obtained postoperatively from a patient (ND) with true hermaphroditism (46,XX). Abs denotes absorption with cells of the indicated sex. Each point represents an average value from these separate tests. C denotes control (including complement, but not antiserum). Serum aliquots were read as coded samples. From Saenger et al. (1976, p. 1238).

38 SAENGER, LEVINE, PANG, NEW

has been described in the neonate (Dennison and Bacsich, 1961), symptoms are usually absent until the advent of puberty. Surgical creation of an artificial vagina is mandatory (Jones and Scott, 1971, pp. 406-420).

2.3. Male pseudohermaphroditism (MPH)

Normal male differentiation requires the secretion of two fetal testicular hormones: testosterone, which promotes and stabilizes the differentiation of the Wolffian system, and antiMüllerian hormone, which induces the regression of the Müllerian ducts. Complete differentiation of male external and internal genitalia also requires peripheral conversion of T to DHT. Whereas antiMüllerian hormone acts only locally, T and DHT display both local and systemic action.

While H-Y antigen, which induces the development of the fetal testis, is located on the Y chromosome, genes regulating testosterone synthesis and metabolism are located on the autosomes. Genes regulating T and DHT receptors are X-linked.

MPH is the term describing 46,XY individuals with ambiguous sexual differentiation. MPH can be caused by defects in testosterone synthesis, testosterone metabolism and androgen action (at the receptor or at the transcriptional level (see Fig. 6). MPH may result in a phenotype indistinguishable from that seen in female pseudohermaphroditism. Accurate delineation of biochemical defects requires, therefore, careful anatomic, endocrinological and genetic studies. A highly desirable pre-

diction of future pubertal development may be possible on the basis of these studies.

2.3.1. Placental and fetal pituitary gonadotropin deficiency. Placental HCG deficiency has not been described. It is conceivable that such a defect can occur; the consequences would be markedly impaired sexual differentiation, since male differentiation until the 20th week is entirely under HCG control.

Prader et al. (1976) invoked prenatal luteinizing hormone deficiency as a possible cause of MPH, hypospadias, micropenis and cryptorchidism. This postulated pathophysiological mechanism is at variance with the concept that fetal gonadotropins assume control of testicular function only after the period of genital differentiation is completed. Detailed evaluation of pituitary function at a later date would appear to be indicated since deficiency of other pituitary hormones (particularly growth hormone and thyroid hormone) has to be ruled out.

2.3.2. Leydig cell agenesis. Berthezène et al. (1976) described a 35-year-old MPH who represents a specific defect in testicular Leydig cell differentiation. The patient had a female phenotype with a shallow vagina. No Müllerian structures were present. Testes were found intraabdominally and vasa deferentia and an epididymis were present. At biopsy the testis contained no recognizable Leydig cells. Serum testosterone was low, luteinizing hormone was elevated, yet follicle stimulating hormone was normal. There was no response to HCG stimu-

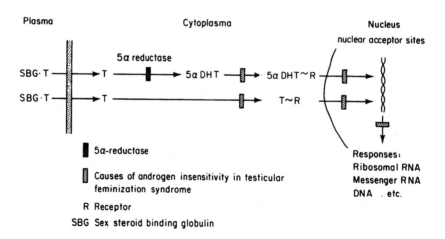

Figure 6. A schematic model for the mechanism of action of androgens. Adapted from Mainwaring (1977).

lation. The testes produced antiMüllerian hormone normally and testostrerone at least during some time in fetal life since Wolffian differentiation was completed. This form of MPH is similar to an animal model in which a luteinizing hormone receptor defect is proposed (Bardin et al., 1973).

2.3.3. Congenital anorchia (vanishing testes syndrome).
Congenital anorchia, or the absence of one or both testes in a 46,XY phenotypically male individual has been estimated to occur in about 1 in 5000 or 1 in 20,000 male births respectively (Goldberg et al., 1974). Familial aggregates have been reported (Hall et al., 1975). According to Jost's work (1972), the testes must have been functional until at least the 16th week of gestation in order to produce normal male internal ducts, Müllerian regression and male external genitalia. A testicular vascular accident producing torsion, infarction and loss of one or both testes is the most appealing explanation for this syndrome. Absence of a testosterone response to

HCG stimulation confirms the bilateral anorchia in these patients. Though the patient is similar to a prepubertal castrate, gonadotropins may not be elevated in early childhood (Winter and Faiman, 1972). If the condition is bilateral, hormonal replacement at puberty is necessary. At puberty, silastic prostheses should be implanted into the scrotum, which is often hypoplastic.

2.4. Deficient testosterone synthesis as a cause of MPH

Five enzymatic deficiencies have been described resulting in MPH. The deficient enzymes are 3-β-hydroxysteroid dehydrogenase, 20,22-desmolase, 17-α-hydroxylase, 17,20-desmolase, and 17-hydroxysteroid dehydrogenase (Fig. 7).

The first three defects result in cortisol as well as testosterone deficiency and are forms of congenital adrenal hyperplasia (CAH). Inhibition of the Müllerian ducts is usually complete in these patients; masculinization of the external genitalia is not.

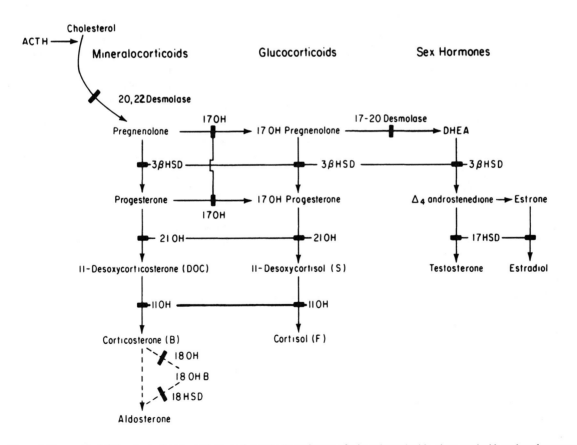

Figure 7. Enzymatic deficiencies in the biosynthetic and metabolic pathways of mineralocorticoids, glucocorticoids and sex hormones.

Different mutational events altering structural or regulatory genes explain the phenotypic variety that these patients display. Even identical mutations may lead to different phenotypes due to variations in gene penetrance and expression (Imperato-McGinley and Peterson, 1976).

2.4.1. Cholesterol desmolase deficiency. Prader and Gurtner (1955) described a male pseudohermaphrodite with severe salt wasting and impaired synthesis of all three classes of adrenal corticosteroids: mineralcorticoids, glucocorticoids and sex steroids. Urinary 17-KS and 17-OHS excretion was low and was not stimulated by ACTH. In this genetic male, female external genitalia with male genital ducts were found at autopsy. The enlarged adrenals were remarkable in that the cortical cells were filled with lipoid material, which prompted the name lipoid adrenal hyperplasia.

Camacho et al. (1968) described a patient with a mild form of cholesterol desmolase deficiency, an enzyme defect early in the biosynthetic scheme, involving the conversion of cholesterol to pregnenolone. Degenhart (1971) produced biochemical evidence that the enzyme involved was the cholesterol 20-α-hydroxylase. This enzymatic deficiency leads to adrenal insufficiency and in affected males the complete masculine differentiation suggests that the defect is also present in the testes. Since the defect impairs aldosterone and DOC secretion, the salt wasting is attributable to the lack of mineralocorticoid secretion. Few patients have survived early infancy (Kirkland et al., 1973). Early recognition and proper treatment should permit survival of these infants as in Addison's disease of infancy.

2.4.2. 3β-Hydroxysteroid dehydrogenase 3β-HSD deficiency. Enzymatic deficiency of 3β-HSD, first described by Bongionvanni (1962), also results in decreased synthesis of all three classes of steroids. There is impaired secretion of aldosterone, cortisol and testosterone which leads to MPH and life threatening salt wasting in infancy. The female with 3-β-HSD defect shows only minimal clitoral enlargement, probably due to the extremely high amounts of DHEA, a weak androgen.

CAH due to 3-β-HSD deficiency must be suspected in a newborn with salt wasting symptoms who has ambiguous genitalia. The inheritance is autosomal recessive. The male with this disorder may resemble the virilized female with salt wasting due to 21-hydroxylase deficiency. The male with 21-hydroxylase deficiency shows no sexual ambiguity. Thus, in a genetic male with salt wasting and complete male differentiation, 3-β-HSD is unlikely. The female with 21-hydroxylase deficiency is more virilized than the female with 3-β-HSD deficiency; labioscrotal fusion has not been reported in 3-β-HSD deficiency. The urine of patients with 3-β-HSD deficiency contains predominantly steroids with a double bond at the fifth position (Δ^5 steroids). Excessive urinary excretion of DHEA and pregnenetriol or elevated DHEA levels in plasma are diagnostic of 3-β-HSD deficiency. The 3-β-HSD enzyme in testes, adrenal and liver may all be under different genetic control. This may result in different degrees of enzymatic deficiency in different organs and may explain the advent of male puberty and breast development as described in some cases of 3-β-HSD deficiency (Parks et al., 1971; Schneider et al., 1975).

2.4.3. 17-α-Hydroxylase deficiency. A defect in 17-α-hydroxylase will result in diminished secretion of all glucocorticoids and sex steroids (Biglieri et al., 1966). The inheritance is autosomal recessive. Cases have been reported in males and females. Patients with a 46,XY karyotype are usually born with ambiguous genitalia. In all cases presented to date there was an overproduction of DOC and B with low aldosterone secretion. Females with this defect manifest sexual infantilism; in males the same defect produces MPH or possibly even a complete normal female phenotype. Hypertension is frequent in this form of MPH. Prominent breast development was the only secondary sex characteristic which occurred at puberty in the male described by New (1970). Lifelong therapy with glucocorticoids is mandatory in males and females with this defect in order to maintain normal blood pressure.

2.4.4. 17,20-Desmolase deficiency. This defect was first described by Zachmann et al. (1972) in three patients – two first cousins and a 'maternal aunt'; suggesting an autosomal recessive or X-linked mode of inheritance. All three patients had a 46,XY karyotype. These three patients shared a familial form of MPH due to a partial defect in conversion of 17α-hydroxyprogesterone and 17-hydroxypregnenolone to C_{19} steroids by testes and adrenals. Only sex steroid biosynthesis is affected in this form of MPH. The patients presented with ambiguous external genitalia and inguinal or intraabdominal testes. All had third degree hypospadias but normal male ductal differentiation. Urinary pregnenetriolone, one of the metabolites of 17-hydroxypregnenolone, was elevated and increased further after ACTH and HCG stumulation. However, testosterone or DHEA excretion did not rise appreciably. In vitro studies with testicular tissue also demonstrated the defect in testosterone biosynthesis. The results were therefore consistent with a deficiency of adrenal and testicular 17,20-desmolase activity. Gynecomastia may occur at puberty though it was not present in Zachmann's patients.

2.4.5. 17-Hydroxysteroid dehydrogenase 17-HSD deficiency.

Deficiency of the 17-HSD enzyme, which also results in decreased testosterone synthesis, is another known cause of MPH. With one exception all previously reported genetic males were assigned to the female sex of rearing at birth because they were so incompletely masculinized (Virdis et al., 1978). Only one patient who presented with sexual ambiguity noted in infancy (Knorr et al., 1973) was given a male sex assignment. The diagnosis was made at or after puberty when signs of virilization appeared.

Common clinical and anatomical features are listed in Table 3.

Table 3. Common clinical and anatomic features in 10 patients with 17-ketosteroid reductase deficiency.

Parameter	Incidence
External genitalia female at birth	9/10
Sex of rearing female	9/10
Clitoral hypertrophy	10/10
Testes in inguinal canal or in labia majora	10/10
Breast development at puberty	5/10
Hirsutism	10/10
Absent Müllerian structures	10/10
Normally developed Wolffian structures	10/10
Leydig cell hyperplasia	10/10
Absent spermatogenesis	8/9

From Virdis et al. (1978).

The hyperplastic Leydig cells in these patients secrete predominantly Δ^4, a testosterone precursor. This could be documented in testicular effluent studies where the Δ^4 testosterone ratio was 96:5 (normal 3:75) (Virdis et al., 1978). Peripheral conversion of Δ^4 to testosterone is apparently still intact; thus Δ^4:T ratio measured in peripheral blood is less elevated (5.8; normal 0.25-1.05) than that in the testicular venous effluent. This suggests that the enzymes controlling 17-HSD in testes and liver are under different genetic control. Conversion of estrone to estradiol is also impaired, but usually to a lesser degree.

Follicle stimulating hormone may be normal while luteinizing hormone is elevated in association with the low serum testosterone levels noted in these patients. Indeed luteinizing hormone is suppressible when T is given therapeutically. The relative lack of intrauterine virilization may be due to efficient aromatization of Δ^4 to estrone in the placenta. Thus very little Δ^4 is available for extratesticular conversion to T (Goebelsmann et al., 1973).

At puberty these patients display heterogeneity in their phenotype. Varying concentrations of circulating estrogens, particularly estradiol, may explain varying degrees of breast development noted in patients with 17-HSD. Increased gonadal Δ^4 and estrone secreted at puberty are converted peripherally to T and estradiol which may explain the simultaneous occurrence of gynecomastia and virilization in some of these patients (Goebelsmann et al. 1973). Data on the T/DHT ratio suggest normal 5-α-reductase activity, though as a consequence of low testosterone levels the absolute DHT concentration is similarly decreased. It has also been shown by Saez et al. (1971) that nitrogen retention in response to testosterone is preserved. Despite the fact that external genitalia are only partially virilized, Wolffian ducts are normal.

The defect in Δ^4 and estrone metabolism is also demonstrable in vitro with testicular incubation studies (Virdis et al. 1978).

Demonstration that Δ^4 is not converted normally to T is necessary for diagnosis in 17-HSD deficiency. Thus, elevated Δ^4:T ratios in peripheral and spermatic blood are diagnostic. Since breasts and virilization develop at puberty, the patients may require treatment to make the puberty conform with the sex of assignment.

2.5. Male pseudohermaphroditism resulting from abnormal testosterone metabolism

2.5.1. 5-α-Reductase deficiency. A form of MPH caused by steroid 5-α-reductase deficiency has been reported by three different groups (Imperato-McGinley et al., 1974; Peterson et al., 1977; Saenger et al., 1978; Walsh et al., 1974). Familial incomplete male pseudohermaphroditism Type II was the term applied by Walsh et al. (1974) to describe the defect in two siblings raised as females. Peterson et al. (1977) investigated a large pedigree in the Dominican Republic with this form of MPH, consisting of 24 families with 38 affected males. This disorder is transmitted by an autosomal recessive gene. Carrier detection is possible. At birth the affected male presents with a clitoris-like phallus. The urethral opening is at the base of the phallus; a urogenital sinus is present. Occasionally, separate urethral and vaginal openings are present on the perineum. The testes may be intraabdominal, in the inguinal canal or in the bifid scrotum. The Wolffian structures are normally differentiated; no Müllerian structures are present (Figure 8). In the pedigree described by Peterson et al. (1977) puberty is associated with development of a male muscular habitus, growth of the phallus and scrotum, voice change, but not with gynecomastia. Adult males with this syndrome describe erections and were found to produce an ejaculate with sperm. They have no facial hair or beard growth, develop no temporal recession of the hair line or acne and on

rectal examination only a small prostate is palpable. Testicular biopsy reveals a normal testis. A short blind ending vaginal pouch can be demonstrated radiographically (Saenger et al., 1978).

Females have the same biochemical defect but are phenotypically normal.

As with other forms of male pseudohermaphroditism, the diagnosis of 5-α-reductase deficiency must be made biochemically since phenotypic heterogeneity does not allow classification based on physical findings. The age of the patient determines the usefulness of the various diagnostic procedures:

1. In young male infants whose testosterone is physiologically high from 10 to 60 days of life (Forest et al., 1976), and in prepubertal children following HCG stimulation, measurement of a high T:DHT ratio can be diagnostic (Pang et al., 1979). In a six-year-old patient with 5-α-reductase deficiency the ratio of T to DHT was 53 (normal <20).

The patients studied by Walsh et al. (1974) had normal circulating T and DHT; however, 5-α-reductase activity in slices of genital skin was deficient. On this basis, Walsh postulated that the male pseudohermophroditism in these patients was due to deficient 5-α-reductase in androgen target tissue only. However, Imperato-McGinley et al. (1974) and Saenger et al. (1978) demonstrated low DHT concentration in sera of patients with 5-α-reductase deficiency.

Whereas Pinsky et al. (1972) and Wilson (1975) reported that the 5-α-reductase defect was demonstrable only in fibroblasts from genital skin,

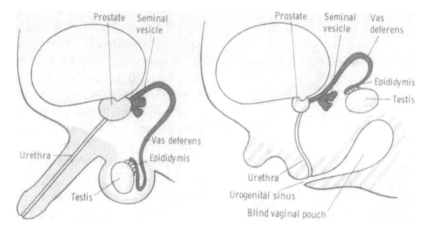

Figure 8. Illustration for the hypothesis for the role of testosterone and dihydrotestosterone in sexual differentiation in utero. Dark stippled area = testosterone-dependent. Light stippled area = dihydrotestosterone-dependent. From Imperato-McGinley and Peterson (1976).

Imperato-McGinley et al. (1974) and Saenger et al. (1978) demonstrated decreased 5-α-reductase activity in skin fibroblasts derived from nongenital skin. Incubation studies using slices of genital skin proved that 5-α-reductase activity is clearly diminished in this target tissue when compared to controls (Saenger et al., 1978). Therefore a spectrum of deficiency of 5-α-reductase may exist. In some cases the enzymatic defect is limited to androgen target tissue leading to normal circulating DHT, whereas in other cases, nongenital skin and even possibly liver cells also have the defect.

2. 5-α-Reductase deficiency is also expressed by an abnormal ratio of T metabolites in the urine. The ratio of etiocholanolone, a 5-β-metabolite, to androsterone, a 5-α-metabolite, is normally less than 1. In patients with this enzyme deficiency, it is more than 5.

3. The percentage conversion of infused radiolabelled testosterone to DHT is one of the most valuable investigative procedures to establish the diagnosis and can be carried out even after castration. T to DHT conversion in normals is $5.3 \pm 3\%$; in two patients with 5-α-reductase deficiency, the conversion was 0.3 and 0.4% (Saenger et al., 1978).

4. Metabolism of cortisol is impaired. Both endogenous and exogenous cortisol are transformed almost exclusively to THF (5-β) and not to allo-THF (5-α). Thus, hepatic biotransformation of both sex steroids and glucocorticoids is impaired in this disease (Saenger et al. unpublished observations).

5. Binding of ³H DHT to cytosol of skin fibroblasts was normal in these patients (Saenger et al., 1978). This finding also proves that this syndrome is more a defect in T androgen metabolism than in androgen binding.

In summary, steroid 5-α-reductase deficiency causes abnormally low conversion of T to DHT, the androgen responsible for masculinizing the external genitalia of the male fetus. 5-α-Reductase deficiency is the first inherited abnormality of steroid metabolism in which the basic defect resides in the hormone-responsive target tissues.

2.6. Female pseudohermaphroditism resulting from fetal testosterone overproduction due to defects of glucocorticoid and mineralocorticoid synthesis

A female fetus will become masculinized if ex-posed to excessive androgens in utero. The degree of masculinization is dependent upon the time of exposure to excessive androgens. If exposed after the 12th week when the vagina has already separated from the urethra only clitoral hypertrophy will occur. If androgens are high before that date the masculinization may be so profound that the urethra is penile.

Since the female fetus does not possess a testis, antiMüllerian hormone is not produced and the female with CAH is born with a normal uterus and Fallopian tubes. Female genital abnormalities are present only in the androgen responsive external genitalia. The usually complete involution of the Wolffian system, despite increased fetal androgen, suggests that the level of androgen necessary for Wolffian development is higher than that produced in CAH. It is possible that only testicular androgens achieved high enough concentration in the region of the Wolffian duct differentiation. The variability in degree of masculinization seen in female pseudohermaphroditism due to CAH has been puzzling endocrinologists for some time. If one assumes initiation of adrenal androgen secretion by the 10th week, why is a urogenital sinus present in some girls whereas in others only clitoral hypertrophy is seen? Variation in the onset and degree of oversecretion of adrenal androgens is a possible explanation.

2.6.1. 21-Hydroxylase deficiency. Impairment of 21-hydroxylation is the commonest enzymatic deficiency observed in CAH, and accounts for approximately 95% of CAH cases (Gregory and Gardner, 1976). The deficiency results in decreased cortisol synthesis; this in turn induces increased ACTH secretion. Consequent to ACTH oversecretion, there is overproduction of cortisol precursors (17-hydroxyprogesterone) and androgens. Measurement of 17-hydroxyprogesterone by a new microfilter paper method permits the rapid screening of newborns for congenital adrenal hyperplasia due to 21-hydroxyplase deficiency (Pang et al., 1977) (Figure 9). This approach uses a 3 mm spot of dried blood similar to that used for screening for phenylketonuria or congenital hypothyroidism. Newborn screening for this form of congenital adrenal hyperplasia is potentially life saving since the first newborn male with salt-wasting disease may go unrecognized until he presents in crisis.

The urinary metabolite of 17-hydroxyproges-terone is pregnanetriol which is excreted in excess. Urinary 17-ketosteroids which include DHEA and the metabolic products of Δ^4 and testosterone, androsterone, and etiocholanolone, are also ex-creted in increased amounts. Although a mild 21-hydroxylase deficiency for mineralocorticoid syn-thesis is probably present in most cases, only one-third of the patients demonstrate overt salt loss and aldosterone deficiency. As a consequence of salt loss, plasma renin activity is elevated in these patients and may be used as an additional guide for optimizing therapy in CAH.

Recent studies suggest that all patients with CAH and elevated level of plasma renin activity, both salt losers and simple virilizers, would benefit from therapy with mineralocorticoids (e.g., 9-α-fluoro-cortisone) and salt for adequate hormonal control of the disease. ACTH levels normalize as renin is suppressed under this regimen (Rösler et al., 1977) (Fig. 10). The salt-wasting form of this disease is life threatening. It must be recognized at birth. Symp-toms may not appear until the 9th to 12th day of life. While the genital ambiguity in girls with CAH im-mediately triggers diagnostic studies, first born males with normal genitalia may go undetected and are therefore at increased risk for rapid virilization and/or salt-wasting crises.

2.6.2. 11-β-Hydroxylase deficiency. A defective

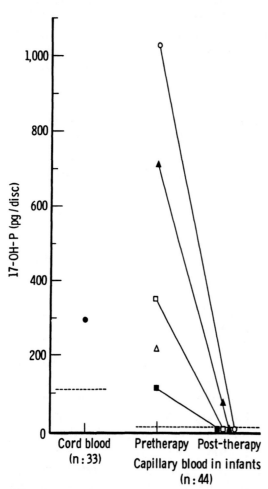

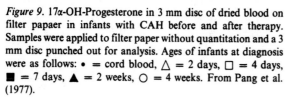

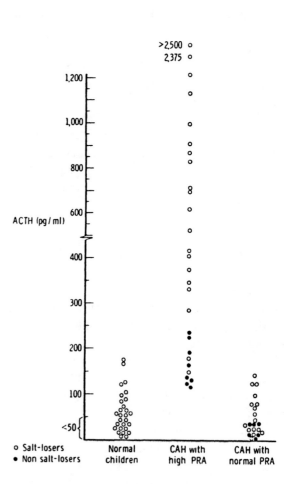

Figure 9. 17α-OH-Progesterone in 3 mm disc of dried blood on filter papaer in infants with CAH before and after therapy. Samples were applied to filter paper without quantitation and a 3 mm disc punched out for analysis. Ages of infants at diagnosis were as follows: • = cord blood, △ = 2 days, □ = 4 days, ■ = 7 days, ▲ = 2 weeks, ○ = 4 weeks. From Pang et al. (1977).

Figure 10. ACTH levels in normal children and in seven patients with CAH treated with constant replacement doses of gluco-corticoids equivalent to 25 mg/m²/day of hydrocortisone. Samples were drawn between 8:00 and 9:00 a.m. Levels of plasma renin activity (PRA) were high during the ad lib, normal and low sodium diets. Normal PRA were achieved by sodium diet and/or additional 9-α-fluorocortisol. From Rösler et al. (1977).

11-β-hydroxylation results in the hypertensive form of CAH. Cortisol synthesis is also decresed. The predominant precursors produced in response to ACTH oversection are compound S and DOC. Their urinary metabolites, tetrahydrodesoxycortisol (tetrahydro-compound S) and tetrahydro-DOC, respectively, are found in markedly increased amounts in the urine. 17-Hydroxyprogesterone and urinary pregnanetriol are not as high as in 21-hydroxylase deficiency. There is overproduction of adrenal androgens (Δ^4, DHEA, DS, T) and increased urinary excretion of their metabolites, 17-ketosteroids (New and Levine, 1973). The most prominent clinical feature of 11-β-hydroxylase deficiency is virilization. As in the simple virilizing form, the external genitalia of the female fetus are masculinized by the excessive fetal adrenal androgens and female pseudohermaphroditism results. The internal female genitalia are normal.

Postnatally, as in 21-hydroxylase deficiency, the excessive androgen production results in rapid somatic growth, advanced epiphyseal maturation, progressive clitoral enlargement, early appearance of facial, axillary and pubic hair, and acne. Without treatment, early epiphyseal closure and short stature result (New and Levine, 1973).

An additional finding in many but not all patients with this form of CAH is hypertension. The hypertension and lack of salt-wasting symptoms are attributed to the excessive DOC production. The absence of hypertension in some has not been explained but it has been shown in animal experiments that exogenous DOC acetate does not always induce hypertension.

Both salt-wasting and non-salt-wasting forms of CAH are transmitted by an autosomal recessive gene (Childs et al., 1956). In a given family, affected individuals usually manifest the same degree of salt-wasting.

Prenatal diagnosis of the most common form of CAH-21-hydroxylase deficiency is possible by measuring 17-β-hydroxyprogesterone concentration in amniotic fluid (Nagamani et al., 1978) (Fig. 11). The incidence of the disease has been estimated recently to be 1 in 10,000 (Pang et al., 1977).

A synopsis of clinical and biochemical findings in CAH and MPH is presented in Table 4.

Close linkage of the 21-hydroxylase deficiency

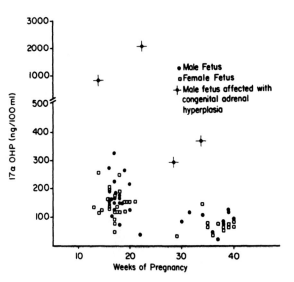

Figure 11. 17-α-Hydroxyprogesterone (OHP) levels in the amniotic fluid of control and affected pregnancies. Adapted from Nagamani et al. (1978).

gene with HLA (the major histocompatibility complex of man) has been established (Dupont et al., 1977; Levine et al., 1978). All patients studied to date were HLA genotypically different from their healthy siblings. When two or more children were affected in the same sibship they were always HLA-B identical. All patients studied to date were HLA genotypically different from their healthy sibs. The studies demonstrate that the gene for congenital adrenal hyperplasia due to 21-hydroxylase deficiency is located very close to the HLA-B locus and can be separated by genetic recombination from the HLA-A locus and from the locus for glyoxalase I-polymorphism and Bf (Pucholt et al., 1979). As a result of these studies, on the basis of HLA genotyping of siblings of an affected patient, it is possible to predict which sex is heterozygous and which sib is genetically unaffected. Subsequent hormonal studies in families of patients with this form of congenital adrenal hyperplasia have corroborated the HLA genotype. Heterozygotes can be identified biochemically by measuring the rise in 17-hydroxyprogesterone and cortisol after ACTH stimulation (Lorenzen et al., 1979). Prenatal diagnosis of the disease in high risk families by HLA typing of cultured amniotic cells has been reported (Pollack et al., 1979). This is the first example in which an enzymatic deficiency of steroid biosynthesis has been shown to be closely linked to HLA.

Table 4. Clinical and laboratory features of various forms of congenital adrenal hyperplasia and male pseudohermaphroditism.

| CLINICAL FEATURES | | | | | | | LABORATORY FEATURES | | | | | | | | | | | |
| Newborn with sexual ambiguity | | Salt wasting | Hyper-tension | Postnatal virili-zation | Pubertal virili-zation | Enzyme deficiency | URINE | | | | | BLOOD | | | | | | |
FEMALE	MALE						17KS	17OH	P'triol	Aldo	E/A	170HP	DHEA	DS	Δ4	T	DHT	T/DHT
0	+	+	0	0	0	Cholesterol desmolase	↓	↓	↓	↓	?	↓	↓	↓	↓	↓	↓	?
+	0	0	0	++	0	21-Hydroxylase mild	↑	nl or ↓	↑	nl	nl	↑	↑	↑	↑	↑	↑	nl
+	0	+	0	++	0	severe	↑	↓	↑	↓	nl	↑	↑	↑	↑	↑	↑	nl
+	0	0	+	+	0	11-Hydroxylase	↑	↑*	↑	↓	?	↑	↑	↑	↑	↑	↑	nl
+	+	+	0	0	+	3-β-HSD	↑**	↓	↓	↓	nl	↓	↑	↑	↓	↓	↓	?
0	+	0	+	0	0	17-Hydroxylase	↓	↓	↓	↑	nl	↓	↓	↓	↓	↓	↓	?
0	+	0	0	0	0	17-20 Desmolase	↓	nl	nl§	?	nl	↑	↓	↓	↓	↓	↓	nl
0	+	0	0	0	+	17 HSD	↑	nl	↑	nl	nl	↑	↑	↑	↑	↓	↓	nl
0	+	0	0	0	+	5-α-reductase deficiency	nl	nl	nl	nl	nl	nl	nl	nl	nl	nl	↓	↑

* Mostly THS.
** Mostly Δ5 17-ketosteroids (e.g. DHEA).
§ Pregnanetriolone markedly elevated.

It should be stressed that adequately treated, patients with 21-hydroxylase deficiency will reach an acceptable adult height and will be fertile (Kirkland et al., 1977).

2.7. Effect of maternal ingestion of androgens and progestins

Masculinization of the external genitalia of female infants has been observed after maternal ingestion of androgens (testosterone and alkylated derivatives), progestins (progesterone and 17-α-hydroxyprogesterone), synthetic progestins (medroxyprogesterone, norethindrone, ethisterone, norethynodryl), and aminoglutethimide (Simpson, 1976, pp 169-176). There is a low risk of fetal virilization from oral contraceptives which contain only small amounts of progestins.

To cause formation of a urogenital sinus these drugs have to be ingested before the 12th week of pregnancy; after that they may only cause clitoral enlargement.

2.8. Sexual ambiguity resulting from abnormal testosterone action

2.8.1. Testicular feminization syndrome – complete and incomplete forms. Individuals with testicular feminization have a karyotype indistinguishable from that of normal males (46, XY) and under the influence of the Y chromosome their gonads differentiate as testes. Nevertheless, since these individuals cannot respond to testosterone, they develop as phenotypic females. The fetal testes of these females apparently secrete antiMüllerian hormone; the development of the Fallopian tubes, uterus and the upper third of the vagina is thus suppressed (Morris and Mahesh, 1963). Patients with testicular feminization are usually detected because they have primary amenorrhea or an inguinal hernia. The incidence is about 1 in 60,000 (Jagiello and Atwell, 1962).

At puberty, affected individuals show normal breast development. External genitalia are unambiguously female. The vagina ends blindly and may be shortened depending on the relative contribution of Müllerian ducts and the urogenital sinus to the formation of the vagina.

The testes may be present in the inguinal canal or in the labia of the newborn. A buccal smear indicates a male pattern. In prepubertal patients the testes are histologically similar to testes of cryptorchid males.

The risk of testicular neoplasia is small in the first two decades. Manuel et al. (1976) estimated that prior to age 25, the risk of neoplasia is 2.6%. Thereafter, the risk increases to 20-30% by age 40-50 years. Therefore testes should remain until pubertal development is completed and be promptly removed thereafter.

Since androgen secretion and formation of DHT is normal in this syndrome (Koo et al., 1977b), a defect in androgen action has to be postulated. It has now been demonstrated that there are at least two genetic variants:

a. The first is characterized by undetectable DHT binding to cytosol of fibroblasts. This is due either to the absence of the receptor protein or alternatively to changes in the receptor structure resulting in a loss of affinity for the steroid. This form of androgen insensitivity results from a mutation of an X-linked gene specifying the DHT receptor (Meyer et al., 1975). A similar defect has been described in androgen insensitive rodents (Attardi and Ohno, 1974).

b. The second variant demonstrates normal cytoplasmic and nuclear binding of DHT and may represent a defect in transcriptional or translational events (Amrhein et al., 1977b).

Amrhein et al. (1977b) point out that it is important for the clinician to recognize these two variants. An XY individual with inguinal testes and completely female external genitalia with undetectable androgen binding may be expected to *feminize* spontaneously at puberty. However, an infant with normal androgen binding may not be completely insensitive to androgens and may therefore *virilize* at puberty. Presently there is unfortunately no way to predict the response of cells in these patients with conserved androgen binding.

Incomplete forms of testicular feminization have been described and probably have a partial defect in cytosol androgen binding (Haning et al., 1978) or gene transcription. The affected individuals have bilateral testes, genital ambiguity, and no Müllerian development. They show varying degrees of masculinization and breast development at puberty. Familial aggregates have been described. The disorder is probably transmitted by an X-linked recessive gene. There is considerable phenotypic variability within a given family. Wilson et al. (1974) concluded therefore that all forms of incomplete testicular feminization result from a single mutant gene that is variably expressed. He suggested calling the disorder male pseudohermaphroditism Type I.

Before arriving at the diagnosis of incomplete testicular feminization, biosynthetic defects of testosterone production must be ruled out.

2.8.2. Reifenstein's syndrome. Reifenstein (1947) originally described a clinical phenotype of hereditary MPH consisting of hypospadias, gynecomastia with incomplete virilization at puberty, and infertility. All individuals were raised as males. Inadequate virilization results, however, not from inadequate testosterone production, as suggested by Bowen et al. (1965), but rather from partial androgen insensitivity (Amrhein et al., 1977a). The patients have normal or elevated testosterone and DHT, elevated LH and normal 5-α-reductase activity. DHT binding studies using fibroblasts demonstrated two genetic variants, partial deficiency of androgen binding and others with normal binding activity. The syndrome is therefore best placed at the most masculine end of the spectrum of incomplete testicular feminization (Imperato-McGinley and Peterson, (1976).

2.9. Hypospadias and micropenis

The two concluding pathological conditions do not, per se, fit into either category of male or female pseudohermaphroditism. Since they frequently give rise to clinical debate as to what sex assignment would be appropriate, they are included in this chapter.

2.9.1. Hypospadias. Maternal ingestion of synthetic progestins has been implicated in the etiology of hypospadias by Aarskog (1970). Animal data by Goldman et al. (1966) provided some experimental support in favor of Aarskog's hypothesis. The etiologic relationship remains unproven and Simpson (1976, p. 223) argues that Aarskog's observations probably represent coincidental associations. Placental insufficiency leading to deficient placental gonadotropin secretion may be another cause of hypospadias (Chen and Woolley, 1971). The incidence of hypospadias as an isolated finding is about 1 in 350 male births (Farkas, 1970). If the meatus is small and opens on the glans or on the penile shaft, the male sex assignment is not in doubt. Perineal hypospadias, especially with a urogenital sinus or a separate vaginal opening, requires detailed genetic, radiological, and endocrine studies; and 5-α-reductase deficiency, 17-HSD deficiency or Reifenstein's syndrome in particular have to be ruled out.

After the birth of one affected child, the recurrence risk of hypospadias is 7-10% (Chen and Woolley, 1971). This disorder is usually of polygenic or multifactorial origin.

2.9.2. Micropenis. Penile morphogenesis and growth begins in the 8th fetal week when HCG stimulates the Leydig cells of the testes. Abnormal penile development prior to the 12th-14th week may also be associated with other anomalies such as hypospadias and chordee. After the 14th week androgen deficiency will result in a small but otherwise normal penis. Smith (1977) compiled a list of problems which can lead to micropenis (Table 5). Reference values for penile length and diameter should be consulted before the diagnosis of micropenis is made (Feldman and Smith, 1975).

Table 5. Types of problems causing micropenis.

ENDOCRINE
1. Primary testosterone deficiency yielding micropenis, with or without incomplete morphogenesis.
   a) Klinefelter's XXY syndrome.
   b) Defects in testicular morphogenesis.
   c) Inborn errors in steroidogenesis of testosterone.
2. End-organ deficiency in responsiveness to testosterone yielding micropenis, usually with incomplete morphogenesis.
3. Hypothalamic-pituitary gonadotropin deficiency with secondary testosterone deficiency yielding micropenis.
4. Pituitary growth hormone deficiency.
5. ? Acquired hormonal suppression or inhibition yielding micropenis with or without incomplete morphogenesis.

NONENDOCRINE
1. Defect in morphogenesis of penis, with no problem in testosterone production or response, usually with incomplete morphogenesis.

From Smith (1977, p. 149).

A course of androgen therapy serves a dual purpose:

a. to evaluate responsiveness of the penis to T therapy. This will aid in predicting pubertal growth response of the penis; and

b. to enlarge the penis to normal size for age.

Smith (1977) recommends testosterone therapy using 25 mg testosterone enanthate i.m. every 3 weeks for 3 months. This course is usually accompanied by an increase in both length and diameter of the penis. Thereafter therapy should be stopped until puberty so as not to cause undesirable acceleration of bone maturation.

This mode of therapy is probably more controllable and more readily reproducible than local testosterone cream application (Immergut et al., 1971).

2.10 Management of patient with ambiguous genitalia

Ambiguous sex in the newborn infant is a medical emergency. The decision as to sex assignment at birth has obvious lifelong implications. A rational approach permits a careful assessment of the problem and a judicious choice of sex assignment.

Early sexual identification can be divided into several aspects, which appear in chronologic order, as shown in Figs 12 and 13. It can be noted that the nursery room sex assignment, which is the key to the child's later gender role, depends on the external genitalia, generally evaluated by an obstetrician's examination in the delivery room. When all aspects

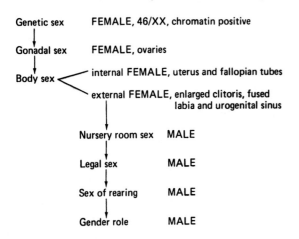

Figure 12. Aspects of sexual identification in a female pseudohermaphrodite given a male sex assignment in error. From New and Levine (1973, p 309).

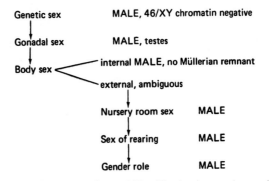

Figure 13. Aspects of sexual identification in a male pseudohermaphrodite with 17-hydroxylase deficiency given a male sex assignment. From New and Levine (1973, p 310).

of identification are the same (isosexual), then the nursery room sex assignment is correct. However, in situations in which all aspects of sexual identification are not alike, the external body sex may be misleading.

A male sex assignment to a female pseudohermaphrodite with CAH due to 21-hydroxylase deficiency would result in the scheme of sexual identification shown in Fig. 12.

The assignment of this infant to the male sex is particularly tragic, since with proper treatment the infant could lead a normal female sex life and be fertile. The error could have been avoided by a systematic approach to the problem of ambiguous genitalia in the newborn. With the ascertainment of female genetic sex by means of buccal smear or karyotype, the diagnosis of female pseudohermaphroditism would have been entertained and the previously discussed laboratory tests applied to make the diagnosis.

Genital surgery according to methods outlined by Jones and Scott (1971) should preferably be completed between 18 and 30 months of age, i.e. the period when a child gains gender awareness. Reconstruction of an adequate vaginal introitus can be postponed until late adolescence.

A scheme drawn up for the male pseudohermaphrodite with 17α-hydroxylase deficiency given a male sex assignment would be as shown in Fig. 13.

The male assignment to such a patient (New, 1970) is tragic because his anatomy prevents him from functioning as a normal male. Thus, in this case, a female sex assignment would have been more rational and compatible with normal female sexual activity. The appearance of the genitalia in an infant with intersex does not indicate the cause of the genital abnormality. The genetic sex, the gonadal sex and the biochemical defect also do not solely govern the sex of assignment. The principles of sex assignment, which have been reviewed by Money (1965; 1970) must be applied in these disorders, as well as in any other chromosomal or genetic disorder which produces intersex. The sex of assignment should be guided by the anatomy of the internal genitalia, the possibility that puberty will conform to the sex of assignment and the capacity for sexual activity and fertility.

ACKNOWLEDGMENTS

The authors wish to acknowledge the USPHS, National Institutes of Health for their partial support of the research investigations reviewed in this chapter by a grant (RR 47) from the General Clinical Research Centers Program of the Division of Research Resources, and by a grant (HD 00072) from the National Institute of Child Health and Human Development. The authors wish to express their appreciation to Vita Amendolagine for her assistance in the preparation of this review.

REFERENCES

Aarskog D (1970) Clinical and cytogenetic studies in hypospadias. Acta Paediatr Scand Suppl 203.

Amrhein JA, Klingensmith GJ, Walsh PC, McKusick VA, Migeon CJ (1977a) Partial androgen insensitivity: the Reifenstein syndrome revisited. N Engl J Med 297: 350.

Amrhein JA, Meyer WJ III, Keenan BS, Migeon CJ (1977b) Androgen receptor studies in androgen insensitivity syndrome in man. In: Lee PA, Plotnick LP, Kowarski AA, Migeon CJ, eds. Congenital adrenal hyperplasia, pp 95-96. Baltimore: University Park Press.

Attardi B, Ohno S (1974) Cytosol androgen receptor from kidney of normal and testicular feminized (TFM) mice. Cell 2: 205.

Baker TG (1963) A quantitative and cytological study of germ cells in human ovaries. Proc R Soc London (Biol) 158: 417.

Bardin CW, Bullock LP, Sherins RJ, Mowscowicz I, Blackburn WR (1973) Androgen metabolism and mechanism of action in male pseudohermaphroditism: a study of testicular feminization. Recent Prog Horm Res 29: 65.

Berthezène F, Forest MG, Grimand JA, Claustrat B, Mornes R (1976) Leydig cell agenesis: a cause of male pseudohermaphroditism. N Engl J Med 295: 969.

Biglieri EG, Herron MA, Brust N (1966) 17-Hydroxylation deficiency in man. J Clin Invest 45: 1946.

Blanchard MG, Josso N (1974) Source of the antiMüllerian hormone synthesized by the fetal testis: Müllerian inhibiting activity of fetal bovine Sertoli cells in tissue culture. Pediatr Res 8: 968.

Bongiovanni AM (1962) The andrenogenital syndrome with deficiency of 3β-hydroxysteroid dehydrogenase. J Clin Invest 41: 2086.

Bowen P, Lee CSN, Migeon CJ, Kaplan NM, Whalley PJ, McCusick VA, Reifenstein EC Jr (1965) Hereditary male pseudohermaphroditism with hypogonadism, hypospadias, and gynaecomastia (Reifenstein's syndrome). Ann Intern Med 62: 252.

Brook CGD, Wagner H, Zachmann M, Prader A, Armendares S, Frenk S, Alemán P, Najjar SS, Slim MS, Genton N, Bozic C (1973) Familial occurrence of persistent Müllerian structures in otherwise normal males. Br Med J 1: 771.

Camacho AM, Kowarski A, Migeon CJ, Brough AJ (1968) Congenital adrenal hyperplasia due to a deficiency of one of the enzymes involved in the biosynthesis of pregnenolone. J Clin Endocrinol Metab 28: 153.

Chen YC, Woolley PV Jr: Genetic studies on hypospadias in males. J Med Genet 8: 153.

Childs B, Grumbach MM, Van Wyk JJ (1956) Virilizing adrenal hyperplasia: a genetic and hormonal study. J Clin Invest 35: 213.

Clements JA, Reyes FI, Winter JSD, Faiman C (1976) Studies on human sexual development III. Fetal pituitary and serum, and amniotic fluid concentrations of LH, HCG FSH. J Clin Endocrinol Metab 42: 9.

Davidoff F, Federman DD (1973) Mixed gonadal dysgenesis. Pediatrics 52: 727.

Degenhart HJ (1971) A study of the cholesterol splitting enzyme system in normal adrenals and in adrenal lipoid hyperplasia. Acta Pediat Scand 60: 611.

De Grouchy J, Lamy M, Aicardi J, Pellerin D (1963) Mosaique XX/XO chez un pseudo-hermaphrodite masculin. Ann Pediatr 39: 789.

Dennison WM, Bacsich P (1961) Imperforate vagina in the newborn: neonatal hydrocolpos. Arch Dis Child 36: 156.

Donahoe PK, Ito Y, Morikawa Y, Hendren WH III (1977) Müllerian inhibiting substance in human testes after birth. J Pediatr Surg 12: 323.

Dupont B, Oberfield SE, Smithwick EM, Lee TD, Levine LS (1977) Close genetic linkage between HLA and congenital adrenal hyperplasia (21-hydroxylase deficiency). Lancet ii: 1309.

Farkas LG (1970) Minor defects of the penis. Microforms or stigmata of hypospadias and epispadias? Plast Reconstr Surg 45: 480.

Federman DD (1967) Abnormal sexual development, pp 58-70. Philadelphia: W.B. Saunders.

Feldman KW, Smith DW (1975) Fetal phallic growth and penile standards for newborn male infants. J Pediatr 86: 395.

Ferguson-Smith MA (1966) Hypothesis: X-Y chromosomal interchange in the etiology of true hermaphrodites and of XX Klinefelter's syndrome. Lancet ii: 475.

Forest MG, De Peretti E, Bertrand J (1976) Hypothalamic-pituitary-gonadal relationships in man from birth to puberty. Clin Endocrinol 5: 551.

Goebelsmann U, Horton R, Mestman JH, Arce JJ, Nagata Y, Nakamura RM, Thorneycroft IH, Mishell DR (1973) Male pseudohermaphroditism due to testicular 17β-hydroxysteroid dehydrogenase deficiency. J Clin Endocrinol Metab 36: 867.

Goldberg LM, Skaist LB, Morrow JW (1974) Congenital absence of testes: anorchism and monorchism. J Urol 111: 840.

Goldman AS, Bongiovanni AM, Yakovac WC (1966) Production of congenital adrenal cortical hyperplasia, hypospadias and clitoral hypertrophy (adrenogenital syndrome) in rats by inactivation of 3β-hydroxysteroid dehydrogenase. Proc Soc Exp Biol Med 121: 757.

Gregory T, Gardner LI (1976) Hypertensive virilizing adrenal hyperplasia with minimal impairment of synthetic route to cortisol. J Clin Endocrinol Metab 43: 709.

Grumbach MM, Van Wyk JJ (1974) Disorders of sex differentiation. In: Williams RH, ed. Textbook of endocrinology, p 442. Philadelphia: W.B. Saunders.

Hall JG, Morgan A, Blizzard RM (1975) Familial congenital anorchia. Birth Defects 11: 115.

Haning RV, Ambani L, Hsia E (1978) Incomplete testicular feminization with multiple congenital abnormalities. Obstet Gynecol 51: 785.

Immergut M, Boldus R, Yannone E, Bunge R, Flocks R (1971) The local application of testosterone cream to the prepubertal phallus. J Urol 105: 905.

Imperato-McGinley J, Guerrero L, Gautier T, Peterson RE (1974) Steroid 5α-reductase deficiency in man. An inherited form of male pseudohermaphroditism. Science 186: 1213.

Imperato-McGinley J, Peterson RE (1976) Male pseudohermaphroditism, the complexities of male phenotypic development. Am J Med 61: 251.

Jagiello G, Atwell JD (1962) Prevalence of testicular feminization. Lancet i: 329.

Jirásek JE (1976) Principles of reproductive embryology. In: Simpson JL, ed. Disorders of sexual differentiation. New York: Academic Press.

Jirásek JE (1977) Morphogenesis of the genital system in the human. In: Blandau JJ, Bergsma D, eds. Morphogenesis and malformation of the genital system, pp 13-39. Birth Defects 13: 2.

Jirásek JE, Raboch J, Uher J (1968) The relationship between the development of gonads and external genitalia in human fetuses. Am J Obstet Gynecol 101: 830.

Jones HW Jr, Scott WM (1971) Hermaphroditism, genital anomalies and related endocrine disorders, 2nd edn. Baltimore: Williams & Wilkins.

Josso N, Picard JY, Tran D (1977) The antiMüllerian hormone. Recent Prog Horm Res 33: 117.

Jost A (1970) Hormonal factors in the sex differentiation of the mammalian foetus. In: Discussion on determination of sex. Philos Trans R Soc Lond (Biol Sci) 259: 119.

Jost A (1972) A new look at the mechanisms controlling sex differentiation in mammals. Johns Hopkins Med J 130: 38.

Jost A, Vigier B, Perchellet JP (1973) Studies on sex differentiation in mammals. Recent Prog Horm Res 29: 1.

Kirkland RT, Keenan BS, Clayton GW (1977) Long-term follow-up of patients with congenital adrenal hyperplasia in Houston. In: Lee PA, Plotnick LP, Kowarski AA, Migeon CG, eds. Congenital adrenal hyperplasia, p 273. Baltimore: University Park Press.

Kirkland RT, Kirkland JL, Johnson C, Horning M, Librik L, Clayton GW (1973) Congenital lipoid adrenal hyperplasia in an eight-year oldphenotypic female. J Clin Endocrinol Metab 36: 488.

Knorr D, Bidlingmaier F, Engelhardt D (1973) Reifenstein's syndrome: a 17β-hydroxysteroid-oxydoreductase deficiency? Acta Endocrinol (Kbh) Suppl 173: 37.

Koo, GC, Wachtel SS, Krupen-Brown V, Mittl LR, Breg WR, Genel M, Rosenthal IM, Borgaonkar DS, Miller DA, Tantravahi R, Schreck RR, Erlanger BF, Miller OJ (1977a) Mapping the locus of the H-Y gene on the human Y chromosome. Science 198: 940.

Koo GC, Wachel SS, Saenger P, New MI, Dosik H, Amorose AP, Dorus E, Ventruto V (1977b) H-Y antigen: expression in

human subjects with testicular feminization syndrome. Science 196: 655.

Levine LS, New MI (1971) Preoperative detection of hidden testes. Am J Dis Child 121: 176.

Levine LS, Zachmann M, New MI, Prader A, Pollack MS, O'Neill GJ, Yang SY, Oberfield SE, Dupont B (1978) Genetic mapping of the 21-hydroxylase deficiency gene within the HLA linkage group. N Engl J Med 299: 911.

Lorenzen F, Pang S, New MI, Dupont B, Chow DM, Levine LS (1979) Hormonal phenotype and HLA-genotype in families of patients with congenital adrenal hyperplasia (21 hydroxylase deficiency). Pediatr Res 13: 1356.

Mainwaring WIP (1977) The mechanism of action of androgens, p 9. New York: Springer-Verlag.

Manuel M, Katayama KP, Jones HW Jr (1976) The age of occurrence of gonadal tumors in intersex patients with a Y chromosome. Am J Obstet Gynecol 124: 293.

Meyer WJ III, Migeon BR, Migeon CJ (1975) Locus on human X chromosome for dihydrotestosterone receptor and androgen insensitivity. Proc Natl Acad Sci USA 72: 1469.

Money J (1965) Psychological evaluation of the child with intersex problems. Pediatrics 36: 51.

Money J (1970) Sexual dimorphism and homosexual gender identity. Psychol Bull 74: 475.

Morillo-Cucci G, German J (1971) Abnormal Y chromosomes and monosomy 45,X: a concept derived from the study of three patients. Birth Defects 7: 210.

Morishima A, Grumbach MM (1969) The interrelationship of sex chromosome constitution and phenotype in the syndrome of gonadal dysgenesis and its variant. Ann NY Acad Sci 155: 695.

Morris J McL, Mahesh VB (1963) Further observations on the syndrome, 'testicular feminization'. Am J Obstet Gynecol 87: 731.

Nagamani M, McDonough PG, Ellegood JO, Mahesh VB (1978) Maternal and amniotic fluid 17α-hydroxyprogesterone levels during pregnancy: diagnosis of congenital adrenal hyperplasia in utero. Am J Obstet Gynecol 130: 791.

New MI (1970) Male pseudohermaphroditism due to 17α-hydroxylase deficiency. J Clin Invest 49: 1930.

New MI, Levine LS (1973) Congenital adrenal hyperplasia. In: Harris H, Hirschhorn K, eds. Advances in human genetics, Vol. 4, p 288. New York: Plenum Press.

Ohno S (1976) Major regulatory genes for mammalian sexual development. Cell 7: 315.

Ohno S (1977) The role of H-Y antigen in primary sex determination. J Am Med Assoc 239: 3.

Pang S, Hotchkiss J, Drash A, New MI (1977) Microfilter paper method for 17α-hydroxyprogesterone radioimmunoassay: its application for rapid screening for congenital adrenal hyperplasia. J Clin Endocrinol Metab 45: 1003.

Pang S, Levine LS, Chow D, Sagiani F, Saenger P, New MI (1979) Dihydrotestosterone and its relationship to testosterone in infancy. J Clin Endocrinol Metab 48: 821.

Parks GA, Bermudez JA, Anast CS, Bongiovanni AM, New MI (1971) Pubertal boy with the 3β-hydroxysteroid dehydrogenase defect. J Clin Endocrinol Metab 33: 269.

Pelliniemi LJ, Niemi M (1969) Fine structure of the human foetal testis. I. The interstitial tissue. Z Zellforsch Mikrosk Anat 99: 507.

Peterson RE, Imperato-McGinley J, Gautier T, Sturla E (1977) Male pseudohermaphroditism due to steroid 5α-reductase deficiency. Am J Med 62: 170.

Pinsky L, Finkelberg R, Straisfeld CI, Zilahi B, Kaufman M, Hall G (1972) Testosterone metabolism by serially subcultured fibroblasts from genital and nongenital skin of individual human honors. Biochem Biophys Res Commun 44: 364.

Pollack MS, Levine LS, Pang S, Sachs G, Merkatz IR, Nitowsky HM, Duchon M, Owens RP, Maurer D, New MI, Dupont B (1979) Prenatal diagnosis of congenital adrenal hyperplasia (21-hydroxylase deficiency) by HLA typing. Lancet i: 1107.

Prader A, Gurtner HP (1955) Das Syndrom des Pseudohermaphroditismus masculinus bei Kongenitaler Nebennierenrinden Hyperplasie ohne Androgen-Überproduktion. Helv Pediatr Acta 10: 397.

Prader A, Illig R, Zachmann M (1976) Prenatal LH deficiency as a possible cause of male pseudohermaphroditism hypospadias, hypogenitalism, and cryptorchidism. Pediatr Res 10: 883.

Pucholt V, Fitzsimmons JS, Reynolds MA, Gelsthorpe K (1979) Location of the gene for 21-hydroxylase deficiency. Pediatr Res 13: 1186/13.

Reifenstein EC Jr (1947) Hereditary familial hypogonadism. Clin Res 3: 86.

Rösler A, Levine LS, Schneider B, Novogroder M, New MI (1977) The interrelationship of sodium balance, plasma renin activity and ACTH in congenital adrenal hyperplasia. J Clin Endocrinol Metab 45: 500.

Saenger P, Goldman AS, Levine LS, Korth-Schutz S, Muecke EC, Katsumata M, New MI (1978) Prepubertal diagnosis of steroid 5α-reductase deficiency. J Clin Endocrinol Metab 46: 627.

Saenger P, Levine LS, Wachtel SS, Korth-Schutz S, Doberne Y, Koo GC, Lavengood RW, German J, New MI (1976) Presence of H-Y antigen and testis in 46 XX true hermaphroditism, evidence for Y-chromosomal function. J Clin Endocrinol Metab 43: 1234.

Saez JM, de Peretti E, Morera AM, David M, Bertrand J (1971) Familial male pseudohermaphroditism with gynecomastia due to a testicular 17-ketosteroid reductase defect. I. Studies in vivo. J Clin Endocrinol Metab 32: 604.

Schneideer G, Genel M, Bongiovanni AM, Goldman AS, Rosenfeld RL (1975) Persistent testicular Δ^5 isomerase-3β-hydroxysteroid dehydrogenase (Δ^5-3β-HSD) deficiency in the Δ^5-3β-HSD form of congenital adrenal hyperplasia. J Clin Invest 55: 681.

Siiteri PK, Wilson JD (1974) Testosterone formation and metabolism during sexual differentiation in the human embryo. J Clin Endocrinol Metab 38: 113.

Simpson JL (1976) Disorders of sexual differentiation. New York: Academic Press.

Singh RP, Carr DH (1966) The anatomy and histology of XO human embryos and fetuses. Anat Rec 155: 369.

Smith DW (1977) Micropenis and its management. In: Blandau RJ, Bergsma D, eds. Morphogenesis and malformation of the genital system. Birth Defects 13: 2.

Van Niekerk WA (1974) True hermaphroditism. New York: Harper & Row.

Virdis R, Saenger P, Senior B, New MI (1978) Endocrine studies in a pubertal male pseudohermaphrodite with 17-ketosteroid reductase deficiency. Acta Endocrinologica 87: 212.

Wachtel SS H-Y antigen and the genetics of sex determination. Science 198: 797.

Wachtel SS, Koo GC, Breg WR, Elias S, Boyse EZ, Miller OJ (1975) Expression of H-Y antigen in human males with two Y-chromosomes. N Engl J Med 293: 1070.

Wachtel SS, Koo GC, Breg WR, Thaler HT, Dillard GM, Rosenthal IM, Dosik H, Gerald PS, Saenger P, New MI, Liebner E, Miller OJ (1976) Serological detection of a Y-linked gene in XX male and XX true hermaphrodites. N Engl J Med 295: 750.

Wachtel SS, Ohno S (1979) The immunogenetics of sexual development. In: Steinberg AG, Bearn AG, Motulsky AG and Childs B, eds. Progress in medical genetics, Vol. 3, p 114. Philadelphia: W.B. Saunders.

Walsh PC, Madden JD, Harrod MJ, Goldstein JL, MacDonald PC, Wilson JD (1974) Familial incomplete male pseudohermaphroditism type 2: decreased DHT formation is pseudovaginal perineoscrotal hypospadias. N Engl J Med 291: 944.

Weiss EB, Kiefer JH, Rowlah UF, Rosenthal IM (1978) Persistent Müllerian duct syndrome in male identical twins. Pediatrics 61: 797.

Wilson JD (1973) Testosterone uptake by the urogenital tract of the rabbit embryo. Endocrinology 92: 1192.

Wilson JD (1975) Dihydrotestosterone formation in cultured human fibroblasts. J Biol Chem 250: 3408.

Wilson JD, Harrod MJ, Goldstein JL, Hemsell DL, MacDonald PC (1974) Familial incomplete male pseudohermaphroditism, type 1. Evidence for androgen resistance and variable clinical manifestations in a family with the Reifenstein syndrome. N Engl J Med 290: 1097.

Wilson JD, Siiteri PK (1973) Developmental pattern of testosterone synthesis in the fetal gonad of the rabbit. Endocrinology 92: 1182.

Winter JSD, Faiman C (1972) Serum gonadotropin concentrations in agonadal children and adults. J Clin Endocrinol Metab 35: 561.

Zachmann M, Völlmin JA, Hamilton W, Prader A (1972) Steroid 17,20-desmolase deficiency: a new cause of male pseudohermaphroditism. Clin Endocrinol 1: 369.

4. THYROID FUNCTION AND MALE REPRODUCTION

K. GILBERG and P.G. WALFISH

Primary thyroid dysfunction is much less common in men than in women. As a result, information on the effects of abnormalities of thyroid function on male reproduction is less available than that for the female. In this chapter, the most recent literature and concepts involving the interaction between thyroid function and male reproduction are reviewed.

1. THYROID PHYSIOLOGY

The cells of the thyroid gland are stimulated to produce thyroxine (T4) and triiodothyronine (T3) upon stimulation by the pituitary with thyroid-stimulating hormone (TSH). This pituitary peptide hormone is, in turn, stimulated by thyrotropin-releasing hormone (TRH), a tripeptide produced in the hypothalamus and secreted into the hypophyseal portal venous system. Feedback control of TSH exists at both the pituitary and hypothalamic levels and feedback of TRH exists at the hypothalamus.

Recently, TRH has become available to test thyroid function and the hypothalamic-pituitary thyroid axis. This test is used as a supplement to established tests of thyroid function.

For a full review of thyroid physiology and thyroid function tests the reader is referred to previous publications on this subject (Bain and Walfish, 1978; Carlson and Hershman, 1975; Larsen, 1975).

2. THYROID DYSFUNCTION AND SEX STEROID METABOLISM

2.1. Androgen metabolism and thyroid function

In hyperthyroidism of both spontaneous and iatrogenic origin, serum testosterone is increased by 2-3 fold compared to euthyroid patients and the metabolic clearance rate of testosterone is decreased by 30-40% (Ruder et al., 1971; Chopra and Tulchinsky, 1974; Southern et al., 1974; Gordon et al., 1969). These changes in testosterone metabolism appear to be due to the concomitant increase in sex hormone binding globulin (SHBG) noted in states of thyroid hormone excess (Olivo et al., 1970). Despite the increase in serum testosterone, the percent unbound fraction of testosterone is decreased and thus, the serum concentration of the absolute 'free' or metabolically active testosterone is normal and the testosterone production rate is not significantly different from that associated with the euthyroid state (Chopra, 1975; Gordon et al., 1969).

Like testosterone, dihydrotestosterone is also bound to SHBG and its total serum concentration is increased in hyperthyroidism (Chopra and Tulchinsky, 1974). Although there have been no reports on the possible effects of hyperthyroidism on the unbound fraction of dihydrotestosterone, it is likely that since it is also bound to SHBG there will be a reduction in the percentage free but a normal absolute free circulating level of dihydrotestosterone.

The increase in serum androstenedione levels observed in hyperthyroidism is thought to occur because of accelerated glandular production rather than changes in binding, although increased conversion from a precursor other than testosterone cannot be excluded as a cause of the elevated level (Southren et al., 1974). The metabolic clearance rate of androstenedione is unchanged in hyperthyroidism and the increased levels of androstenedione observed in the presence of thyroid hormone excess favour the enhanced conversion of androstenedione to testosterone. In addition to the above changes, hyperthyroidism influences the activity of 5-α-reductase to enhance the conversion of androgens to androsterone and to reduce the synthesis of etiocholanolone (McGuire and Tomkins, 1959).

Androgen metabolism has been less well studied in states of thyroid hormone deficiency. Although serum testosterone has been reported to be either normal or decreased, the plasma production rate of testosterone is within normal limits (Gordon et al., 1969). SHBG is decreased in hypothyroidism (Olivo et al., 1970) and the metabolic clearance rate of testosterone is increased with the predominant pathway involving the conversion from androstenedione to testosterone. The hypolipidemic effect of androsterone and its low levels in hypothyroidism have been postulated to be a factor in the known associated hypercholesterolemia often observed in this condition (Hellman et al., 1959).

The above mentioned alterations observed in the concentrations of androgen and SHBG as well as the effects on metabolic clearance rates and conversion ratios that are observed in both the hypothyroid and hyperthyroid state returned to normal with the attainment of euthyroidism (Gordon et al., 1969; Olivo et al., 1970).

2.2. Estrogen metabolism and thyroid function

Plasma 17-β-estradiol levels are increased in males with hyperthyroidism (Chopra and Tulchinsky, 1974). The metabolic clearance rate of estradiol is decreased and the production rate of estradiol is normal (Ridgway et al., 1975), probably secondary to a mechanism similar to that affecting testosterone metabolism. In the urine, the amount of 2-methoxy compounds is increased while that of estriol is decreased (Brown and Strong, 1965; Fishman et al., 1962).

The increased 17-β-estradiol levels have been thought to be the cause of the increase in SHBG noted in hyperthyroid human patients. However, a recent study has suggested that the increase in SHBG is a direct effect of thyroid hormone itself because cortisol binding globulin, an indicator of estrogen excess, is not increased in hyperthyroidism (Ridgway et al., 1975). This same study has shown that the highest SHBG levels are present in those

patients with the lowest production rates and lowest plasma levels of estradiol. Other workers have recently noted a simultaneous reduction not only in serum triiodothyronine (T3) levels but also a decline in plasma SHBG concentrations following the administration of propranolol to hyperthyroid subjects, leading to their speculation that the plasma SHBG levels may represent an objective biochemical marker of tissue response to thyroid hormone (Conti et al., 1978).

17-β-estradiol is the major metabolically active estrogen in the human male. Approximately 75% of the 17-β-estradiol in men is derived from the peripheral conversion of androgens. It has been demonstrated that in hyperthyroid subjects of both sexes, the conversion of both androstenedione and testosterone to estrone is increased while that of testosterone to estradiol is unchanged (Southren et al., 1974). In addition, the conversion of androstenedione to estradiol is increased in the male only. Since the plasma concentration of androstenedione is increased in only the male, whereas the production rate of androstenedione is increased in both sexes, this suggests that the increased estradiol levels in hyperthyroidism must result mainly from increased peripheral conversion to estradiol from androstenedione rather than from increased glandular secretion of estradiol (Southern et al., 1974).

The authors are not aware of any reported studies to date on the effects of hypothyroidism on estrogen metabolism in the male.

2.3. Estrogen-testosterone ratio and thyroid function

In an attempt to elucidate the mechanism involved in the production of gynecomastia noted in some hyperthyroid subjects, the ratio between androgen and estrogen levels was evaluated by Chopra and Tulchinsky (1974). They determined that total serum testosterone, dihydrotestosterone and unbound testosterone levels were not different in hyperthyroid males with or without gynecomastia. In addition, the ratio of total serum estradiol to testosterone in the 15 hyperthyroid males studied, while slightly higher, was not significantly different from the ratio obtained in euthyroid males. However, the ratio of unbound (free) estradiol to unbound (free) testosterone in the hyperthyroid subjects was almost twice that of the normal men.

Among the 15 hyperthyroid males studied, those four with gynecomastia had the highest ratios of unbound estradiol to unbound testosterone and had significantly higher levels of total and unbound estradiol, suggesting that increased tissue perfusion by estradiol may be an important factor in the development of gynecomastia in hyperthyroid males. However, within the same study, there were other hyperthyroid males with comparably elevated ratios of unbound estradiol to testosterone that occurred in the absence of clinical gynecomastia (Chopra and Tulchinsky, 1974). Therefore, an increased free estradiol to testosterone ratio cannot solely explain the gynecomastia that is present in some hyperthyroid males.

2.4. Hypothalamic-pituitary-testicular axis and the influence of thyroid function

Serum gonadotropin levels may be increased in men with either spontaneous or iatrogenically induced hyperthyroidism (Chopra and Tulchinsky, 1974; Ruder et al., 1971). Since unbound serum testosterone is normal in hyperthyroid males and unbound estradiol is increased in these same subjects, the presence of an increased serum LH suggests the possibility of a supra-normal set-point in the feedback system involving the hypothalamic-pituitary-testicular axis as well as a possibility of concomitant limitation of testosterone secretion in the hyperthyroid male, (Chopra, 1975; Chopra and Tulchinsky, 1974). Alternatively, the elevation of the serum LH may reflect enhanced hypothalamic gonadotropin releasing hormone activity secondary to the alterations in androgen and estrogen secretion that occur in the hyperthyroid male.

No reports have appeared as yet to document the effects of hyperthyroidism on the maturation of the hypothalamic-pituitary-testicular axis in man. Our own personal clinical observations suggest that hyperthyroidism may facilitate the early onset of puberty. By comparison, hypothyroidism has been well documented as being associated with either a delay of puberty or the paradoxical onset of precocious puberty. These effects of hypothyroidism will be discussed later in the chapter. There has been little documentation of the possible alterations that occur in serum gonadotropin levels either in the basal state or following gonadotropin releasing hor-

mone administration. Such information in both pre-pubertal and post-pubertal males with either hyperthyroidism or hypothyroidism would be of interest.

TSH binding sites have been demonstrated in the interstitial tissue of the guinea pig testes which are distinct from human chorionic gonadotropin (HCG) and luteinizing hormone (LH) binding sites (Davies et al., 1978). Both the testicular and thyroidal TSH binding sites appear to have a similar degree of cross-reactivity for HCG suggesting that testicular function may be influenced by TSH stimulation. The ability of HCG to inhibit TSH binding to thyroidal TSH receptors may be the cause of the thyroid stimulating property of HCG postulated to occur in association with both clinical and laboratory indices of hyperthyroidism noted in the presence of some cases of hydatidiform moles and choriocarcinoma (Davies et al., 1978; Higgins et al., 1975).

3. GONADAL DYSFUNCTION AND THE THYROID

3.1. Experimental animal studies

The sex of the rat appears to influence its thyroid gland such that (a) the relative weight of the gland is higher in adult female rats, (b) the volume fraction of colloid is higher in female rats, (c) the volume fractions of epithelium and epithelium to colloid ratios are higher in male rats, and (d) the follicular cells of the thyroid are taller in males than in females (Malendowicz et al., 1977). Both the height of the follicular cells of the thyroid and the volume fractions of the epithelium are reduced by orchidectomy and aging and are restored by testosterone replacement. Such observations confirm a previous report by van Rees et al. (1965), who demonstrated that orchidectomy induced a decrease in both serum and pituitary TSH levels in the rat which was reversed by testosterone therapy. From these studies, it has been postulated that either there is a greater secretion of thyrotropin (TSH) in the male rat or, alternatively, that the male rate thyroid gland is more sensitive to circulating TSH than is that of the female (Malendowicz et al., 1977).

The effects of age and testicular function on the

pituitary-thyroid system in male rats has also been studied by Chen and Walfish, (1978, 1979). Their results have indicated that the aged male rat has a lower serum total thyroxine (T4), total triiodothyronine (T3) and free (unbound) T3 and total serum testosterone concentrations in comparison with young male rats. Although the basal TSH levels were slightly increased, thereby suggesting primary thyroidal dysfunction, there was a decrease in the TSH response to thyrotropin releasing hormone (TRH) in the aged male rat. From these observations, it was concluded that these age specific factors were likely to be due not only to a reduction in thyroid gland function and plasma T4 protein binding, but also secondary to a concomitant hypo-responsiveness of the aged male rat pituitary-thyrotrope to TRH stimulation. These studies also demonstrated that in young rats, orchidectomy decreased basal T4 and TSH levels as well as the TSH response to TRH, which was reversed by treatment with pharmacologic doses of testosterone propionate. Similar but lesser effects on pituitary-thyrotrope response were observed in old rats following orchidectomy except that the basal T4 which was already low failed to decrease further significantly. Such studies have demonstrated a significant influence of testicular function on the pituitary-thyroid system of the male rat.

3.2. Clinical disease states

3.2.1. Klinefelter's syndrome.
Initial reports of thyroid function in patients with Klinefelter's syndrome noted an impaired radioactive iodine uptake (Barr et al., 1960; Carr et al., 1961; Davis et al., 1963; Plunkett et al., 1964; Zuppinger et al., 1967). Subsequently, other investigators reported a possible impairment in the TSH response to TRH stimulation with a further blunting of this response after therapy with testosterone (Ozawa and Shishiba, 1975; Cheikh et al., 1975). However, further independent studies on six patients with Klinefelter's syndrome (Burman et al., 1975) and ten patients with Klinefelter's syndrome as well as one male patient with a 46XX chromosomal abnormality (Yap et al., 1978) could not confirm the results of the previous investigators since normal basal TSH and normal TSH responses to TRH stimulation were present. Hence, although an increased incidence of insensitivity of the pituitary TSH response to exogenous TRH stimulation may be present as compared to the normal population, it appears to be neither a consistent nor a conclusively proven feature of Klinefelter's syndrome. In addition, the absence of elevated levels of serum thyroid hormone antibodies in Klinefelter's syndrome is in contrast to the high incidence of these antibodies noted in Turner's syndrome, thereby decreasing the likelihood of an associated risk for autoimmune chronic thyroiditis and concurrent hypothyroidism in Klinefelter's syndrome (Ferguson-Smith et al., 1966; Vallotton and Forbes, 1967).

3.2.2. Myotonia dystrophica.
The most frequent endocrine abnormality noted in association with the neurologic disorder of myotonia dystrophica is gonadal failure (Sagel et al., 1975). While concurrent thyroidal dysfunction has been frequently suspected Sagel et al. (1976) in a study of 12 patients (8 males and 4 females) with myotonia dystrophica, noted normal thyroidal function in all and a normal TSH response to TRH in five of the seven patients tested. In the other two patients, the serum TSH response after TSH showed a continuing rise to reach a peak response at 60 minutes instead of 20 minutes, thereby suggesting the possibility of a hypothalamic-hypothyroid mechanism accounting for this response. From their studies, the authors concluded that the hypothalamic-pituitary-thyroid axis was intact in the majority of both male and female patients with myotonia dystrophica.

3.2.3. Concurrent gonadal and thyroidal hypofunction.
Concurrent failure of gonadal and thyroid function may occur secondary to hypothalamic-pituitary disease regardless of etiology. However, the less common co-existence of multiple endocrine deficiencies, which are all due to concurrent primary failure of endocrine gland function has also been documented and may occur on the basis of an autoimmune mechanism (Irvine, 1975; Volpe, 1977). To our knowledge, there has been only one case reported to date documenting polyendocrine glandular failure associated with hypergonadotrophic hypogonadism in a male (Weinberg et al., 1976). This patient had been followed for many years and in addition to the hypogonadism, also had evidence

of primary hypoparathyroidism, hypoadrenalism, and hypothyroidism, as well as diabetes mellitus and alopecia totalis. Although testicular biopsy was not performed on this patient and anti-testicular antibodies were not available, it is possible that the primary testicular failure which occurred in this male was on an autoimmune basis similar to the autoimmune premature ovarian failure noted in women with multiple endocrine deficiencies (Anderson et al., 1968; Irvine et al., 1968, 1969; Volpe, 1977).

3.2.4. Concurrent gonadal and thyroidal hyperfunction. In 1937 a syndrome entitled polyostotic fibrous dysplasia (McCune-Albright syndrome) was described. This syndrome is characterized by disseminated, brown, non-elevated pigmented areas on the skin in addition to endocrine hyperfunction. The endocrinopathies described included sexual precocity, hyperthyroidism, hyperparathyroidism, acromegaly and Cushing's syndrome (DiGeorge, 1975). This disease occurs more commonly among girls than boys and sexual precocity occurs in 1/3 of the affected girls but is rare among boys. Hyperthyroidism is the second most common of the complicating endocrinopathies after sexual precocity and is often associated with either single or multiple adenomas arising in the thyroid gland. While the mechanism of the sexual precocity appears to be on a hypothalamic-pituitary basis, no such common mechanism has been established in the initiation of the hyperthyroid syndrome which is usually associated with the adenomas of the thyroid gland.

4. THYROID DYSFUNCTION AND GONADAL AND BREAST FUNCTION IN MEN

4.1. Hyperthyroidism

4.1.1. Gynecomastia. The clinical occurrence of gynecomastia in males with hyperthyroidism had only been sporadically noted until a 1974 study in which breast biopsies were performed on 18 hyperthyroid males (Becker et al., 1974). Of these 18, 15 had histologic evidence of gynecomastia, whereas only 8 had clinical evidence of gynecomastia or mastodynia. Histologically, the abnormal breast tissue was of four types: (a) epithelial hyperplasia with periductal edema and tortuous ducts, (b)

epithelial hyperplasia only, (c) epithelial hyperplasia with periductal sclerosis and (d) periductal sclerosis only. Since these patients were not followed with serial biopsies into a euthyroid remission, it is known to what degree the gynecomastia regressed histologically. However, in a previous report of three patients with gynecomastia, serial biopsies were performed and a recession in the height of the epithelium with less branching and decreased denseness of the tissue occurred despite the persistence of intracellular glycogen (Becker et al., 1968).

The increased total estradiol, increased unbound estradiol and increased unbound estradiol to testosterone ratio which occur in hyperthyroid subjects result in a greater than normal amount of available estrogen being present to influence breast tissue. These factors may be among those accounting for gynecomastia but are probably not the only ones causing this condition in hyperthyroidism (Chopra and Tulchinsky, 1974). Moreover, no definite relationship has been established to date between the degree of gynecomastia and the severity of the hyperthyroidism, the age of the patient, the size of the goiter or the presence or absence of exophthalmos (Becker et al., 1974).

4.1.2. Male infertility. Because most hyperthyroid males consult a physician with complaints relative to their primary disease process rather than to alterations in fertility, few studies have been conducted regarding possible changes in spermatogenesis during hyperthyroidism. The coincidental presentation, within a short period of time, of both hyperthyroidism and impaired semen analyses in three young males has been recently reported (Clyde et al., 1976). All three of these men had elevated gonadotropin levels as well as impaired spermatogenesis with return to normal of the LH, FSH and semen analyses after the restoration of the euthyroid state with propylthiouracil therapy.

The possible mechanisms involved in the suppression of spermatogenesis in hyperthyroid males have not yet been established. Theoretically, the commonly observed increase in serum LH levels should stimulate testicular Leydig cell production of testosterone and this high local concentration of testosterone should improve rather than impair spermatogenesis. Since this does not appear to be the case, the suppression of spermatogenesis in these patients may be mediated by other non-specific factors related to their hyperthyroidism such as increased body temperature, increased metabolic rate or excessive stress (Clyde et al., 1976). Further studies are necessary to determine whether abnormalities of semen analyses are consistently present in hyperthyroidism in order to further determine the precise influence of thyroid hormone excess on spermatogenesis.

Radioactive iodine therapy for hyperthyroidism has been questioned as a possible cause of chromosomal damage to germinal epithelial cells. It has been previously determined that the administration of an average therapeutic dose of 131-I radioactive iodine to hyperthyroid subjects produces a gonadal radiation dose of approximately 0.2 rads per mCi (Robertson and Gorman, 1976).

The only chromosomal abnormality produced by radioactive iodine administration to hyperthyroid subjects reported to date is that of a change in the peripheral lymphocyte chromosomes when examined by Q-banding. The commonest aberrations produced are translocation of the dicentric and tandem types and the incidence of these abnormalities appears to increase proportionally with the dose of radioactive iodine administered (Haglund et al., 1977). Although these abnormalities occur in circulating lymphocytes, no such effects have been demonstrated for spermatocytes to date and, in view of the low average gonadal radiation dose used in the therapy of hyperthyroidism, it is our view that there is not likely to be any significantly greater genetic abnormality occurring from radioactive iodine therapy when compared to the cumulative radiation effects received from standard diagnostic X-ray procedures.

4.2. Hypothyroidism

4.2.1. Abnormal sexual maturation. Hypothyroidism in the pre-pubertal child has been thought to retard both somatic and sexual development with the degree of retardation depending upon the duration of hypothyroidism, its severity and its age of onset. Replacement therapy with exogenous thyroid hormones has generally produced increased growth and normalization of sexual development.

Occasionally, pre-pubertal children with hypothyroidism may present with the unexpected finding of precocious puberty (Van Wyk and Grumbach, 1960; Franks and Stempfel, 1963; Barnes et al., 1973; Costin et al., 1972; Lee and Blizzard, 1974). In untreated hypothyroid girls with sexual precocity and markedly elevated serum TSH levels, serum gonadotropins have also been found to be elevated (Lee and Blizzard, 1974). In some of these girls, breast development and galactorrhea have occurred in association with elevated serum prolactin levels (Costin et al., 1972; Van Wyk and Fisher, 1977; Van Wyk and Grumbach, 1960). These cases of precocious puberty puzzled investigators until a study of 54 children (38 females and 16 males) with hypothyroidism, in which Barnes et al. (1973) contended that since somatic development is retarded in hypothyroidism, the comparison of development with chronologic age is invalid. By using bone age as a measure of somatic age they found that advanced iso-sexual development was present in 56% of the boys and 58% of the girls. Among the males assigned to the advanced sexual development group, enlargement of the testes with thinning and rugation of the scrotum without any other evidence of secondary sexual development was noted. Testicular biopsies on two males showed increased seminiferous tubule growth with little change in the Leydig cells. Also, enlargement of the sella turcica was noted on the X rays of some of these patients. With initiation of thyroxine replacement, rapid regression or stabilization of the features of advanced sexual maturation occurred despite simultaneous rapid somatic growth. These children later underwent puberty at the appropriate age (Barnes et al., 1973).

4.2.2. Male sexual function. Little information is available on the effects of hypothyroidism on male sexual function when the onset of the hypothyroidism occurs post-pubertally. Although loss of libido is a known clinical observation, to our knowledge no systematic studies relative to the effects of hypothyroidism on human male sexual function have as yet been reported. By comparison, females may have secondary menstrual irregularities, particularly menorrhagia, with associated increases in serum prolactin levels and infertility which revert to normal with thyroid hormone replacement therapy. No such observations have as yet been reported in the male.

Using the rationale that the metabolism of biogenic amines may be altered in hypothyroidism and that TRH may modify synaptic transmission in the hypothalamic areas responsible for the control of sexual function, oral TRH has been administered to impotent males in an attempt to improve their symptomatology (Benkert et al., 1976). These workers determined that such therapy failed in a double blind study to produce a significant improvement in sexual function when compared to the control placebo group and, therefore, TRH therapy does not appear to have any role in the management of impotence.

4.2.3. Male infertility. In a study of 1294 consecutive cases of male infertility, it was found that only 0.8% were due to thyroid dysfunction (Dubin and Amelar, 1971). Since hypothyroidism is less common in men than is hyperthyroidism, only a small percentage of hypothyroid males would be expected to have fertility problems secondary to this condition alone. Nevertheless, both L-thyroxine and triiodothyronine have been used empirically by some groups in the therapy of both

impotence and impaired spermatogenesis as documented by semen analysis (Jakobovits, 1970; Taymor and Selenkow, 1958) and have produced controversial reports on the value of such therapy. In addition, testicular biopsies have been obtained in men with prolonged hypothyroidism and although abnormalities were present, no report on the reproductive capacity of these men was made (DelaBalze et al., 1962). Thus, the scientific evidence indicating that the administration of thyroid hormone preparations to euthyroid men will improve the semen analysis and fertility is lacking (Arrata et al., 1969). Therefore, with the recent availability of sensitive tests of thyroid hypofunction such as the serum thyroxine and TSH assays for confirmation of overt hypothyroidism and the TRH provocative test for TSH and T3 responses for the detection of early subclinical hypothyroidism (Bain and Walfish, 1978), the authors, in agreement with the conclusion of others (Amelar and Dubin, 1977), recommend that empiric therapy with thyroid hormone preparations in the treatment of male infertility and impotence, in the absence of documented thyroidal hypofunction, be discouraged.

REFERENCES

Amelar RD, Dubin L (1977) The management of idiopathic male infertility. J Reprod Med 18: 191.

Anderson JR, Goudie RB, Gray K, et al. (1968) Immunological features of idiopathic Addison's disease: an antibody to cells producing steroid hormones. Clin Exp Immun 3: 107.

Arrata WSM, Arronet GJ, Dery JP (1969) The subfertile male. Fertil Steril 20: 460.

Bain J, Walfish PG (1978) The assessment of thyroid function and structure. Otolaryn Clin N Am 11: 419.

Barnes ND, Hayles AB, Ryan RJ (1973) Sexual maturation in juvenile hypothyroidism. Mayo Clin Proc 48: 849.

Barr ML, Shaver EL, Carr DH, Plunkett ER (1960) The chromatin positive Klinefelter syndrome among patients in mental deficiency hospitals. J Ment Defic Res 4: 89.

Becker KL, Mathews MJ, Higgins GA Jr, Mohanadi M (1974) Histologic evidence of gynecomastia in hyperthyroidism. Arch Pathol 98: 257.

Becker KL, Winnacker JL, Mathews MJ, Higgins GA Jr (1968) Gynecomastia and hyperthyroidism. An endocrine and histological investigation. J Clin Endocrinol Metab 28: 277.

Benkert O, Horn K, Pickardt CR, Schmid D (1976) Sexual impotence: studies of the hypothalamic-pituitary-thyroid axis and the effect of oral thyrotropin-releasing factor. Arch Sex Behav, 5: 275.

Brown JB, Strong JA (1965) The effect of nutritional status and thyroid function on the metabolism of oestradiol. J Endocrinol 32: 107.

Burman KD, Dimond RC, Noel GL, Earll JM, Frantz AG, Wartofsky L (1975) Klinefelter's syndrome: examination of thyroid function and the TSH and prolactin responses to thyrotropin releasing hormone prior to and after testosterone administration. J Clin Endocrinol Metab 41: 1161.

Carlson HE, Hershman JM (1975) The hypothalamic-pituitary-thyroid axis. Med Clin N Am 59: 1045.

Carr DH, Barr ML, Plunkett ER, Grumbach MM, Morishima A, Chu HY (1961) An XXXY sex chromosome complex in Klinefelter subjects with duplicate sex chromatin. J Clin Endocrinol Metab 21: 491.

Cheikh I, Hamilton BP, Hsu TH, Wiswell JG (1975) Response of TSH and prolactin to TRH in Klinefelter's syndrome (abstract). Endocrinology (Suppl) 96: A153.

Chen HJ, Walfish PG (1979) Effects of age and testicular function on the pituitary-thyroid system in male rats. J Endocrinol 82: 53.

Chen HJ, Walfish PG (1978) Alterations in pituitary-thyroid axis function in the aged male rat. Program 60th Annual Meeting of the Endocrine Society, Miami, Florida, June, 1978, p 266 (Abstract).

Chopra IJ (1975) Gonadal steroids and gonadotropins in hyperthyroidism. Med Clin N Am 59: 1109.

Chopra IJ, Tulchinsky D (1974) Status of estrogen-androgen balance in hyperthyroid men with Graves disease. J Clin Endocrinol Metab 38: 269.

Clyde HR, Walsh PC, English RW (1976) Elevated plasma testosterone and gonadotropin levels in infertile men with hyperthyroidism. Fertil Steril 27: 662.

Conti A, Staub JJ, Huber P, Mueller Y (1978) Reduction of

SHBG and T3 induced by propranolol in hyperthyroidism. Ann Endocrinol (Paris) (9th Annual Meeting of the European Thyroid Assoc) P 56A.

Costin G, Kershnar AK, Kogut MD, Turkington RW (1972) Prolactin activity in juvenile hypothyroidism and precocious puberty. Pediatrics 50: 881.

Davies TF, Rees-Smith B, Hall R (1978) Binding of thyroid stimulators to guinea pig testis and thyroid. Endocrinology 103: 6.

Davis TE, Canfield CJ, Herman RH, Goler D (1963) Thyroid function in patients with aspermiogenesis and testicular tubular sclerosis. N Engl J Med 268: 178.

DelaBalze FA, Arrilloga I, Mancini RE et al. (1962) Male hypogonadism in hypothyroidism. A study of six cases. J Clin Endocrinol Metab 22: 212.

DiGeorge AM (1975) Albright syndrome: is it coming of age? J Pediatr 87: 1018.

Dubin L, Amelar RD (1971) Etiologic factors in 1294 consecutive cases of male infertility. Fertil Steril 22: 469.

Ferguson-Smith MA, Anderson JR, Froland A, Gray KG (1966) Frequency of autoantibodies in patients with chromatin-positive Klinefelter's syndrome and their parents. Lancet ii: 566.

Fishman J, Hellman L, Aumoff B, Gallagher TF (1962) Influence of thyroid hormone on estrogen metabolism in man. J Clin Endocrinol Metab 22: 389.

Franks RC, Stempfel RS (1963) Juvenile hypothyroidism and precocious testicular maturation. J Clin Endocrinol Metab 23: 805.

Gordon GG, Southern AL, Tochimoto S, Rand JJ, Olivo J (1969) Effects of hyperthyroidism and hypothyroidism on the metabolism of testosterone and androstenedione in man. J Clin Endocrinol Metab 29: 164.

Haglund U, Lundell G, Zech L, Ohlin J (1977) Radioiodine administration in hyperthyroidism: a cytogenetic study. Hereditas 87: 85.

Hayles AB (1976) Precocious sexual maturation in juvenile hypothyroidism. Fertil Steril 27: 1220.

Hellman L, Bradlow HL, Zumoff B, et al. (1959) Thyroid adrenal interrelations and the hypocholesterolemic effect of androsterone. J Clin Endocrinol Metab 19: 936.

Higgins HP, Hershman JM, Kenimer JG, Patillo RA, Bayley TA, Walfish PG (1975) The thyrotoxicosis of hydatidiform mole. Ann Intern Med 63: 307.

Irvine WJ (ed.) Autoimmunity in endocrine disease. Clin Endocrinol Metab 4: 227.

Irvine WJ, Chan MMW, Scarth K (1969) The further characterization of autoantibodies reactive with extra-adrenal steroid producing cells in patients with adrenal disorders. Clin Exp Immun 4: 489.

Irvine WJ, Chan MMW, Scarth L, Kolb FO, Hartog M, Bayliss RIS, Drury MI (1968) Immunological aspects of premature ovarian failure associated with idiopathic Addison's disease. Lancet ii: 883.

Jakobovits T (1970) The treatment of impotence with methyl-testosterone and thyroid (100 patients: a double blind study). Fertil Steril 21: 32.

Larsen PR (1975) Tests of thyroid function. Med Clin N Am 59: 1063.

Lee PA, Blizzard RM (1974) Serum gonadotropins in hypothyroid girls with and without sexual precocity. Johns Hopkins Med J 135: 55.

Malendowicz LK, Parchimiwicz L, Ruchalski M, Suda P,

Walczak M (1977) Sexual dimorphism in the thyroid gland. II. Morphometric studies on the effects of post-pubertal gonadectomy and gonadal hormone replacement on the rat thyroid gland. Endokrinologie 69: 329.

McGuire JS Jr, Tomkins GM (1959) The effects of thyroxine administration on the enzymatic reduction of D4-3 ketosteroids. J Biol Chem 234: 791.

Olivo J, Southern AL, Gordon GG, Tochimoto S (1970) Studies of the protein binding of testosterone in plasma in disorders of thyroid function. Effect of therapy. J Clin Endocrinol Metab 31: 539.

Ozawa Y, Shishiba Y (1975) Lack of TRH-induced TSH secretion in a patient with Klinefelter's syndrome: a case report. Endocrinol Japonica 22: 269.

Plunkett ER, Rangecroft G, Heagy FG (1964) Thyroid function in patients with sex chromosomal anomalies. J Ment Defic Res 8: 25.

Ridgway EC, Longcope C, Maloof F (1975) Metabolic clearance and blood production rates of estradiol in hyperthyroidism. J Clin Endocrinol Metab 41: 491.

Robertson JS, Gorman CA (1976) Gonadal radiation dose and its genetic significance in radiation therapy of hyperthyroidism. J Nucl Med 17: 826.

Ruder H, Corvol P, Mahovdeau JA, Ross, JT, Lipsett MB (1971) Effects of induced hyperthyroidism on steroid metabolism in man. J Clin Endocrinol Metab 33: 382.

Sagel J, Distiller LA, Morley JE, Isaacs H (1975) Myotonia dystrophica: studies on gonadal function using luteinizing hormone releasing hormone (RH). J Clin Endocrinol Metab 40: 1110.

Sagel J, Distiller LA, Morley JE, Isaacs H (1976) Letter: normal thyrotropin-releasing hormone response in myotonia dystrophica. Arch Neurol 33: 520.

Southren AL, Olivo J, Gordon GG (1974) The conversion of androgens to estrogens in hyperthyroidism. J Clin Endocrinol Metab 38: 207.

Taymor ML, Selenkow HA (1958) Clinical experiences with L-triiodothyronine in male sterility. Fertil Steril 9: 560.

Vallotton MB, Forbes AP (1967) Autoimmunity in gonadal dysgenesis and Klinefelter's syndrome. Lancet i: 648.

van Rees GP, Noach EL, van Dieten JAM (1965) Influence of testosterone on the secretion of thyrotropin in the rat. Acta Endocrinol 50: 155.

Van Wyk JJ, Fisher DA (1977) In: Rudolph AM, Barnett HL, Einhorn AH, eds. Pediatrics, 16th edn, pp 1163-1693. New York: Appleton-Century-Crofts.

Van Wyk JJ, Grumbach MM (1960) Syndrome of precocious menstruation and galactorrhea in juvenile hypothyroidism. An example of hormonal overlap in pituitary feedback. J Pediatr 57: 416.

Volpe R (1977) The role of autoimmunity in hypoendocrine and hyperendocrine function. Ann Intern Med 87: 86.

Weinberg V, Kraemer FB, Kammerman S Case reports: co-existence of primary endocrine deficiencies. A unique case of male hypogonadism associated with hypoparathyroidism, hypoadrenocorticism and hypothyroidism. Am J Med Sci 272: 215.

Yap PL, Renton WB, Price WH, Fyffe JA, Lidgard GP (1978) Response to thyrotropin releasing hormone in Klinefelter's syndrome. Clin Endocrinol 8: 237.

Zuppinger K, Engel E, Forbes AP, Mantooth L, Claffey J (1967) Klinefelter's syndrome. A clinical cytogenetic study in twenty-four cases. Acta Endocrinol (Kbh) Suppl 113: 5.

5. MALE REPRODUCTIVE FUNCTION IN DIABETES MELLITUS

B.S. LEIBEL and P.R. GARNER

1. HISTORICAL DEVELOPMENTS

Diabetes mellitus can interfere with male reproduction by altering semen quality or by disrupting normal coital function. However, contrary to early evidence, both testicular steroidogenesis and testosterone metabolism are probably unaltered by the diabetic state.

Histologically, atrophic changes in the testes of men with diabetes mellitus were noted initially in the pre-insulin years (Koch, 1910), with an increase in total interstitial tissue and tubular degeneration. This was attributed initially to decreased pressure within the testicular tissue, when tubules shrank in volume. Later, note was made of increased thickness of the tubular basement membrane, and disrupted spermatogenesis (Warren and Le Compte, 1952), but the tissue was taken from autopsy specimens whose clinical courses had varied. Early reports of testicular biopsy material, taken from diabetics with gonadal dysfunction, suggested a wide spectrum of pathology. Most biopsies showed some pathological changes, (Schöffling et al., 1959), prominent amongst which are tubular atrophy and canaliculi basement membrane thickening. Spermatogenesis was also often affected, with significant decreases seen in spermatogonia, spermatocytes I, spermatids and spermatozoa. Again an increase in interstitial tissue was noted with a relative increase in Sertoli cell concentration. The Leydig cell population was usually unaltered when compared with normal controls.

Surprisingly, contrary to these earlier surveys, more recent biopsy evaluation of impotent diabetics described *normal* testicular histology (Oakley, 1950). Using both light and electron microscopy, no change in either Sertoli cell or Leydig cell populations was noted (Rivarola et al., 1970).

Initial histological findings, however, were enough to stimulate interest in other areas of male reproduction. Three main aspects have been carefully examined, namely alterations in semen quality, possible changes in steroidogenesis, and impotence and ejaculatory failure.

2. THE ROLE OF INSULIN AND CARBOHYDRATES METABOLISM IN THE CONTROL OF SPERMATOZOAN METABOLISM AND SEMEN QUALITY

The major energy producing pathway in human spermatozoa is glycolysis. Spermatozoan motility can be maintained solely from this energy source without respiratory metabolism. Under both aerobic and anaerobic conditions the rate of glycolysis is very similar. To drive this glycolytic pathway, spermatozoa require exogenous hexoses, which are converted to lactic acid (MacLeod and Freund, 1958). Fructose, glucose and mannose can be utilized by spermatozoa and motility is maintained at physiological concentrations of these substrates (Peterson and Freund, 1969).

Of these hexoses, fructose is found in semen in the highest concentration, with a mean of 300 mg/100 ml (MacLeod and Freund, 1958). The concentration of glucose is much lower, with values varying between 5 and 10 mg/100 ml (Peterson and Freund, 1971). In spite of this low concentration, the affinity constant for glucose is approximately 30 times greater than that for fructose. It has been estimated that over 50% of sugar used by spermatozoa is in fact glucose, and the concentration of the hexose in semen is maintained by breakdown of semen polysaccharides (Peterson and Freund, 1971). Human semen has a high enzymatic com-

J. Bain and E.S.E. Hafez (eds.), Diagnosis in andrology, 61-74. All rights reserved.
Copyright © 1980 by Martinus Nijhoff Publishers bv, The Hague/Boston/London.

ponent including polysaccharidases and glycosidases (Sheth et al., 1970).

The functional pathway for glucose utilization is the Embden-Myerhoff pathway, and there is strong evidence that glycolysis in mammalian spermatozoa is primarily under nucleotide control (Hoskins, 1975). Activation of phosphofructokinase is increased by cyclic AMP. However, the naturally occurring activators of spermatozoan adenyl cyclase are not known. In man, the effect of insulin on spermatozoan metabolism and motility is uncertain (Eliasson et al, 1969). Prostaglandins, catecholamines and estrogens seem to be without effect (Hicks et al., 1972), but extracts of follicular fluid can stimulate spermatozoan oxygen uptake and motility. Spermatozoa in normal ejaculates are highly motile and natural activators of adenyl cyclase must therefore occur in human semen.

Although the role of insulin in spermatozoa metabolism is uncertain, the seminal plasma from normal fasting subjects has an insulin concentration of 19 ± 3 μU/ml, which is twice the normal fasting serum concentration (Hicks et al., 1973). Hicks noted the addition of glucose to human spermatozoa inhibited oxygen uptake, which could be reversed by insulin. When glucose or fructose was used as substrate, hexose utilization by spermatozoa also increased markedly (Hicks et al., 1973). However, other workers have *not* been able to demonstrate any effect of insulin on spermatozoal hexose utilization (Eliasson et al., 1969; Paz et al., 1977). The addition of insulin in vitro to washed spermatozoa from diabetic and non-diabetic men had no affect on oxygen and glucose uptake, or on lactate production and spermatozoal motility.

Thus, although there is no dispute that immunoreactive insulin levels are higher in seminal plasma than serum, the lack of effect on addition of further insulin in vitro to spermatozoa has been attributed to the fact that fructose utilization is not insulin dependent. In view of this, other mechanisms have been suggested by which insulin could affect semen quality. Indirect evidence suggests a role for insulin in both prostatic and seminal vesicle secretion. Insulin deficient animals have a remarkable reduction in both accessory gland secretion and fertility (Paz et al., 1977b), and the parallel condition can be seen in insulin deficient men (Rubin, 1962).

The metabolic activity of the spermatozoa in-

creases during passage through the epididymis. There is a significant increase in fructolysis and also in carnitine content. The latter may aid glycolysis and lactate oxidation (Pasillas, 1973). As the spermatozoa progress toward the cauda epididymis, there is an increase in cyclic AMP content, which may contribute to their increased motility (Hoskins, 1973).

3. ALTERATION IN SEMEN QUALITY IN DIABETES MELLITUS

Early studies of the ejaculate in patients with diabetes mellitus suggested that sperm motility was impaired (Klebanow and MacLeod, 1960). Although sperm count and spermatozoa morphology did not appear to deviate from the normal range, motility was impaired in 50% of cases. Juvenile-onset diabetics also demonstrated decreased spermatozoan motility when assessed by the sperm velocity test (Bartak et al., 1975). However, this group also noted a significant increase in abnormal forms which they postulated may have contributed to the decreased motility.

It is difficult to compare the data of various authors, as methods of assessing semen quality, particularly motility, vary considerably. However, Neubauer attempted to correlate the results from single groups containing 10 to 40 diabetics (Table 1) Semen analysis with a decreased total count occurred between 9 and 45% of cases. Decreased seminal fluid volume (less than 2.5 ml) occurred in 50% of cases. Decreased motility with less than 6% forward progressing sperm, was found in 73-100% of cases (Neubaueer et al., 1972). However these abnormalities should be interpreted with care. No correlation was made between semen quality and

Table 1. Semen quality in diabetes mellitus (after Neubauer et al., 1972).

Aspect	% cases reported
Decreased total count ($<50 \times 10^6$)	9—45
Decreased seminal fluid volume (<2.5 ml)	50
Decreased spermatozoal motility ($<6\%$ forward progression)	73-100

age, or duration of diabetes mellitus, or association with other diabetic sequelae.

In conclusion, impaired motility continues to be the most consistent finding (Spellacy, 1976), although hypospermatogenesis has been reported in diabetic men by (Schöffling, 1965; Schöffling et al., 1963; Foglia et al., 1963).

There is also a change in the Spermatogenic Activity Test in diabetes mellitus. This test is based on the selective accumulation of high-energy phosphates in tissues with marked mitotic activity (Czerniak, 1962). Accumulation of ^{32}P as tracer is parallel to metabolic activity, and produces selective uptake of ^{32}P in testis, bone marrow and malignant tumours. In diabetic patients, the uptake of ^{32}P into the testes is decreased when compared with controls suggesting an alteration in spermatogenesis (Panayotov et al., 1974).

4. THE HYPOTHALAMIC-PITUITARY-TESTICULAR AXIS IN DIABETES MELLITUS

The effect of diabetes mellitus on testicular steroidogenesis and hypothalamic-pituitary control has also been a controversial area. Initial data from diabetic animals suggested that glycogen infiltration of the pituitary gland could interfere with normal pituitary function (Dixit and Lazarow, 1962). Deficient glucose utilization of the pituitary gland in diabetic rats has also been described (Goodner and Freinkel, 1961). These studies suggested that the pituitary was an insulin-sensitive gland, and serve to raise the question whether testicular dysfunction seen in diabetes mellitus could be related to abnormal gonadotropin release or synthesis.

Early data using bioassays suggested that urinary gonadotropin levels were low in poorly controlled diabetics. However, no relationship between levels of urinary gonadotropins, steroidogenesis and sper matogenesis was sought (Bergqvist, 1954; Drudi and Dornetti, 1958). Urinary gonadotropic excretion was also found to be diminished in impotent diabetics, whereas diabetic subjects with normal potency tended to have normal excretion patterns (Schöffling, 1965). In spite of the inadequacy of the early bioassay methods, the interest in these findings lies mainly in the absence of high gonadotropin

levels in any of the series. This obviously lessened support for primary hypogonadism being the cause of gonadal and sexual dysfunction in diabetes mellitus.

Basal LH and FSH levels are normal in diabetes mellitus (Distiller et al., 1975). Interest has been focussed more recently on the application of the LH-RH Test to diabetic men, with some conflicting data. Distiller found that the mean LH response to LH-RH was significantly reduced at the thirty minute level when compared with controls. This low incremental change of LH response to LH-RH has been found in diabetics with or without impotence. Whether this is a reflection of abnormal LH synthesis, or abnormal release at a pituitary level is unclear. The limitations of the LH-RH Test restrict further speculation, and other workers have found normal incremental change in both LH and FSH (Schally et al., 1971).

In conclusion, therefore, the early bioassay reports of 'low' gonadotropin levels in diabetes mellitus have not been confirmed by radioimmunoassay. The limitation of both types of assay await confirmation by a sensitive bioassay method. LH-RH testing has demonstrated both low incremental and normal LH response and requires further elucidation. The overall suggestion is that impotence related to diabetes mellitus may not have an endocrine basis, but present dynamic testing may be too crude to assess subtle changes.

5. ANDROGEN METABOLISM IN DIABETES MELLITUS (TABLE 2)

Studies of androgenic function in diabetic males have also suffered the rigors of inaccurate assays. Early results of steroid analyses carried out in diabetes mellitus were expectedly variable. Decreased 17-ketosteroid excretion was noted in impotent diabetics (Miller and Mason, 1945), but well controlled diabetics had normal excretion patterns (Schöffling, 1965). Chromatographic fractionation of 17-ketosteroids has produced equally divergent data although there is some suggestion of an increase in adrenal androgen production in diabetes (Pond, 1954). This correlates well with animal work demonstrating adrenal hypertrophy following castration (Schöffling et al., 1961). Confirmation using accurate adrenal androgen production and clearance rates is obviously needed.

Plasma testosterone levels are similar in impotent diabetics, and diabetics with normal potency, when compared with normal men (Ellenberg, 1971; Faerman et al., 1972; Kolodny et al., 1974; Rivarola et al., 1970). The significance of these normal testosterone levels when related to sexual potency is discussed later in the chapter. However, in spite of the normal plasma testosterone levels, changes in free testosterone fractions and testosterone binding capacity have been noted (Geisthövel et al., 1975). Free testosterone levels were lower in diabetics with potency disturbances when compared with diabetics of normal sexual function. Testosterone binding capacity was also increased in the former group. However, these findings are contrary to LH-RH resting results in controls in impotent diabetics where plasma testosterone and sex-hormone binding globulin capacities were similar (Wright et al., 1976).

Leydig cell response to HCG stimulation is normal, if single dose (5000 units) HCG stimulation is used (Faerman et al., 1972). However, if a three-day HCG stimulation test is used, the response may be blunted both in diabetic men with or without normal potency (Geisthövel et al., 1975) In vitro steroid biosynthesis by testicular tissue has also been assessed in patients with diabetes mellitus (Faerman et al., 1972) Percentage conversion of pregnenolone to testosterone, androstenedione, pro-

gesterone and 17-α-hydroxyprogesterone appears to be similar to that seen in the normal testis. The normal in vitro steroidogenesis seen in diabetes mellitus correlates well with the morphological picture. In diabetes mellitus, the morphology and subcellular characteristics of the Leydig cells are generally normal (Faerman et al., 1972).

In summary, testicular steroidogenesis and testosterone production rates are not impaired in diabetics with impotence or with normal sexual function. Plasma androgen levels are also normal, suggesting no change in testosterone metabolic clearance rates. The controversy over free testosterone concentrations and sex-hormone binding globulin concentrations must be clarified. The significant lack of correlation of impotence in the diabetic male with any endocrine abnormality is discussed later.

6. GLUCOSE TOLERANCE TESTING IN IDIOPATHIC OLIGOSPERMIA

The application of oral glucose tolerance testing, and provocative glucose tolerance testing to the infertile male has been unrewarding. No difference in standard oral glucose tolerance testing, or prednisone-provoked glucose tolerance testing in azoospermic, oligospermic or normal males has been noted (Goldman et al., 1970). There has been a suggestion that prednisone-provoked glucose tolerance testing produces a decrease in carbohydrate

Table 2. The hypothalamic-pituitary-testicular axis in diabetes mellitus. Comparison of diabetics with normal sexual function, impotence, and controls.

Test	Diabetics with normal sexual function	Impotent diabetics	Source
1. Urinary gonadotropins	Normal	Normal	Schöffling (1965)
2. Basal plasma LH and FSH	Normal	Normal	Distiller et al. (1975)
3. LRH test – incremental LH	Normal	Normal	Distiller et al. (1975)
	Low	Low	Mortimer et al. (1973)
4. Incremental FSH	Normal	Normal	Distiller et al. (1975)
5. 17-Ketosteroids	Normal	Normal	Schöffling et al. (1961)
6. Plasma testosterone	Normal	Normal	Kolodny et al. (1974)
			Faerman et al. (1972)
7. Free testosterone	Normal	Low	Geisthövel et al. (1975)
	Normal	Normal	
8. HCG stimulation test	Normal	Normal	Faerman et al. (1972)
Single dose – 3-day	Blunted	Blunted	Geisthövel et al. (1975)
9. In vitro testosterone biosynthesis	Normal	Normal	Faerman et al. (1972)

tolerance in the impotent male, but this requires validation. At present, therefore, there is no indication for routine investigation of carbohydrate metabolism in the infertile male.

7. THE EFFECT OF MATERNAL DIABETES MELLITUS ON FETAL TESTICULAR DEVELOPMENT

Many investigators have underlined the importance and influence of certain complications of pregnancy on the number of Leydig cells in the fetal and neonatal testis (Zondek and Zondek, 1967). Hyperplasia of testicular interstitial cells was initially noted in a full-term stillborn fetus of a diabetic mother (Bayer, 1942), but the pregnancy had also been complicated by pregnancy-associated hypertension. This finding has been confirmed by other workers in up to 40% of neonatal testes of babies born to diabetic mothers (Driscoll et al., 1960). In a survey of Leydig cell population in various medical problems of pregnancy the highest number of Leydig cells was noted in a 37-week-old fetus of a diabetic mother (Zondek and Zondek, 1962). A postulated cause for such Leydig cell hyperplasia is the occurrence of high HCG levels secondary to placental hypertrophy in diabetes mellitus. To date no correlation between maternal serum or urinary HCG levels and fetal Leydig cell hyperplasia has been noted.

8. DISEASES PRESENTING WITH ASSOCIATED HYPOGONADISM AND DIABETES MELLITUS

Diabetes mellitus and male hypogonadism co-exist in many disease states (Table 3). An important point is that hypogonadism appearing in a patient with diabetes mellitus may not be due to the

Table 3. Diseases with associated hypogonadism and diabetes mellitus.

Hemochromatosis
Klinefelter's syndrome
Myotonic muscular dystrophy
Werner's syndrome
Alström's syndrome
Cushing's syndrome
Acromegaly

diabetes per se. There are several possible mechanisms behind this association. In some disorders both pancreatic and testicular function is impaired by the same disease process. In others, a genetically controlled association seems likely, but not proven. In acromegaly and Cushing's disease both carbohydrate intolerance and hypogonadism are secondary to pituitary dysfunction.

The first report of the association of hemochromatosis and multiglandular insufficiency appeared in 1912 (Claude and Sourdel, 1912). The incidence of hypogonadism in hemochromatosis varies between 1.7% (Finch and Finch, 1955) and 70% (Stocks et al., 1968). The nature of the hypogonadism has been attributed to destruction of the anterior pituitary by iron deposition, to hemosiderin deposition in the testis, and to hepatic dysfunction. No relationship has been noted between patients with hypogonadism and those with diabetes mellitus, suggesting that this occurrence is not interdependent. However, hypogonadism has been related to the presence of atrophy of subcutaneous fat at insulin injection sites (Dymock et al., 1971). As the duration of insulin therapy is significantly longer in those with fat atrophy, there appears to be a time element involved in the development of both fat atrophy and hypogonadism in hemochromatosis.

Isolated reports of diabetes mellitus in Klinefelter's syndrome have appeared over the last two decades (Lamotte et al., 1965; Rohde, 1963; Yodaiken et al., 1960). Interest in this association stems mainly from a cytogenic-psychiatric investigation of patients with sex chromosome abnormalities (Nielsen et al. 1969). In this survey it was noted that 10% of parents of patients with Klinefelter's syndrome had diabetes mellitus. This incidence has been confirmed in later series (Menzinger et al., 1966) and is similar to the rate of occurrence of diabetes in families of patients with Turner's syndrome (Forbes and Engel, 1963). Chromatin-positive Klinefelter's syndrome is reported to have a high incidence of diabetes mellitus (Nielsen et al., 1969). Thirty-nine percent have a diabetic glucose tolerance curve and 19% of their mothers have overt diabetes mellitus. The incidence of diabetes is lower in chromatin-negative Klinefelter's syndrome and the XYY syndrome. The diabetes in all types is usually maturity-onset in type, and generally mild.

However, unlike the typical maturity-onset diabetic, diabetics with Klinefelter's syndrome demonstrate a brisk and prolonged rise in plasma insulin levels after glucose ingestion. This response is similar to that seen in diabetics secondary to other diseases, such as acromegaly. However, no significant changes in growth hormone levels have been noted in Klinefelter's syndrome, in either the fasting or stimulated state (Nielsen et al., 1969).

The high frequency of overt diabetes in the mothers of Klinefelter's syndrome, and in the syndrome itself, suggested that the disposition towards diabetes and chromosomal non-disjunction may be genetically connected. The majority of Klinefelter mosaic 46XY/47XXY have a diabetic glucose tolerance curve, and the incidence is also higher in 48XXXY and 49XXXXY patients. The etiology of this relationship however, remains controversial. Reports of high levels of auto-antibodies against insulin and pancreatic tissue in Klinefelter's syndrome (Charvat et al., 1967) have not been confirmed (Nielsen et al., 1969). It has been suggested that the increased frequency of abortions and congenital abnormalities in children of diabetic fathers as well as diabetic mothers, might be due in part to diabetes-induced non-disjunction (White & Hunt, 1943). Certainly this theory supports well the suggestion that it is the genetic constitution for diabetes mellitus that is transmitted, with the disease itself increasing the risk on-disjunction.

Hypogonadism and diabetes mellitus also coexist in myotonic muscular dystrophy. Eighty percent of patients with this disorder have testicular atrophy (Drucher et al., 1962). Pubertal development is often normal, and testicular damage occurs at varying times during adult life. The testes are small and soft, reflecting hyalinization, and fibrosis of the seminiferous tubules. Leydig cell function is usually normal. Unlike Klinefelter's syndrome, clinical evidence of androgen deficiency, gynecomastia, longleggedness are infrequently encountered. Glucose intolerance and hyperinsulinemia are frequently present (Huff and Lebovitz, 1968). The disorder is inherited as an autosomal dominant, but a common genetic basis for the diabetes mellitus and hypogonadism is purely speculatory.

Werner's syndrome was first described in 1904 by Otto Werner in his thesis 'Cataract in Combination with Scleroderma'. In addition to the characteristic skin changes and premature graying of the hair, both hypogonadism and a tendency to diabetes mellitus occur frequently. Over 50% of Werner's syndrome have an abnormal glucose tolerance curve. The majority have infantile testes and gynecomastia. However, gonadotropin levels vary widely and on the data available cannot be classified into hypo- or hypergonadotropic hypogonadism. No correlation between the severity of the diabetes and hypogonadism has been noted (Epstein et al., 1966).

Alstrom's syndrome may present with the combined features of childhood blindness, nerve deafness, obesity, diabetes mellitus and male hypogonadism. Surprisingly, there is often normal secondary sexual characteristic development. The syndrome is transmitted as an autosomal recessive (Alstrom et al., 1959). Diabetes occurs in 90% of males assessed (Goldstein et al., 1970). One-third of these males had associated primary hypogonadism, with small testes, low serum testosterone and elevated gonadotropins. Hyalinization of the seminiferous tubules was found on biopsy. The primary biochemical defect remains unknown. However, on the basis of membrane thickening and hyalinization of connective tissue in kidneys, pancreas, testes and skin, the primary defect may involve a genetic alteration common to the membranes of these tissues. These examples suggest that the association of diabetes mellitus and hypogonadism in the male in many diseases is more than coincidental.

9. COITAL FUNCTION DIABETES MELLITUS

Sexual potency may be defined as a firm penile erection of sufficient duration to achieve vaginal admission with subsequent orgasm. More than 90% of sexual impotence in the general population is estimated to be of psychogenic origin (Masters and Johnson, 1976; Strauss, 1950). Nevertheless, it is possible by a number of observations and measurements to distinguish organic from psychological impotence (Weiss, 1972; Stekel, 1927; Hastings, 1963).

Since Rollo (1797) recorded sexual impotence in diabetes, it has become increasingly apparent that there is an increased incidence of this disorder in diabetes mellitus (Kolodny et al., 1974; Schöffling et al., 1963). Beginning with observations by Van Noorden in 1903 (Von Noorden, 1903). who commented on the high incidence of impotence in diabetes, and by Naunyn in 1906 (Naunyn, 1906), who listed impaired potency as an early symptom of the disease, there have been more recent studies (Schöffling et al., 1963) that indicate the average prevalence at approximately 50% of all male diabetics, which is considerably greater than that of the average population (Kinsey et al., 1948). The magnitude of the problem will become evident when it is realized that in the United States of America there are 750,000 impotent diabetic males, 200,000 in Britain and 75,000 in Canada (Cooper, 1972).

The precise underlying cause or causes of impotence in diabetes remains unknown. From a scientific point of view, knowledge of the neural, vascular, muscular and hormonal physiology of erection which involves the pooling and trapping of blood in the corpora of the penis is incomplete. The large amount of indirect data which has been accumulated to support one or other causal relationship must be regarded as speculative allegation.

The stimuli for erection maybe classified as either psychogenic or reflexogenic. The former consist of auditory, visual, olfactory, gustatory, tactile and imaginative stimuli, all and each of which arouse the erotic centre of the brain. This in turn can be suppressed by hostility and guilt.

Reflexogenic erection is caused by two kinds of stimuli, namely interoceptive such as those which emanate from a full bladder or rectum and exteroceptive an example of which is the tactile sensation caused by stroking the penis. While it is not clear how exteroceptive and interoceptive stimuli can inhibit erection, it is apparent that they do act synergetically to produce erections.

10. NEUROANATOMY OF ERECTIONS

In man, efferent neural impulses for erection are thought to arise from parasympathetic fibres in sacral spinal cord root S2, S3 and S4 although the role of S2 has been questioned. These are the same spinal roots that provide the efferent (parasympathetic) supply to the detrusor muscle of the urinary bladder and to the rectum and colon. Thus the same pelvic nerves from the sacral segments of the spinal cord control erection, defecation and micturition.

Injury to the spinal cord or to the pelvic nerves may alter one of these functions without affecting the others, which indicates that although these pathways are anatomically similar they are not identical. Also, it has been demonstrated in cats that removal of the sacral spinal cord eliminated reflexogenic erection (Root and Bard, 1947). Nevertheless, psychogenic erection occurred in these animals via sympathetic pathways in the thoracic cord communicating with the higher brain centres. For example, in the absence of the sacral cord, stroking the penis failed to produce an erection while a female in estrus resulted in a full erection with coitus.

Similar observations were made clinically by Kuhn (1950) in a patient with an injury that necessitated severing all anterior and posterior spinal roots below L1. In this man the entire pelvic region had been denervated and reflexogenic erections could not be elicited. Nevertheless, he still had erections associated with erotic psychic stimuli.

Other studies in men who have suffered spinal cord injuries (Bors and Comarr, 1960; Zeitlin et al., 1957). have helped clarify the neuroanatomy of spinal centers for erection. Transections of the cord well above the sacral level usually left reflexogenic erections intact but eliminated psychogenic erections. But bilateral pudendal nerve destruction eliminates the afferent limb of the sacral reflex and prevents reflexogenic erection. Conversely, about one fourth of patients who suffered complete lower motor neuron lesions of the sacral cord were able to have psychogenic but not reflexogenic erections (Bors and Comarr, 1960). In patients with incomplete spinal cord lesions both psychogenic and reflexogenic erections can occur. From these data it is evident that an intact outflow from the thoracolumbar cord estimated to originate around T_{12}-L_1 can mediate psychogenic erections in patients with complete destruction of the sacral cord. Bilateral sympathectomy in man (Ross, 1953; Whitelaw and Smithwick, 1951) does not appear to have any consistent effect on erectile function. The thoracolumbar sympathetic outflow has been found to contain both adrenergic vasoconstrictor and cholinergic vasodilator fibres (Bacq, 1935), and presumably the dilator fibres are stimulated by erotic psychogenic stimuli.

Knowledge of the cerebral localization of penile erections in man is fragmentary but it appears to be located in the region of the ansa lenticula (Meyers, 1962). Temporal lobe lesions in man have been associated with loss of erections but normal libido (Hierons and Saunders, 1966).

It is clear from the foregoing evidence that in cases of complete impotence of neurological origin both the sacral and the thoraco-lumbar centres must be compromised.

11. NEUROPATHY AND IMPOTENCE

Fearman et al. (1974) analyzed the autonomic nervous fibres of the corpora cavernosa of the penis by light microscopy in impotent diabetics and normal non-diabetic controls. Unfortunately their study did not include a third group, namely potent diabetics. Of the five diabetic subjects, four showed

morphological changes including hyperargentophilia, beaded and spindle-shaped thickenings, and argentophilic microangiopathy. None of the non-diabetic controls and only one of the diabetics showed any lesion. This study lends indirect support to the concept that impotence in the diabetic is due to a neurological lesion of the nerve fibres that control erection.

The electrophysiological peripheral neuropathy may be graded according to its anatomical extent. When this grading is compared with the associated symptoms and clinical signs of neuropathy, it is evident that the abnormality is often subclinical (Buck et al., 1976). Whereas all 60 diabetic subjects in this study had electrophysiological signs of peripheral neuropathy, only 30% had corresponding symptoms or clinical signs, although 80% had some symptoms of neuropathy. Sixty percent complained of impotence and 48% had bladder symptoms. Neuropathic abnormalities were demonstrable in

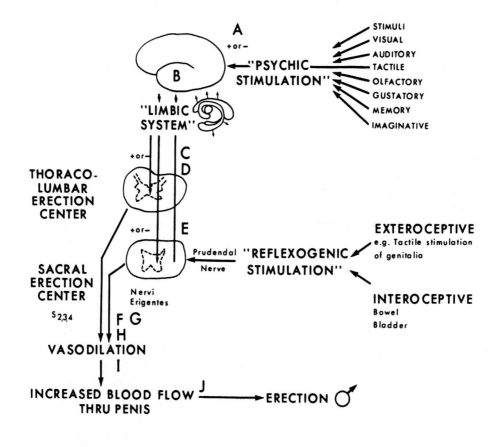

Figure 1. Human penile erection.

all eleven newly diagnosed diabetics. They did not find a correlation between patients with abnormal bladder function and those with nerve conduction defects in the limbs. Patients with abnormal vascular reflexes have a more marked disturbance of motor conduction in the legs than patients with normal vascular responses (Ewing et al., 1973).

It is often assumed that in a large proportion of diabetics, impotence is directly related to autonomic neuropathy that has affected fibres serving erection (Baron, 1974). The evidence for this mechanism is indirect, depending as it does on bladder dysfunction which shares the same nerve supply as the penis as well as the micturition and erection reflex centers being located in the same sacral segments. This is wholly circumstantial evidence since it is not a direct examination of erectile dysfunction.

The bladder abnormality consists of large capacity hypotonia insensitivity. In addition there is excessive residual volume and poor urine flow rate. Impotence involved more than 60% of the cases with bladder dysfunction (Buck et al., 1976; Ellenberg, 1971). The coexistence of anatomic nervous dysfunction, particularly that involving the urinary bladder and impotence in the diabetic male, has received attention by several investigators (Bors and Commarr, 1960; Pick, 1970). It has not yet been explained why a significant number of diabetics in each group with neurogenic disease of the bladder and often with more widespread neuropathy escape sexual impotence. Conversely, why are some impotent diabetics free from any visceral evidence of autonomic neuropathy?

A series of 42 diabetic patients with symptoms of autonomic neuropathy (Ewing et al., 1973) were objectively assessed using the Valsalva and hand-grip tests. Fifteen patients who had impotence as the *only* manifestation suggestive of diabetic autonomic neuropathy, had less abnormal vascular reflexes than the remainder of the patients who had other features of diabetic autonomic neuropathy. There were no differences in age, or in duration of the diabetes between the two groups. In view of the almost normal vascular reflexes in patients with impotence alone, this study suggests that either impotence is an *early* feature of autonomic neuropathy, or is independent of the disorder.

In a study of 35 impotent diabetic men aged 33 to 78 nocturnal penile tumescence (NPT) was measured and compared to 35 age-matched control subjects (Karacan et al., 1978). Electroencephalographic and other measurements showed that the diabetic men as a group exhibited a significant reduction in NPT and in the number and amount of full erections, which suggests that their impotence was organogenic. It would have been interesting to know that results of these tests on age-matched potent diabetics.

12. HEMODYNAMICS OF PENILE ERECTION

The hemodynamics of penile erection has been reviewed (Weiss, 1972). The actual transformation of the penis from a flaccid to an erect state is a vascular phenomenon. Blood reaches the penis via terminal branches of the right and left internal pudendal arteries. These vessels carry blood to the 'erectile tissues' of the penis, which consist of two corpora cavernosa lying side by side on the dorsal aspect of the penis and the corpus spongiosum surrounding the urethra. The erectile tissues are composed or irregular sponge-like systems of vascular spaces interspersed between the arteries and veins (Alvarez-Morujo, 1967). When the penis is flaccid, the vascular spaces contain very little blood and are virtually collapsed. During erection the vascular spaces are transformed into large cavities distended with blood at relatively high pressure (Henderson and Roepke, 1933).

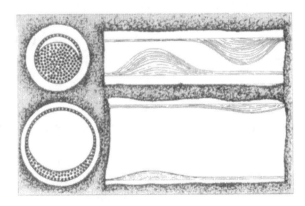

Figure 2. Diagram of the function of the Ebner pads at rest (top) and during erection (bottom).

The distension of the penis with blood during erection is brought about by the opening of anastomoses between the arterioles and vascular spaces in the erectile tissues. Conti (1952) described valve-like structures called Ebner pads or 'polsters' containing smooth muscle located at the anastomoses between the arterioles and the vascular spaces. The polsters cause blood to be shunted away from the corpora cavernosa directly into the veins when the penis is flaccid. The polsters are under the control of the autonomic nervous system (fibers from the sacral and thoraco-lumbar erection centers) and relax when impulses for erection are transmitted, thereby allowing a greatly increased volume of blood to flow into the vascular spaces of the erectile tissues (Newman et al., 1964). The rate of arterial inflow is temporarily greater than the rate of venous outflow, thus causing the characteristic increase in penile volume during erection. A steady-state is eventually reached, where the rates of inflow and outflow are equal and the penis ceases to enlarge but remains rigid (Hotchkiss and Fernandez-Leal, 1957).

Polsters are also present in the veins draining the erectile tissue, leading to the speculation that these polsters contract when the arteriolar polsters dilate, thereby promoting turgescence by diminishing the venous outflow (Garrett and Rhamy, 1966). But Newman et al. (1964) believed that venous blockade is not necessary for human penile erection and probably does not occur. Also, observations of humans (Bors and Comarr, 1960; Newman et al., 1964), and animals (Dorr and Brody, 1967; Hart and Kitchell, 1966; Henderson and Roepke, 1933) have shown that the ischio- and bulbo-cavernosus muscles do not play an essential role in penile erection.

If the psychic or reflexogenic stimuli that elicited the erection are not adequately sustained, detumescence of the penis normally occurs within a few moments. It is not known whether this is merely due to diminution of the cholinergic (vasodilator) impulses that open the polsters or whether an active vasoconstrictor impulse is also involved. It is thought that when ejaculation takes place erection subsides promptly because the sympathetic impulses that facilitate emission of semen also cause constriction of the vessels supplying blood to the erectile tissues of the penis (Kuntz, 1953). Persis-

tence of such impulses after ejaculation might explain the well-known latent period between ejaculation and the ability to have another erection.

Ruzbarsky and Michal (1976) studied the morphological changes in the arterial bed of the penis with aging in post mortem material of 30 subjects ranging in age from 19 to 85 years with a mean of 57 years. Fifteen of the cases were diabetic with an average duration of 13 years. The pathological findings of diabetics and non-diabetics were the same but the penile vasculature in diabetics showed a higher density and increased progression of lesions over age-matched controls. It would appear, therefore, that diabetes mellitus accelerates the aging process in the penile vasculature and that these changes might well explain the impotence that occurs with aging and more particularly that which occurs with diabetes.

Canning et al. (1963) palpated the penile pulse as an indicator of vascular sufficiency and found that 31 out of 451 subjects so examined who did not have a measurable pulse had significantly diminished potency. Indeed the association of pelvic vascular insufficiency as seen in Leriche's syndrome has long been known to be accompanied by impotence. Abelson (1974) modified an ultrasonic Doppler method for measuring blood pressure in infants to measure penile blood pressure. In addition, they studied the penile pulses in all subjects which included normal and impotent diabetic males.

Pulses were present in all 29 normal subjects but of the 15 impotent male diabetics 6 had no penile pulses. Unfortunately among these six patients there were other complicating factors which confused the issue. Penile blood pressure was measurable in 4 of the 6 impotent patients without penile pulses.

They found the mean blood pressure in the penis to be higher than that in the arm or leg of the normals due to a higher diastolic reading. In the diabetic impotent group blood pressure either could not be obtained or was significantly lower than normal. Of the fifteen impotent diabetics 11 had neuropathy and 4 had peripheral vascular disease.

13. HORMONAL ASPECTS OF ERECTION

As outlined previously in the section on the pituitary-testicular axis in diabetes, impotence in diabetic males does not correlate with any endocrine abnormality. More recent studies of testosterone levels and testosterone biosynthesis by testicular homogenates in vitro have not shown any abnormalities of androgen production in impotent diabetic men (Wright et al., 1976). In vitro steroid biosynthesis by testicular homogenates is normal, as is the morphology of the interstitial tissue and subcellular characteristics of Leydig cells (Faerman et al., 1972). However, alterations in bladder motility were seen in all but one of these impotent diabetics. Motor nerve conduction velocity was abnormal in all of the subjects. Faerman concluded that in all of their patients, androgenic function was normal and therefore impotence could not be attributed to hormonal deficiency.

Emission of semen following orgasm was found to be decreased or absent in many diabetic patients (Klebanow and MacLeod, 1960). Calcification of the vas deferens does not appear to be the explanation for this symptom. Neuropathy affecting the sympathetic nerve supply of the vas deferens and seminal vesicles preventing the contraction of otherwise normal muscle fibers is a plausible explanation, but so far has no scientific support.

14. DIAGNOSIS AND TREATMENT OF IMPOTENCE

From an etiological point of view, sexual impotence may be predominantly constitutional, psychogenic or organic (Cooper, 1972). The first exists in otherwise normal people who never throughout their lifetime experience much sexual drive or responsiveness. To a varying degree, they have an untroubled indifference to the entire subject. By contrast, psychogenic impotence is alleged to be selective, transient, occurring in certain situations and at certain times. Unless it is due to a congenital lesion, organic impotence will evolve from previous competence in association with some pathological lesion. In assessing the differences between the kinds of impotence it should be realized that in every case the three types co-exist and complicate each other to a greater or lesser degree.

The clinician's task is to discover the relevant etiologies in each patient in order to institute rational treatment. Abnormalities of spermatogenesis, sperm count, sperm motility and seminal volume are of doubtful relevance to sexual potency. A variety of causes of impotence must be considered, such as drugs including estrogens, antidepressants, tranquilizers, certain hypotensive agents and alcohol. Lesions of the spinal cord such as those caused by pernicious anemia, syringomyelia, myelitis and multiple sclerosis and spinal cord tumor are frequently accompanied by impotence without loss of libido (Leavens, 1964).

Neuropathy, particularly of the visceral type, as well as degenerative vascular disease may coexist and actually cause impotence in the presence or absence of diabetes and therefore should be considered in the differential diagnosis of impotence.

Clinically, impotence in diabetes develops in three ways. Most commonly, it appears after the diabetes has been present for several years, but sometimes, it may be one of the earliest if not the first symptom of the disease. Finally, it may occur in a transient form while the diabetes is out of control. Characteristically, the mode of onset of all three of the developmental forms of impotence occurs in a male who was previsouly sexually competent.

Impotence due to lack of control of the diabetes is largely a reflection of the fluid and electrolyte disturbance with corresponding changes in metabolic substrates. It should be remembered that there may be an endocrine basis for the impotence besides the diabetes. When diabetic impotence is due to neurological disease there is no known prophylactic agent or therapeutic remedy and the prognosis is poor.

There is no correlation between the occurrence of impotence and the control, duration or severity of the diabetes. Impotence may be the first manifestation of diabetes mellitus (Rubin and Babbott, 1958). Impotence is related to the kind of treatment used, be it diet alone, diet and insulin, or diet and oral hypoglycemic agents (Kolodny et al., 1974).

Typically, the onset of impotence is gradual, usually progressing over a period of six months to a year with an interval during which firmness of erection is diminished but not completely lost.

Libido persists in spite of the absence of potency in diabetes, but it may diminish in intensity secondary to the disappointment of inadequacy (Ellenberg, 1971). This latter observation may make the diagnosis of the cause of the impotence more difficult.

Since there is no abnormality of androgen production in impotent diabetic men, there is no reason to expect that such therapy would prove helpful (Cooper, 1972; Ismaeil, 1970; Ismail et al., 1970). Ellenberg (1971) administered testosterone therapy to 45 impotent diabetic males without apparent benefit even though the therapy was adequate both

in duration and dosage. These conclusions are supported by others (Kolodny et al., 1973; and Cooper et al., 1972).

At the present time there is no specific cure for male diabetic impotence. Psychotherapeutic counselling (Merrill and Swanson, 1976; Scott et al., 1973; Wright et al., 1976) and mechanical prostheses will benefit a few patients but the large majority will have to await more enlightenment on the subject.

REFERENCES

Abelson D (1974) Diagnostic value of the penile pulse and blood pressure: a Doppler study of impotence in diabetics. J Urol 113: 636.

Alstrom CH, Hallgren B, Nillson LB et al. (1959) Retinal degeneration combined with obesity, diabetes mellitus and neurological disorders. Acta Psychiatr Neurol Scand 34 Suppl 129: 1.

Alvarez-Morujo a (1967) Terminal arteries of the penis. Acta Anat (Basel) 67: 387.

Bacq XM (1935) Recherches sur la physiologie et la pharmacologie du système nerveux autonome. XII. Nature cholinergique et adrénergique des diverses innervations vasomotrices du pénis chez le chien. Arch Intern Physiol Biochem 41: 311.

Bartak V, Jositko M, Horackova M (1975) Juvenile diabetes and human sperm quality. Int J Fertil 20: 30.

Bayer J (1942) Die Hypertrophie der Pankreasineln bei Neugenbarenen Diabetischer Mütter in ihrein Beziehung zu den anderen Regulatoren des Zucherstoffwechsels. Virch Arch Path Anat 308: 659.

Bergqvist N (1954) The gonadal function in male diabetes. Acta Endocrinol (Kbh), Suppl 18: 1.

Bors E, Comarr AE (1960) Neurological disturbances of sexual function with special reference to 529 patients with spinal cord injury. Urol Survey 10: 191.

Buck AC, Reed YK, Siddiq GD (1976) Bladder dysfunction and neuropathy in diabetes. Diabetologia 12: 251.

Charvat J, Engelberth O, Jezkova Z et al. (1967) Autoprotilatky u Klinefelterova Syndromu. Cas Lek Cesk 106: 36.

Claude H, Sourdel M (1912) Hémosidérose viscérale et insuffisance pluriglandulaire. Bull Soc Méd Hôp Paris 28:32.

Cooper AJ (1972) Diagnosis and management of 'Endocrine impotence'. Br Med J 2: 34.

Czerniak P (1962) P^{32} studies of spermatogenesis in man. Establishment of a spermatogenic activity test. Am J Roentgenol 88: 327.

Distiller LA, Sagel J, Morley JE et al. (1975) Pituitary responsiveness to LH-RH in insulin-dependent diabetes mellitus. Diabetes 24: 378.

Dixit PK, Lazarow A (1962) Effect of hyperglycaemia and hypoglycaemia on the glycogen content of the pituitary and adrenal glands of normal, subdiabetic and diabetic rats. Endocrinology 71: 745.

Dorr LD, Brody MJ (1967) Hemodynamic mechanisms of erection in the canine penis. Am J Physiol 213: 1526.

Driscoll SG, Benirschke K, Curtis GW (1960) Neonatal deaths among infants of diabetic mothers. Post-mortem findings in ninety-five infants. Am J Dis Child 100: 818.

Drucher WD, Blane WA, Rowland LP et al. (1962) The testis in moytonic muscular dystrophy: a clinical and pathological study withh a comparison with the Klinefelter syndrome. J Clin Endocrinol Metab 23: 59.

Drudi C, Dornetti F (1958) Sul comportamento della escrezione gonadotropa nel diabete mellito giovanile. Folia Endocrinol. (Roma) XI: 708.

Dymock IW, Cassar J, Pyke DA et al. (1971) Observations on the pathogenesis, complications and treatment of diabetes in 115 cases of haemochromatosis. Am J Med 52: 203.

Ellenberg M (1971) The neurologic factor. Impotence in diabetes. Am Intern Med 75: 213.

Eliasson R, Murdock RN, White IG (1969) The metabolism of human spermatozoa in the presence of prostaglandin E. Acta Physiol Scand 72: 379.

Epstein CJ, Martin GM, Schultz AL et al. (1966) Werner's syndrome. Medicine 45: 177.

Ewing DJ, Burt AA, Campbell IW (1973) Vascular reflexes in diabetes autonomic neuropathy. Lancet.

Faerman I, Glocer L, Fox D (1974) Impotence and diabetes. Diabetes 23: 971.

Faerman I, Vilar O, Rivarola MA et al. (1972) Impotence in diabetes. Studies of androgenic function in diabetic impotent males. Diabetes 21: 23.

Finch SC, Finch CA (1955) Idiopathic haemochromatosis: an iron storage disease. Medicine 34: 381.

Foglia VG, Borghelli FR, Chieri RA (1963) Sexual disturbances in the diabetic rat. Diabetes 12: 231.

Forbes AP, Engel E (1963) The high incidence of diabetes mellitus in 41 patients with gonadal dysgenesis and their close relatives. Metabolism 12: 428.

Garrett RA, Rhamy DE (1966) Priapism: management with a corpus-saphenous shunt. J Urol 95: 65.

Geisthövel W, Niedergerke V, Morgner KD et al. (1975) Androgen status of male diabetics. Med Klin 70: 1417.

Goldman JA, Schecter A, Echerling B (1970) Carbohydrate metabolism in infertile and impotent males. Fertil Steril 21: 397.

Goodner CJ, Freinkel N (1961) Studies of anterior pituitary tissue in vitro: effects of insulin and experimental diabetes mellitus upon carbohydrate metabolism. J Clin Invest 40: 261.

Hastings D (1963) Impotence and Frigidity pp 56-66. Boston: Little, Brown.

Hart BL, Kitchell RL (1966): Penile erection and contraction of penile muscles in the spinal and intact dog. Am J Physiol 210: 257.

Henderson VE, Roepke MH (1933) On the mechanism of erection. Am J Physiol 106: 441.

Hicks JJ, Martinez-Manautou J, Pedron N et al. (1972) Metabolic changes in human spermatozoa related to capacitation. Fertil Steril 23: 172.

Hicks JJ, Rojas L, Rosando A (1973) Insulin regulation of spermatozoa metabolism. Endocrinology 92: 833.

Hierons R, Saunders M (1966) Impotence in patients with temporal-lobe lesions. Lancet ii: 761.

Hoskins DD (1975) Adenine nucleotide mediation of fructolysis and motility in bovine epididymal spermatozoa. J Biol Chem 248: 1135.

Hotchkiss RS, Fernandez-Leal J (1957) The nervous system as related to fertility and sterility. J Urol 78: 173.

Huff TA, Lebovitz HE (1968) Dynamics of insulin secretion in myotonic dystrophy. J Clin Endocrinol Metab 28: 992.

Karacan I, Salis PJ, Ware JG et al. (1978) Nocturnal penile tumescence and diagnosis in diabetic impotence. Am J Psychiatry 135: 2.

Kinsey AC, Pomeroy WB, Martins CE (1948) Sexual behaviour in the human male. Philadelphia: WB Saunders.

Klebanow D, MacLeod J (1960) Semen quality and certain disturbances of reproduction in diabetic men. Fertil Steril 11: 255.

Koch K (1910) Zwischenzellen und Hodenatrophie. Virch Arch Path Anat 202: 376.

Kolodny RC, Kahn CB, Goldstein HH et al. (1974) Sexual dysfunction in diabetic men. Diabetes 23: 306.

Kuhn EA (1950) Functional capacity of the isolated human spinal cord. Brain 73: 1.

Kuntz A (1953) The autonomic nervous system, 4th edn, pp 295-296. Philadelphia: Lea & Febiger.

Lamotte M, Labrousse C, Perrault MA et al. (1965) Polyarthrite rhumatoide sévère, diabète insulino-résistant syndrome de Klinefelter. Sem Hôp Paris 41: 525.

MacLeod J, Freund M (1958) Influence of spermatozoal concentration and initial fructose level on fructolysis in human semen. J Appl Physiol 13: 501.

Masters WH, Johnson VE (1976) Principles of the new sex therapy. Am J Psychiatry 133: 548.

Menzinger G, Falluca F, Andreani D (1966) Klinefelter's syndrome and diabetes mellitus. Lancet ii: 747.

Merrill DC, Swanson DA (1976) Experience with the Small-Carrion penile prosthesis. J Urol 115: 277.

Meyers R (1962) Three cases of myclonus alleviated by bilateral ansotomy, with a note on postoperative alibido and impotence. J Neurosurg 19: 71.

Miller S, Mason HL (1945) The excretion of 17-ketosteroids by diabetics. J Clin Endocrinol Metab 5: 220.

Mortimer CH, Besser GM, McNeilly AS et al. (1973) Lutinising hormone and follicle stimulating hormone-releasing hormone test in patients with hypothalamic-pituitary-gonadal dysfunction. Br Med J 4: 73.

Naunyn B (1906) Der Diabetes Mellitus. Vienna: Alfred Holder.

Neubauer M, Demisch K, Schöffling K (1972) Diabetische Sexualstörungen. Sexualmedizin 1: 242.

Newman HF, Northrup JD, Devlin J (1964) Mechanism of human penile erection. Invest Urol 1: 350.

Nielsen J, Johansen K, Yde H (1969) The frequency of diabetes mellitus in patients with Klinefelter's syndrome of different chromosome constitutions and the XYY syndrome. J Clin Endocrinol Metab 29: 1062.

Oakley WG (1950) In Discussion of Strauss EB. Brit Med J 1: 697.

Panayotov D, Protich M, Strashimirov D (1974) Spermatogenic activity test in diabetic patients. Rev Roum Med 12: 193.

Paz G, Homomai ZT, Ayalon D et al. (1977a) Immunoreactive insulin in serum and seminal plasma of diabetic and non-diabetic men and its role in the regulation of spermatozoal activity. Fertil Steril 28: 836.

Paz G, Sofer A, Homomai ZT et al. (1977b) Seminal plasma and prostatic fluid compositions and their interrelations with sperm quality. Int J Fertil 22(3): 140.

Peterson RN, Freund M (1969) Glycolysis by washed suspensions of human spermatozoa. Biol Reprod 1: 238.

Peterson RN, Freund M (1971) Factors affecting fructose utilisation and lactic acid formation by human semen. The role of glucose and pyruvic acid. Fertil Steril 23: 639.

Pond MH (1954) 17-Ketosteroid fractionation. Studies by a microchromatography technique in endocrine disorders. J Endocrinol 10: 202.

Rivarola MA, Faerman I, Jadzinsky M et al. (1970) Plasma testosterone levels in diabetic men with and without normal sexual potency. In Abstracts of Excerpta Medica, VIIth Congress of International Federation of Diabetes, Buenos Aires, Argentina, August 1970, p 38.

Rhode RA (1963) Chromatin positive Klinefelter's syndrome. J Chron Dis 16: 1139.

Rollo J (1797) An account of two cases of diabetes mellitus: with remarks, as they arose during the progress of the cure. London: C. Dilly.

Ross SS (1953) An investigation in sterility after lumbar ganglionectomy. Br Med J 1: 247.

Root WS, Bard P (1947) The mediation of feline erection through sympathetic pathways with some remarks on sexual behaviour after deafferention of the genitalia. Am J Physiol 151: 80.

Rubin A (1962) Studies on human reproduction. IV. Diabetes mellitus and seminal deficiency. Am J Obstet Gynecol 83: 200.

Rubin A, Babbott D (1958) Impotence and diabetes mellitus. JAMA 8: 498.

Ruzbarsky V, Michal V (1976) Morphologic changes in the arterial bed of the penis with aging. Invest Urol 1976.

Schally AV, Arimural A, Kastin AJ (1971) Gonadotrophin releasing hormone: one polypeptide regulates secretion of luteinizing and follicle stimulating hormones. Science 173: 1036.

Schöffling K (1965) Hypogonadism in male diabetic subjects in the nature and treatment of diabetes mellitus. In: Liebel BS, Wrenshall GA, eds. Excerpta Medica Foundation ICS 84: 505.

Schöffling K, Federlin K, Ditschuneit H et al. (1954) Über die Keimdrusenfunktion bei mänlichen Zuckerkranken. 6. Symposium der Deutschen Gesellschaft für Endokrinologie Kiel, p 376. Springer: Berlin.

Schöffling K, Federlin K, Ditschuneit H et al. (1963) Disorders of sexual function in male diabetics. Diabetes 12: 519.

Schöffling K, Federlin K, Ditschuneit H, Pfeiffer EF (1963) Disorders of sexual function in male diabetics. Diabetes 12: 519.

Schöffling K, Pfeiffer EF, Robe C et al. (1961) Steroidhormon-Untersuchungen bei Diabetikern mit sekundarein Hypogonadismus. Dtsch Med Wochenschr 86: 819.

Scott FB, Bradley WE, Timm G (1973) Management of erectile impotence. Use of implantable inflatable prosthesis. Urology 2: 80.

Sheth AR, Gunaga KP, Rao SS (1970) Occurrence of amylo-1,6-glucosidase in human seminal plasma. J Reprod Fertil 22: 77.

Spellacy WN (1976) Carbohydrate metabolism in male infertility and female infertility. Fertil Steril 27: 1132.

Stekel W (1927) Impotence in the male, Vol. 2, pp 118-174. New York: Liveright.

Strauss EB (1950) Impotence from a psychiatric standpoint. Br

Med J 1: 697.

Von Noorden C (1903) Die Zuckerkrankheit und ihr Behandling. Berlin: August Hirschwald.

Warren S, Le Compte PM (1952) The pathology of diabetes mellitus, p 208. Philadelphia: Lea & Febiger.

Weiss HD (1972) The physiology of human penile erection. Am Intern Med 76: 793.

White P, Hunt H (1943) Pregnancy complicating diabetes: report of clinical results. J Clin Endocrinol Metab 3: 500.

Whitelaw GP, Smithwick RH (1951) Some secondary effects of sympathectomy: with particular reference to disturbance of sexual function. N Engl J Med 245: 121.

Wright MB, London DR, Holder G et al. (1976) Luteinizing release hormone tests in impotent diabetic males. Diabetes 25: 975.

Yodaiken RE, Levin NW, Sandler A (1960) A case of Klinefelter's syndrome complicated by diabetes and diabetic glomerulosclerosis. S Afr Med J 34: 547.

Zeitlin AB, Cottrell TL, Lloyd FA (1957) Sexology of the paraplegic male. Fertil Steril 8: 337.

Zondek LH, Zondek T (1967) Leydig cells of the fetus and newborn in various complications of pregnancy. Acta Obstet Gynecol Scand 46: 392.

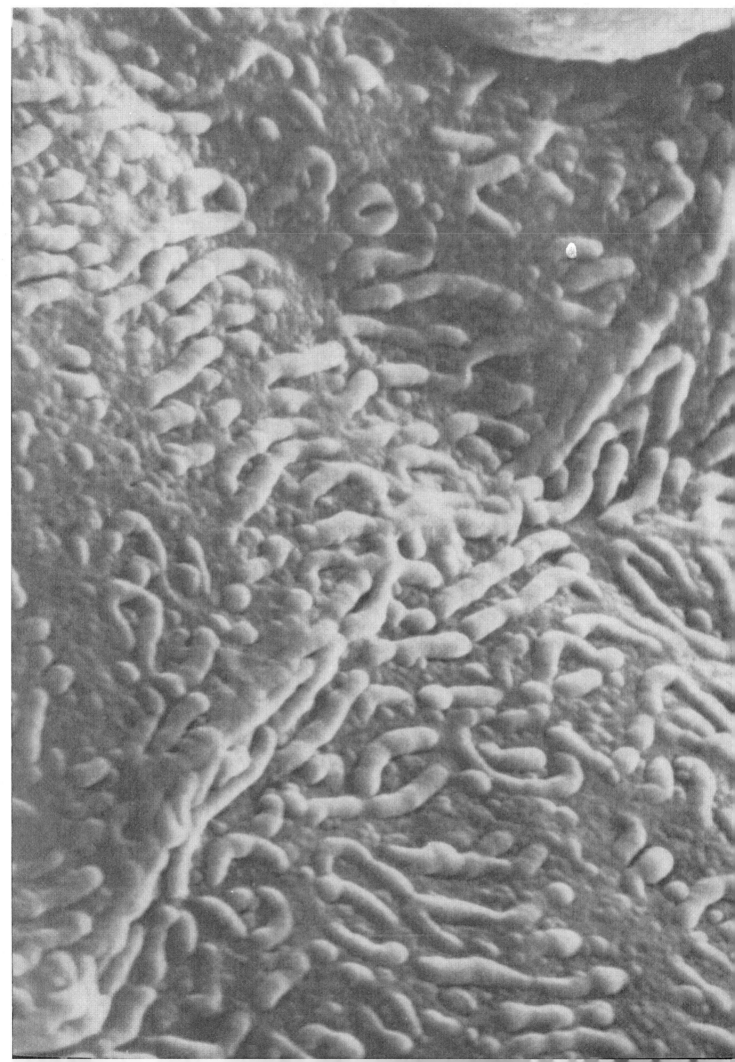